Human Autonomy in Cross-Cultural Context

Cross-Cultural Advancements in Positive Psychology

Volume 1

Series Editor:

ANTONELLA DELLE FAVE
Università degli studi di Milano, Italy

Editorial Board:

MARTIN E.P. SELIGMAN
Positive Psychology Center, University of Pennsylvania, USA
MIHALY CSIKSZENTMIHALYI
Quality of Life Research Center, Claremont Graduate University, USA
BARBARA L. FREDRICKSON
University of North Carolina at Chapel Hill, USA

ALAN WATERMAN
The College of New Jersey, USA
ROBERT A. EMMONS
University of California, Davis, USA

The aim of the *Cross Cultural Advancements in Positive Psychology* book series is to spread a universal and culture-fair perspective on good life promotion. The series will advance a deeper understanding of the cross-cultural differences in well-being conceptualization. A deeper understanding can affect psychological theories, interventions and social policies in various domains, from health to education, from work to leisure. Books in the series will investigate such issues as enhanced mobility of people across nations, ethnic conflicts and the challenges faced by traditional communities due to the pervasive spreading of modernization trends. New instruments and models will be proposed to identify the crucial components of well-being in the process of acculturation. This series will also explore dimensions and components of happiness that are currently overlooked because happiness research is grounded in the Western tradition, and these dimensions do not belong to the Western cultural frame of mind and values.

For further volumes:
http://www.springer.com/series/8420

Valery I. Chirkov · Richard M. Ryan ·
Kennon M. Sheldon
Editors

Human Autonomy in Cross-Cultural Context

Perspectives on the Psychology of Agency, Freedom, and Well-Being

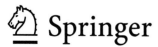 Springer

Editors
Dr. Valery I. Chirkov
Department of Psychology
University of Saskatchewan
Campus Drive 9
S7N 5A5 Saskatoon
SK, Canada
v.chirkov@usask.ca

Richard M. Ryan
Department of Psychology
Psychiatry & Education
University of Rochester
Rochester, New York
NY 14627, USA
ryan@psych.rochester.edu

Dr. Kennon M. Sheldon
Department of Psychology
University of Missouri
McAlester Hall 112
Columbia
MO 65211, USA
SheldonK@missouri.edu

ISSN 2210-5417
ISBN 978-90-481-9666-1
DOI 10.1007/978-90-481-9667-8
Springer Dordrecht Heidelberg London New York

e-ISSN 2210-5425
e-ISBN 978-90-481-9667-8

© Springer Science+Business Media B.V. 2011
No part of this work may be reproduced, stored in a retrieval system, or transmitted in any form or by any means, electronic, mechanical, photocopying, microfilming, recording or otherwise, without written permission from the Publisher, with the exception of any material supplied specifically for the purpose of being entered and executed on a computer system, for exclusive use by the purchaser of the work.

Printed on acid-free paper

Springer is part of Springer Science+Business Media (www.springer.com)

Contents

1 Introduction: The Struggle for Happiness and Autonomy in Cultural and Personal Contexts: An Overview 1
Valery I. Chirkov, Kennon M. Sheldon, and Richard M. Ryan

Part I A Theoretical Context of Human Autonomy, People's Well-Being, and Happiness

2 Positive Psychology and Self-Determination Theory: A Natural Interface 33
Kennon M. Sheldon and Richard M. Ryan

3 A Self-Determination Theory Perspective on Social, Institutional, Cultural, and Economic Supports for Autonomy and Their Importance for Well-Being 45
Richard M. Ryan and Edward L. Deci

4 Dialectical Relationships Among Human Autonomy, the Brain, and Culture 65
Valery I. Chirkov

Part II Human Autonomy Across Cultures and Domains of Life: Health, Education, Interpersonal Relationships, and Work

5 The Role of Autonomy in Promoting Healthy Dyadic, Familial, and Parenting Relationships Across Cultures 95
C. Raymond Knee and Ahmet Uysal

6 Do Social Institutions Necessarily Suppress Individuals' Need for Autonomy? The Possibility of Schools as Autonomy-Promoting Contexts Across the Globe 111
Johnmarshall Reeve and Avi Assor

7 Physical Wellness, Health Care, and Personal Autonomy 133
Geoffrey C. Williams, Pedro J. Teixeira, Eliana V. Carraça, and Ken Resnicow

8 **Autonomy in the Workplace: An Essential Ingredient to Employee Engagement and Well-Being in Every Culture** 163
   Marylène Gagné and Devasheesh Bhave

Part III Human Autonomy in Modern Economy, Democracy Development, and Sustainability

9 **Capitalism and Autonomy** 191
   Tim Kasser

10 **Economy, People's Personal Autonomy, and Well-Being** 207
   Maurizio Pugno

11 **The Development of Conceptions of Personal Autonomy, Rights, and Democracy, and Their Relation to Psychological Well-Being** 241
   Charles C. Helwig and Justin McNeil

12 **Personal Autonomy and Environmental Sustainability** 257
   Luc G. Pelletier, Daniel Baxter, and Veronika Huta

Index 279

Contributors

Avi Assor Department of Education, Ben-Gurion University, Beer-Sheva 84105, Israel, assor@bgumail.bgu.ac.il

Daniel Baxter University of Ottawa, Ottawa, ON, Canada K1N 6N5, daniel.e.baxter@gmail.com

Devasheesh Bhave Department of Management, John Molson School of Business, Concordia University, Montreal, QC, Canada H3G 1M8, dbhave@jmsb.concordia.ca

Eliana V. Carraça Faculty of Human Kinetics, Technical University of Lisbon, Lisbon, Portugal, ecarraca@fmh.utl.pt

Valery I. Chirkov Department of Psychology, University of Saskatchewan, Saskatoon, SK, Canada S7N 5A5, v.chirkov@usask.ca

Edward L. Deci Department of Clinical and Social Sciences in Psychology, University of Rochester, Rochester, NY 14627, USA, deci@psych.rochester.edu

Marylène Gagné Department of Management, John Molson School of Business, Concordia University, Montreal, QC, Canada H3G 1M8, mgagne@jmsb.concordia.ca

Charles C. Helwig Department of Psychology, University of Toronto, Toronto, ON, Canada M5S 3G3, helwig@psych.utoronto.ca

Veronika Huta University of Ottawa, Ottawa, ON, Canada K1N 6N5, vhuta@uottawa.ca

Tim Kasser Department of Psychology, Knox College, Galesburg, IL 61401, USA, tkasser@knox.edu

C. Raymond Knee University of Houston, Houston, TX 77024, USA, knee@uh.edu

Justin McNeil Department of Psychology, University of Toronto, Toronto, ON, Canada M5S 3G3, mcneil.justin@gmail.com

Luc G. Pelletier School of Psychology, University of Ottawa, Ottawa, ON, Canada K1N 6N5, Luc.Pelletier@uOttawa.ca

Maurizio Pugno Department of Economic Sciences, University of Cassino, Cassino, FR I-03043, Italy, m.pugno@unicas.it

Johnmarshall Reeve World Class University Project Group, Department of Education, Korea University, Seoul 136-701, Korea, reeve@korea.ac.kr

Ken Resnicow Faculty of Human Kinetics, University of Michigan, Ann Arbor, MI 48109, USA, kresnic@umich.edu

Richard M. Ryan Department of Clinical and Social Sciences in Psychology, University of Rochester, Rochester, NY 14627, USA, ryan@psych.rochester.edu

Kennon M. Sheldon Department Psychology, University of Missouri, Columbia, MO 65211, USA, SheldonK@missouri.edu

Pedro J. Teixeira Faculty of Human Kinetics, Technical University of Lisbon, Lisbon, Portugal, pteixeira@fmh.utl.pt

Ahmet Uysal University of Houston, Houston, TX 77024, USA, auysaleuh.edu

Geoffrey C. Williams Department of Medicine, Center for Community Health, University of Rochester, Rochester, NY 14607, USA, Geoffrey_Williams@URMC.Rochester.Edu

About the Authors

Avi Assor is a Professor and former Head of the Educational and School Psychology program in Ben Gurion University, Israel. His research focuses on processes affecting children's autonomous internalization of values. In addition, he is involved in the development and assessment of school reforms aimed at enhancing students and teachers' basic psychological needs, intrinsic motivation and caring for others. He has published in *Journal of Personality and Social Psychology, Child Development, Journal of Educational Psychology, Journal of Personality, Journal of Educational Administration,* and *Learning and Instruction.*

Daniel Baxter is a PhD student in the Experimental Psychology Program at the University of Ottawa, Canada. He is conducting his graduate studies under the supervision of Dr. Luc G. Pelletier. His research is unanimously point toward environmental psychology and the promotion of proenvironmental behaviours. More specifically, his work focuses on the effects of motivation on needs satisfaction and proenvironmental behaviour occurrence, frequency, and persistence. He is also interested in the effects of cognitive dissonance on proenvironmental attitudes and behaviours. In addition, he is interested in research using resource dilemmas and the different factors that can facilitate and/or undermine cooperative and sustainable behaviours.

Devasheesh Bhave (PhD, Carlson School of Management, University of Minnesota, USA) joined the John Molson School of Business at Concordia University in 2008. His current research interests focus on electronic performance monitoring, specifically related to performance and job design issues. He is also interested in processes related to emotional regulation in the workplace and its relationship with individual monetary and non-monetary outcomes. His research is published or is forthcoming in the *Journal of Applied Psychology, Personnel Psychology,* and *Journal of Occupational and Organizational Psychology.*

Eliana V. Carraça, a Sport Sciences specialist (MSc), is currently a doctoral student at the Technical University of Lisbon, Faculty of Human Kinetics, in Portugal. Her research interests focus on the role of body image and physical self-perceptions in the context of physical activity promotion and obesity treatment. In particular, she is interested in exploring the role of different body image dimensions, identifying pretreatment correlates of body image, as well as correlates of change and mediation effects of body image during behaviour change interventions. Eliana presents her work regularly in major international conferences and is an author of several peer-review articles.

Valery I. Chirkov is an Associate Professor of Psychology at the University of Saskatchewan, Canada. He studies the topics of human autonomy, autonomous agency and people's well-being in different cultures. He also conducts research and theorizes in the area of psychology of immigration and acculturation. The concept of human autonomous motivation, its nature and consequences for people's functioning and well-being stands at the centre of his thinking and studies. His recent publications include: Chirkov V. I. (2009). Critical psychology of acculturation: What do we study and how do we study it, when we investigate acculturation? *International Journal of Intercultural Relations, 33*(2), 94–105; Chirkov, V. I. (2007). Culture, personal autonomy and individualism: Their relationships and implications for personal growth and well-being. In G. Zheng, K. Leung & J. G. Adair (Eds.), *Perspectives and progress in contemporary cross-cultural psychology.* (pp. 247–263). Beijing: China Light Industry Press; Chirkov, V. I. (2006). Multiculturalism and human nature: A psychological view. In D. Zinga (Ed.), *Navigating multiculturalism: Negotiating change* (pp. 33–57). Cambridge: Cambridge Scholar Press.

Edward L. Deci is the Helen F. and Fred H. Gowen Professor in the Social Sciences at the University of Rochester, USA. For 40 years Deci has been engaged in a program of research on human motivation, much of it with Richard M. Ryan, that has led to and been organized by self-determination theory. He has published ten books, including: *Intrinsic Motivation* (1975) and *Intrinsic Motivation and Self-Determination in Human Behavior* (co-authored with R. M. Ryan, 1985). A grantee of NIH, NSF, and IES, and a fellow of APA and APS, he has lectured at more than 90 universities around the world.

Marylène Gagné (PhD University of Rochester) is the Royal Bank of Canada Professor in Work Motivation at the John Molson School of Business, Concordia University in Montreal, Canada. Her research examines how organizations, through their structures, cultures, rewards, tasks, and managerial/leadership styles, affect people's motivational orientations, and also examines the consequences of these orientations for individual and organizational performance, and for individual mental health. She has won research awards, serves on the review boards of four journals in her field, and has published in the *Journal of Organizational Behavior, The Journal of Personality and Social Psychology,* and *Motivation and Emotion* among others. Her recent publications include: Gagné, M., & Deci, E. L. (2005). Self-determination theory as a new framework for understanding organizational behavior. *Journal of Organizational Behavior, 26,* 331–362; Gagné, M., & Forest, J. (2008). The study of compensation systems through the lens of self-determination theory: Reconciling 35 years of debate. *Canadian Psychology, 49,*

225–232; Gagné, M. (2009). A model of knowledge sharing motivation. *Human Resource Management, 48,* 571–589.

Charles C. Helwig is Professor of Psychology at the University of Toronto, Canada. His research examines the development of moral and social judgments from the preschool years through adulthood, with a focus on the development of moral concepts related to societal issues and social institutions, such as freedoms, civil liberties, and democracy. He has investigated children's understandings of democratic decision-making and rights not only in the context of society at large but in other social contexts such as the family, the school, and the peer group, and in cross-cultural research conducted in China and Canada. His recent publications are: Helwig, C. C. (2006). Rights, civil liberties, and democracy across cultures. In M. Killen & J. G. Smetana (Eds.), *Handbook of moral development* (pp. 185–210). Mahwah, NJ: Erlbaum; Lahat, A., Helwig, C. C., Yang, S., Tan, D., & Liu, C. (2009). Mainland Chinese adolescents' judgments and reasoning about self-determination and nurturance rights. *Social Development, 18,* 690–710; Helwig, C. C. (2006). The development of personal autonomy throughout cultures. *Cognitive Development, 21,* 458–473.

Veronika Huta is a faculty member at the School of Psychology of the University of Ottawa, Canada. She conducts research on the ways in which people pursue well-being, focusing primarily on the difference between hedonic pursuits (seeking enjoyment and relaxation) and eudaimonic pursuits (seeking excellence and virtue). Her work is also focused on extending the assessment of well-being beyond the concepts of positive affect, negative affect, and life satisfaction, with a special interest in the experiences of meaning, vitality, and elevation. She is currently writing the first comprehensive book on eudaimonia research. In addition, she teaches graduate courses in positive psychology, univariate and multivariate statistics, and advanced statistics such as hierarchical linear modeling.

Tim Kasser is Professor of Psychology at Knox College in Galesburg, Illinois, USA. He has authored dozens of scientific book chapters on materialism, values, goals, consumer culture, well-being, and ecological sustainability. His first book, *The high price of materialism,* was published in 2002; his second book (co-edited with Allen D. Kanner), *Psychology and consumer culture,* was released in 2004; and his third book (co-authored with Tom Crompton), *Meeting environmental challenges: The role of human identity,* was released in 2009. Kasser is actively involved with non-profit groups that work against the commercialization of children and towards a more inwardly rich lifestyle than what is offered by consumerism. He lives with his wife, two sons, and assorted animals in the Western Illinois countryside.

C. Raymond Knee is an Associate Professor of social psychology at the University of Houston, USA. He studies close relationships and interpersonal processes from a motivation perspective that incorporates personality, developmental, and situational influences on optimal individual and relational health. He is serving as an Associate Editor for *Personality and Social Psychology Bulletin*, and for *Personal*

Relationships. He publishes almost exclusively with his current and former graduate students and greatly values his role as a mentor.

Justin McNeil received his BA from Cape Breton University and his MA from the University of Toronto. His research interests focus on issues of adolescent autonomy, decision-making power, and engagement, particularly in a school setting. He has also conducted research on volunteerism, particularly how students in mandatory volunteer programs balance issues of prosocial, moral behaviors against their own desires for personal choice.

Luc G. Pelletier is Professor of Psychology, and Chair of the School of Psychology, University of Ottawa, Ontario, Canada. His research activities focus on how people regulate their behaviors and integrate a wide variety of behaviors, including pro-environmental behaviors, into their life style; why people sometimes fail in their attempts to regulate their actions despite being highly motivated; and the influence of persuasive communication on the motivation for different activities.

Maurizio Pugno (M.Phil. Cambridge, UK) is Professor of Economics at the University of Cassino, Italy. His research mainly focuses on human capital, economic growth, and well-being. He has recently edited the book *Capabilities and happiness* (with L. Bruni, F. Comim; Oxford University Press), and he has published articles on job satisfaction, on economics and SDT, and on the decline of social capital in the US. He is a coordinator of the research center *Creativity and motivation* (University of Cassino).

Johnmarshall Reeve is a WCU Professor in the Department of Education at Korea University, Seoul, South Korea. He received his PhD from Texas Christian University and completed postdoctoral work at the University of Rochester. Professor Reeve's research interests center on the empirical study of all aspects of human motivation and emotion, though he particularly emphasize student motivation, student engagement, and teachers' motivating styles. He has published 50 journal articles and book chapters in outlets such as the *Journal of Educational Psychology* and 3 books including *Understanding motivation and emotion*. He sits on two editorial boards and serves as the Associate Editor for *Motivation and emotion*.

Ken Resnicow is a Professor in the Department of Health Behavior and Health Education at University of Michigan School of Public Health, USA. His research interests include: the design and evaluation of health promotion programs for special populations, particularly chronic disease prevention for African Americans; tailored health communications; understanding the relationship between ethnicity and health behaviors; substance use prevention and harm reduction; training health professionals in motivational interviewing. Much of his work is informed by Chaos Theory, Complexity Science, and Self Determination Theory. He has published over 190 peer-reviewed articles and book chapters and has served on numerous advisory panels and review groups.

About the Authors

Richard M. Ryan is Professor of Psychology, Psychiatry, and Education at the University of Rochester, USA, and the Director of Clinical Training. He is a widely cited researcher and theorist in the areas of human motivation and well-being, having published over 250 articles and books on topics from materialism to video games. He is the co-developer (with Edward L. Deci) of Self-Determination Theory, an internationally influential framework for the study of motivation (www.selfdeterminationtheory.org). Ryan has lectured in more than 60 universities around the globe, and received numerous honors from professional organizations, including being an Honorary Member of the German Psychological Society (DGP), a James McKeen Cattell Fellow, and a visiting scientist at the Max Planck Institute for Human Development. He is also a practicing clinical psychologist, and Editor-in-Chief of the journal *Motivation and emotion*.

Kennon M. Sheldon is Professor of Psychology at the University of Missouri, USA He studies motivation, goals, and happiness, with over 150 peer-reviewed journal articles to his credit. Sheldon is active in the positive psychology movement, having won a prestigious Templeton Prize in 2002 and having served as book review editor for *Journal of Positive Psychology* since 2006. He is the lead editor of the forthcoming book *Designing positive psychology: Taking stock and moving forward* (Oxford University Press), and sole author of the book *Optimal human being: An integrated multi-level perspective* (Erlbaum). He has delivered international addresses in Sweden, Israel, Croatia, Portugal, Austria, Australia, and the Netherlands, among others.

Pedro J. Teixeira is an Assistant Professor of Nutrition, Physical Activity, and Obesity at the Technical University of Lisbon, Faculty of Human Kinetics, the largest Sport Science academic institution in Portugal. At the Exercise and Health Laboratory, he leads a research group focused on behavioural issues in obesity treatment and physical activity, and psychosocial predictors of obesity and weight control. For the past 6 years, he has led a long-term randomized clinical trial testing the application of self-determination theory to weight control. Pedro Teixeira has published 2 books, nearly 50 peer-reviewed articles, and several book chapters. He has been involved as an investigator in NIH- and European Commission-funded projects, including the Portuguese National Weight Control Registry. He is the current Vice-President of the Portuguese Obesity Society and a former Executive Committee member of the International Society for Behavioral Nutrition and Physical Activity.

Ahmet Uysal is a graduate student in social psychology at University of Houston, USA. He is interested in self and defensive processes. His recent research focuses on the consequences of self-concealment from a self-determination theory perspective, and the application of self-determination theory to the perception and acceptance of acute and chronic pain. His dissertation will be defended by the time this book is in print, and he has a faculty position in his native country of Turkey awaiting him.

Geoffrey C. Williams is currently the Director of the Healthy Living Center at the University of Rochester in Rochester, New York, USA. He is also a Professor of

Medicine, Psychiatry and Psychology. Dr. Williams has both an M.D. and a PhD in Health Psychology. Dr. Williams has 20 years of practice experience in academic internal medicine and training as a health psychologist. He has contributed to the development of the Self-Determination Theory (SDT) model for health behavior change. Dr. Williams has focused much of his research career on SDT and its application in interventions for health-related motivation, tobacco dependence treatment and other health behaviors that are difficult to change. He has been the recipient of numerous grants including research support from the National Cancer Institute, the National Institute on Drug Abuse, the National Institute of Diabetes and Digestive and Kidney Diseases, Small Business Innovation Research and the National Institute of Mental Health. He has published over 50 peer-reviewed articles as well as one book and numerous book chapters. He has also presented at over 50 major national professional meetings. Williams, G. C., McGregor, H. A., Sharp, D., et al. (2006) Testing a Self-Determination Theory Intervention for Motivating Tobacco Cessation: Supporting Autonomy and Competence in a Clinical Trial. *Health Psychology, 25,* 91–101.

Chapter 1
Introduction: The Struggle for Happiness and Autonomy in Cultural and Personal Contexts: An Overview

Valery I. Chirkov, Kennon M. Sheldon, and Richard M. Ryan

Why Are We Writing This Book?

Despite the amazing advances in science, technology, and engineering to explain, conquer, and transform nature, human bodies, and their brains, life in the modern world has not become less challenging and problematic. Contrary to humanity's unending quest to lead happy and satisfying lives, only a proportion of people in the world can state that they have attained this goal.[1] People too often remain devastating and self-destructive, destroying not only the environment around them, but also themselves and fellow citizens. Terrorism, genocide, hate crimes, and irresponsible governmental and corporate actions have created disasters and problems for millions of people around the world. On the personal level people do not care enough about their own health and well-being, and scientists lack sufficient knowledge of why people still suffer from obesity, unhealthy lifestyles, family and child abuse, drug dependency, and criminal behavior. It is expected that modern social and human sciences can provide at least some insights about where to look for the causes of and remedies for these problems. In this work we examine what psychology can offer to clarify the quandary of the problems we see in people's lives around the globe.

The main thesis that we want to defend in this book is that people's happiness and well-being are inseparable from their experience of personal and motivational autonomy in pursuing freely chosen life-goals, actions, and behaviors. We consider this axiom to be universal and applicable to people from all cultural communities. As we will argue, the feeling of autonomy and self-determination is what makes us most fully human and thus most able to lead deeply satisfying lives – lives that are meaningful and constructive – perhaps the only lives that are worth living.

In this chapter we will first present the thoughts of such contributors to this topic as Socrates, Stoic philosophers, Spinoza, and Kant, and then try to reconcile their ancient admonitions with the recommendations derived from the empirical tradition

---

V.I. Chirkov (✉)
Department of Psychology, University of Saskatchewan, Saskatoon, SK, Canada S7N 5A5
e-mail: v.chirkov@usask.ca

[1] To observe the distribution of happiness around the world visit www.mapofhappiness.com and http://www.worldlifeexpectancy.com/world-happiness-map

of modern psychology, represented mostly by self-determination theory (SDT). In addition to a brief history of Western thoughts concerning the relations between happiness and human autonomy, we will provide an account of how these relations are reflected in the Confucian teaching in Ancient China and how they are accounted for in modern South Asian societies. We will also take a look at the problems that the issue of autonomy has experienced in mainstream psychology, and consider the challenges to the notions of autonomy brought by the determinist and constructionist approaches in social and cultural psychology. This introduction will conclude with a summary of the subsequent chapters.

A Brief History of the Views Regarding the Importance of Autonomy for Human Happiness

Starting with the Ancient thinkers, followed by the Christian theologians and then by the Renaissance and later philosophers, scholars have responded differently to the problem of how people should live in a world full of choices, and how to guide them to experience the fullness of life, a life that could be recalled without shame on one's death bed. It is not a big stretch to say that for the majority of philosophical and religious doctrines that have emerged in different countries and at different times, the quest for happiness, in one form or another, is a dominant consideration. And at least one universal commonality can be discovered in these many theories: as soon as a discourse touches the topic of people's happiness and a good life, the topic of their autonomy and freedom inevitably emerges (McMahon, 2004). In this review, we will try to demonstrate that for many of the great thinkers on this topic, human happiness and personal autonomy are inseparable themes.

A historian, McMahon (2006), who provided an exhaustive account of the history of happiness in the Western world, stated that it was from Ancient Greece that the first explicit theories of happiness emerged. At the dawn of this civilization, people were mostly concerned with mere survival and, if the question of happiness had ever been raised, happiness was treated as something that happens to people, something over which they have no control. Happiness in early Greece was left to gods and fortune. Socrates was the first thinker who announced that happiness can be achievable, that it could be set up as a personal life goal. Even more, he stated that people can reach it through their own efforts. These two statements were revolutionary, bringing people's hope to become masters of their own lives and even of their happiness. "…It was Socrates who was the first to consider in detail what would draw the 'sleepless and laborious efforts' of all subsequent philosophers: the 'question of the necessary conditions for happiness," (2006, p. 24). Socrates was also the first to separate the desire for sensual pleasure, the mere enjoyment and satisfaction of the senses and biological drives, from a much larger and more fundamental desire of people for some higher ends of their lives, accompanied by a deep understanding of life and the place they occupy in it. This latter interpretation of happiness was later labeled *eudaimonia* and was contrasted with pure hedonic sensual and biological pleasures. Another word that Greeks used as a synonym of eudaimonia was *makarios* (μακάριος), which means *blessed* or *happy* (de Heer, 1969). An important observation made by McMahon is that it was a democratic style of governance in Greece's city-states that made this discourse about the achievable happiness possible. "Although it would be reductive to say that Athenian democracy was the cause of the emergence of happiness as a new and apparently realizable human end, it was nevertheless in Athens, democratic Athens, that individuals first put forth that great, seductive goal, daring to dream that they might pursue – and capture – happiness for themselves (p. 23)." He elaborated further on the relations between the nature of Greek society and ideas that its members produced and the goals they exercised. "Surely we may admit some connection between context and concept, between a society in which free men had grown accustomed, through rational inquiry and open deliberation, to decide matters for themselves, and the efforts to extend the sway of self-rule ever further, even to the long-standing domain of the gods" (2006, p. 23). This conclusion is important for the point of view supported in this volume that autonomy is an essential condition for striving for individual happiness, but the emergence of autonomy depends on favorable and facilitating social and cultural conditions; in this case the democratic political organization. Social context is crucially important for people to discover, appreciate, and utilize their capacity for autonomous actions based on self-determined rational reasoning. This and related ideas about the facilitating or detrimental role the social-cultural milieu may play in people's personal and motivational autonomy are intensively elaborated in the following chapters.

Aristotle extended Socrates's teaching into a philosophical investigation of the nature of eudaimonia, and his views have captured the minds of thinkers for centuries (Engstrom & Whiting, 1996; May, 2010; Ryan, Huta, & Deci, 2008; Ryff & Singer, 2008; Waterman, Schwartz, & Conti, 2008). He connected happiness with living a life which is driven by reason, well-justified virtues, and moral values (McMahon, 2004). But it was Stoic philosophers, following the ideas of Socrates and starting with Zeno of Cytium, who actually paved the road for the practical implementations of virtuous living (Strange & Zupko, 2004). They developed further the ideas that happiness is an attainable life goal as well as the highest desire of any human being; that the achievement of eudaimonic happiness brings people satisfaction and contentment that are incomparable in their depth and pleasure with the mere sensual pleasures; that it is people's autonomy, meaning a self-governance by rational reasoning in choosing goals, making decisions, and setting moral values, that lies at the core of people's happy, virtuous, and tranquil lives; and that it is people's capability for rational thinking and reflective reasoning that makes both autonomy and happiness possible.

It is fair to say that the Ancient Greeks stated and elaborated in considerable detail several important theses that were picked up by the scholars of happiness and well-being that followed them: The theses that happiness is a highly desirable and achievable end of people's lives; that real human happiness – eudaimonia – is more than the sum of bodily and sensual pleasures, but rather it extends to moral virtues and the exercise of rational reasoning in one's life; that autonomy is a fundamental condition for happy living; and, finally, that social, political, economic, and cultural contexts play important roles in eliciting and promoting, or hindering, the manifestation and functioning of autonomy and through it, happiness.

In the first millennium after the death of Christ, the Greek perspective on eudaimonic living was gradually replaced by early and then medieval Christianity, both of which offered very different perspectives on the nature of happiness. According to the orthodox Christian doctrine, people cannot find happiness in this world, it can be reached only in the afterworld and only if they devotedly served God during their lives. Happiness became an unreachable (at least in this life) dream-like passion for Christians (McMahon, 2006). As the idea of an achievable happy life disappeared from the scholars' and theologians' discourses, the idea of personal autonomy responsible for happiness's achievement vanished also. If happiness is not realistically achievable, then there is no necessity for personal autonomy or freedom.[2] The Christian's prescription for happiness was to some extent unique: this faith recommended embracing suffering, because those who suffer the most in this life will be fully rewarded in their afterlife. There is also another aspect of Christianity's rejection of the link between autonomy and happiness. Christian theologians professed that people fail to live happily by their own will and by their own light; that they are incapable of governing their own lust, greed, and hatred. People are incapable of being masters of their own selves. Thus, they are predestined to suffer on the Earth, and only after that, if they serve God, they will be rewarded with full happiness. Thus, human autonomy and freedom were sometimes considered enemies of people's salvation. Happiness was placed beyond people's personal control: "God alone, through his grace, could transform and heal us" (McMahon, 2006, p. 105). Thus, as was the case in Ancient Greece, happiness became receivable only as a gift from God.

It was the Renaissance that brought back the notion of happiness and, together with it, the idea of self-development through one's own will. In the early fifteenth century, an Italian philosopher, Giovanni Pico della Mirandola, wrote his famous "On the Dignity of Man." This book is considered by many to be the manifesto of the Renaissance. According to his view, human beings were "brimming with possibility and potential, able to chart the course of their lives for themselves without stumbling under the accumulated weight of Christian superstition" (McMahon, 2006, p. 145). Thus, humankind started moving in its thinking and actions from misery and suffering to dignity and, from there, to happiness on earth.

It was Spinoza in the seventeenth century who returned to the idea that there were important connections between people's earthly happiness and autonomy. Thus, as

---

[2]It is fair to acknowledge that the doctrines of Christianity are, of course, more multiple and complex than this summary allows us to present it (Dumont, 1985; Hollis, 1985). For example, Lukes (1973) claimed that it was St. Thomas Aquinas and later Martin Luther, who emphasized humans' capability for personal autonomy. It was mediaeval Christianity with its *substantia individua rationalis* which was responsible for carving the fundamentals of the modern Western ideology of individualism (Lukes, 1973) without which personal autonomy could not flourish. But it must be noted: neither of these authors and doctrines linked human autonomy to happiness.

in post-Socratic Greece, these two concepts appeared together again. *Autonomy*, *reason*, *virtue*, and *power* are the main ingredients of Spinoza's prescription for happiness. Spinoza, actually, did not use the term "autonomy," but employed the concepts of "activity" and "human freedom" instead, which he contrasted with "passivity" and "servitude." "For Spinoza, to be active is to be the source of our own actions and not to be impelled by forces that are external to us" (Uyl, 2003, p. 38). Activity (=autonomy), according to Spinoza, is determined by "adequate causes," the causes that are clearly understood by an actor with regard to their origin and consequences. This understanding is reached through people's reason and rational thinking. Passivity (=being controlled) is determined by "inadequate causes," causes whose origin, mechanisms, and consequences are not fully understood and reflected upon by an actor. People are passive if, in their lives and actions, they are governed by forces that they do not fully understand and that predominantly come from "outside" of their selves. Reason has several meanings in Spinoza's writings: it is an ability to explain events by logical thinking, as well as the knowledge of the axioms that reflect the essence of things in the world, and lastly it is a cause of actions. Reason is a fundamental human capacity that brings people power. "...True virtue is nothing other than living solely in accordance with the guidance of reason" (Spinoza, 2000, p. 253). A virtuous life, according to Spinoza, is driven not by emotions that happen to people without their adequate understanding of them, and not by unreflected external demands, but by a reason which is supplied by knowledge about Nature and one's place in the world order. By being autonomous and through exercising their reason, people acquire power over their lives and this is a "true virtue" worth living. Therefore, for Spinoza, by perfecting their reasoning and rational thinking, people form adequate ideas about their lives that facilitate their ability to be active, autonomous agents. This autonomy gives people the power to live happy and virtuous lives.

Although Kant has rarely been considered a happiness theoretician, his philosophical investigations also tapped into the problem of human happiness (Engstrom & Whiting, 1996; Guyer, 2000). For Kant, as Guyer (2000) proposed, happiness, both for individuals and for communities, is available only when people's lives and actions are products of freedom and autonomy. Kant also believed that people achieve great pleasure in pursuing happiness through their own efforts. For Kant, "it is only through our own freedom, rather than nature, that we may systematize and maximize human happiness" (Guyer, 2000, p. 98). And it is the free use of reason that actually provides the conditions for happiness. In his essay "On Practical Philosophy," Kant said:

> ...the human being... is determined by nature to be himself the author of his happiness and even of his own inclinations and skills, which make possible this happiness. From this he infers, that he has to order his actions not in accordance with instincts but in accordance with concepts of his happiness which he himself makes. ... He will therefore have as his foremost object himself as a freely acting being in accordance with this independence and self-mastery, so that his desires will harmonize among themselves with the concept of happiness and not with instincts, and in this form consists the conduct that is appropriate to the freedom of a rational being. ...In the same way he will become aware that his happiness depends on the freedom of other rational beings... (cf. Guyer, 2000, p. 102–103).

In this quotion Kant clearly articulated several points that are important for us. First, that human beings can be the authors of their own happiness and that happiness is achievable in people's lives. Second, that people have to autonomously create their own ideal of their happiness and to subordinate all their capacities, inclinations, and desires to reach this goal of personal happiness. Kant also expressed another fundamental idea: that people need to be aware that their happiness depends on the freedom of other rational human beings. Therefore, in order to achieve universal happiness, people have to behave in such a way that will allow other people to be the free creators of their own happiness too. This statement removes Kant's propositions from the conflict with egotistical individualism: Rational human beings need to understand that their individual happiness is achievable only as a part of the happiness of the larger collectivity of people. In conclusion, we may say that Kant helped revive the ancient ideas that personal earthly happiness is achievable through our own efforts as free and rational human beings. His most important new contribution to the teaching of happiness was the idea that a person cannot reach this happiness alone or at the expense of the happiness of other people. An individual can achieve his or her own happiness only by providing the conditions for other people's autonomous pursuits of their happiness.

Above we presented a brief history of Western ideas concerning the relation of autonomy and happy and good lives. But what about the Eastern world, which has its own noteworthy truths and prescriptions for people's lives and social actions? In the next section we will look at just a few relevant ideas from China, another great civilization of the Ancient times, as well as modern India.

Autonomy and the Good (Moral) Life in the Confucian Ethics

The role autonomy plays in the Confucian's understanding of a good and moral life has recently been a topic of considerable scholarly interest (Chan, 2002; Cheng, 2004; Elvin, 1985; Wong, 2008). Upon examining the discussions in the literature, a few summary points seem clear. First, as in the Greek philosophy, happiness and the nature of the good life were frequently considered and debated. In Confucianism, similar to Aristotle's notions, a good life (this mostly means a moral life, and not so much a happy one) is a virtuous one. The main virtues were "dao," "ren," and "lu." As Yu (2009) pointed out, *dao* plays a role in ancient Chinese ethics analogous to the role played by *eudaimonia* or "flourishing" in ancient Greek ethics. *Ren* is translated as "goodness" and "benevolence" with the meaning of "a sensitive concern for others" (Elvin, 1985, p. 165). This paramount moral virtue allows the establishment of relational harmony, which is considered by the Confucian ethics to be one of the most important aspects of the good/moral life. Second, the way of reaching this goodness is by following *lu*— rituals —which, according to Confucius, carve the moral goodness of a man, like a sculptor's knife carves an image of a stone. Placing *ren* and *lu* at the center of its ethics made the Confucian teaching a relational one where maintaining harmonious relationships stands at the center of the good life.

1 Introduction

The question of autonomy in this ethical system is a complex one. "The crucial conflict that developed here [in Ancient China] was between those who emphasized the relative autonomy of man's inner being and those who thought that what was significant in a personality was the creation of social forces working on it from outside, especially education and/or rewards and punishments" (Elvin, 1985, p. 164). As Elvin stated, it was a philosopher Moh Dyi (fifth century BC) who was one of the first to articulate the ideas that will be later labeled "vertical collectivism" (see Chapter 4). The logic of his argument was the following: "Before the formation of government there had been chaos, each person having his own particular morals and his particular values for words" (Elvin, 1985, p. 165). In the context of our discourse, this means that ancient people failed to exercise their autonomy efficiently, as pursuing personal moral values and goals created nothing but chaos. The remedy for this problem was found in a centralized government: "It was the duty of the head of each family, each community, and each state to unify the values of those beneath him" (Elvin, 1985, p. 165). Thus, the vertical centralization of individuals' values-making became one of the central ideas of the later Confucian's teachings on morality. It is fair to say that, at those Ancient times in China, individualistic ideas also existed. According to Elvin, the philosophy of individualism was strongly elaborated by Yang Ju in the fourth century BC. "His doctrine was to act 'for himself'. Personal pleasure was real and fame inane. Social institutions were a form of torture" (Elvin, 1985, p. 165). Yang Ju compared people's inability to pursue their inclinations and to strive for true pleasure with being in a prison.

History shows that the vertical collectivistic ideas have won their primacy in Chinese moral and ethical philosophy. It is fair to say that Chinese philosophers and thinkers were well aware of the existence of human reflective consciousness and the inner world of self-directed thoughts and actions, the phenomenon, factors which belong to the domain of personal autonomy. The fact is that most of them believed that human autonomy could not bring an orderly and good life to people. So they created an ideological/moral system that de-emphasized the value of personal autonomy and discouraged its intensive practice. But even this powerful collectivistic ideology could not ignore people's capability and need for autonomy completely. Several modern interpreters of Confucianism (Chan, 2002; Cheng, 2004; Chong, 2003; Wong, 2008) accept the presence and the value of personal autonomy in this teaching. They refer to the concept *zhi* which means "the will of the self" or "a choice and decision the self makes in view or in recognition of an ideal value or a potential reality that can be achieved through one's efforts" (Cheng, 2004, p. 131). The *zhi*, or the free will of the self, is based on people's self-awareness and reflective reasoning. Following the argumentation of Chan (2002), we can provide the following examples, which could be interpreted as manifestations of autonomy or *zhi* within the Confucian ideological system.

Confucianism encourages its devotees to voluntarily endorse and willingly submit themselves to the matters of first importance, such as political authority, right moral values, and traditions and rituals (Chan, 2002, p. 286). In the language of psychology, this process of voluntarily endorsing external regulations is called *internalization* (Wallis & Poulton, 2001), the process that plays a central role in the conceptual underpinning of many psychological theories including self-determination theory (Grolnick, Ryan, & Deci, 1997). Both Confucius and his famous follower Mencius (third century BC) distinguished people who endorsed morality for its own sake and took delight in acting morally – sages and gentlemen – and "honest village people" who "...follow no moral principle of their own, but only the popular trend. They appear to be virtuous, but they are not really acting for morality's sake" (Chan, 2002, p. 286–287). Confucius despised such people, calling them "the enemy of virtue." This indicates that Confucianism "...understands that a moral life has to be led from inside, by an agent who is voluntarily motivated by morality" (Chan, 2002, p. 287). The phenomenon described here is conceptualized in self-determination theory as the internalization of behavioral regulation and the distinction between its autonomous and controlled forms (Ryan & Deci, 2000b). When people are controlled by external social forces in their following of moral values and behaviors, they turn themselves into the puppets of these forces and do not represent genuine moral individuals. Only the autonomous acceptance of moral virtues and behavior through internalization makes people fully moral human. Thus, Confucianism accepts that the truly moral (good) life is possible only if people are autonomously motivated by their *zhi* to lead that kind of life, and this is an obvious argument for the thesis that, even in vertically collectivistic China, autonomy (in the above presented aspects) is a necessary condition for a good life (Chong, 2003).

Another example of an implicit endorsement of the importance of autonomy came from a Confucius suggestion to not follow various rites blindly just because they are followed by the majority. Rather, as this sage suggested, "one should adopt a reflective moral attitude to examine the ethical reason behind a rite and to determine whether that rite is appropriate" (Chan, 2002, p. 288). As Chan articulated, Confucius was fully aware that "[R]ites as norms of conduct are often too general to give precise guidance in the making of concrete moral decisions. There may be novel situations, borderline cases, and hard cases (where some rites are in conflict with others) that call for reflective judgment and moral discretion" (Chan, 2002, p. 288). Western philosophers consider this reflective judgment and moral discretion the core of human agentic autonomy. This example represents a fundamental attribute of human autonomy: its reflective nature, in which people can reflect on the conditions of their lives, their motivation behind their behaviors, and make choices of what to do and why to do it. In SDT (Deci & Ryan, 2002), this highest form of autonomy is conceptualized as the integrated form of motivational regulation. Therefore, Confucianism does not deny the necessity and capacity of people to exercise their autonomy through reflective reasoning, while being fully emerged into the ideology of rituals and relational dependence.

The previous discussion is related to another example of the Confucianism endorsement of autonomy as a basis of a moral, virtuous, and good life in a group. This is how Chan presented it: "It is possible that what the agent regards as morally right may not be shared by others. It is also possible that the agent may find other people's ways of doing things wrong" (p. 289). In this case, Confucians tell agents to stand firm on the moral position that they reflectively endorse – to act on their independent will. "Confucius says, 'The Three armies can be deprived of their commanding officers, but even a common man cannot be deprived of his will [zhi].'... The idea of a great man having an independent will and sticking to it against all odds presupposes the belief that one should act on one's own best understanding of morality. A great man is one who forms an independent moral will and takes control of his own moral life. In moral life he follows nothing but the moral principles that he reflectively endorses and the moral will that he develops" (Chan, 2002, pp. 289–290). The ancient Greeks would likely agree that this is a description of personal autonomy in its purest form. We may conclude that despite many controversies and complexities surrounding the issue of personal autonomy in Chinese philosophy, the ideas of personal autonomy and self-determination hold an important place in this system of thinking.

But what about the relational ethics of Confucianism that are based on *ren* and *li* and constitute the essence of the ideology of collectivism? The basic thesis of this system, as it is often presented in modern cross-cultural research, is a subordination of individual interests, goals, and even identity to the collective interests and goals. A more thorough analysis shows that there is a room for personal autonomy even within this thesis. As Wong (2008) suggested, this ideology in its essence does not require the complete subordination of individual interests to the collective ones and relations between them are more dialectical. It emphasizes "the mutual dependence between the individual and the group" and provides moral guidance for people regarding where to direct their will. Specifically, it recommends that a person "make the group's interests part of his or her own interests," but it also emphasizes that "the group depends on the individual and must make that individual's interests part of the group's interests" (Wong, 2008). Therefore, the complete implementation of this ideology is impossible without people's autonomous reflections and reasoning about their own interests, the interests of their group, and the decisions based on these reflections (see also Chong, 2003). Thus, as we may see, the idea of human autonomy can fairly comfortably coexist with Chinese collectivistic ideology, although not in such explicit and easily recognizable forms as within Western individualism. Autonomy in this ideology is also an inseparable part of a moral and virtuous life.

Autonomy, Agency, and Happiness in the South Asian Cultural Context

Mauss stated that in his opinion, India was the first civilization to recognize the self as an individual conscious entity (Sanderson, 1985). Later, as Sanderson (1985) suggested, this self was rejected as an undesirable worldly consciousness. Because of this it was not surprising to us to experience difficulties in discovering literary sources on the views of Hinduism (not to mention Shaivism, Jainism, Vaishnavism, and Sikhism) on self-determination and personal autonomy and their relations to happiness and the good life. In this section, we will reflect more on the discussions among cultural anthropologists, sociologists, practicing psychoanalysts, and psychologists who have studied Indian and other South Asian cultural contexts regarding the role human autonomy plays in the lives of people in these countries (Ali & Haq, 2006; Devine, Camfield, & Gough, 2008; Ewing, 1991; Mines, 1988; Roland, 1988; Singer, 1972).

The starting point of these accounts is the conventionally accepted proposition that personal autonomy and individualism are devalued in India, that individual is subordinated to the caste and familial interests and guiding principles, and that individuals' motivation can only be explained in terms of external forces in the form of caste rules and kinship ideologies. The bottom line of the conventional understanding is that the hierarchical organization of Indian society proscribes psychological autonomy (see Mines, 1988). This thesis reflects the dominant and normative ideologies of Indian society, but somehow it has been unjustifiably extended to the understanding of motivation behind people's individual lives and actions, the domain where individual psychological autonomy actually exists and functions. Do Indians reflect on their lives and behaviors? Do they choose their actions based only on the ideological prescriptions, or can they exercise their own freedom of choice and action? Do they have the ability to critically evaluate the existing normative instructions and reason their own directions in life? Do they have the capacity to feel themselves masters of their actions, to enjoy the intrinsic values of their self-determination? These questions, because their explicit denial of the most essential features of human rational consciousness, may even look offensive to representatives of the Indian civilization, but the sad fact is that, based on the modern social science model, these questions are legitimate, and despite their counterintuitive nature they should be answered in a systematic fashion. These questions also imply that according to the above-mentioned collectivistic doctrine Indians' behavior and motivation should be explained exclusively in terms of the social and cultural systems of which the individual is a member, and this explanation is driven by the assumptions "that (1) all the social cultural systems of which an individual is a member, and all aspects of each system, are equally relevant for a particular individual, and (2) the specific behavior of individual members of a "system" replicates the generic characteristics of the system without significant variations or nonsystematic traits" (Singer, 1972, p. 285).

To answer the above questions, some social scientists have analyzed individual cases either in the context of Indians' individual life histories (Mines, 1988), individual psychotherapy (Roland, 1988), in the family context (Ewing, 1991, in Pakistan), or within the industrial entrepreneurial activity in India (Singer, 1972). The goal of these analyses was to provide empirical evidence that "when Indians [and the representatives of other familial and collectivistic societies] talk privately about their lives they frequently depict themselves as active agents, pursuing private goals and making personal decisions that affect the outcome of their lives" (Mines, 1988, p. 568). Anthropologist Mines strongly argued against what he labeled ethnosociological and the social psychological approaches to understanding the Indian notion of personhood, which de-emphasizes the role of individual autonomy and self-determination in Indians' highly hierarchical and collectivist culture. According to

Mines, ethnosociologists believe that the individual is submerged in the social whole and as a result of this "Individual happiness and the autonomy that produces it are irrelevant; the emphasis is on the collective whole, on a collective man" (p. 569). The socio-psychologists emphasize instead the consequences of "the psychological and behavioral adjustments Indians must make because their hierarchical social system rewards compliance and punishes autonomy" (p. 570). Indian social psychologists, according to Mines, argued that, on the one hand, all humans experience themselves as separate from others with their own unique needs, goals, and interests, but, on the other hand, the Indian culture demands the fusion of an individual with family, caste, and class. Because of this polarity, Indians face a dilemma of either "conforming and giving up the individuality or with rebellion and receiving condemnation" (p. 570). Both these approaches, in Mines's opinion, have inherent weaknesses with regard to understanding how Indians manage their personal responsibilities for their lives, how they make and reflect upon their self-determined life decisions and the actions that pursue their personal goals and interests. These weaknesses stems from the inclination of both approaches to provide "cultural explanations of motivation generated primarily by ideological interpretations" (p. 569) instead of idiosyncratic accounts of personal motivation and the role of self-determination in it.

Based on an analysis of 23 life histories of Indians ranging from 23 to 83 years in age, Mines concluded that the issue of personal autonomy is relevant and important to Indians. He discovered that Hindu individuals develop personal goals separate from the goals of their encompassing social groups. For some of his interviewees, these goals were opposed by their families, whereas for others they were congruent. They also reported acts of rebellion that went against the normative prescriptions of family, caste, and/or hierarchy. One of the fundamental reasons for this rebellion was "strongly felt dreams for autonomy" (Mines, p. 573). As Mines mentioned, many of these rebels were "vitalized by their actions" and reported a feeling of responsibility for their lives which was grounded "in a sense of being able to make decisions that determine one's life course in ways that the individual sees as important" (Mines, p. 574). Thus, "they have become their own decision makers" (Mine, p. 575), demonstrating one of the essential forms of personal autonomy. These interviewees reported their concerns with their own needs, their personal circumstances, and their personal goals, which, when reflected upon, all together provided them with the basis for their autonomous decisions. Mines reported an interesting observation that most of the acts of autonomous agency were performed by his interviewees at later stages of their lives, whereas young people were much more strongly restricted by the cultural norms of obedience to hierarchy. Mines rightfully concluded that "the hierarchical-collectivist view generated a distorted picture of the person and of motivation, because the person is depicted as passively trapped within the frame the model describes without any mechanism for generating change" (Mine, p. 576). Contrary to this view, he defends the position that Indians can clearly identify their self-interests and exercise control over life-important decisions, thus they fight for their autonomy and the feeling of responsibility for their lives.

Psychoanalyst Roland (1988) treated Indian patients and, based on this experience, reflected on the role personal autonomy plays in Indians' lives. He distinguished three aspects of the Indians' psychological self: familial, spiritual, and individualized, and stated that their selves consist of mostly familial and spiritual components with only a small portion of the individualized component. He agreed that the issue of autonomy was one of the most deeply rooted sources of problems and conflicts that urban middle-class men, whom he mostly treated, brought to his office. He observed that these patients were habitually socialized to make major life decisions only after consultations with extended family elders, and that this upbringing nearly paralyzed his patients' ability to make autonomous decisions which was needed to manage their lives in a self-determined fashion. Issues of personal autonomy vs. compliance with their father's expectations emerged saliently in the cases of his male patients. Roland's observations of and conversations with his clients revealed to him the two layers of their inner functioning: personal and socio-cultural levels. The personal level is the level where his clients' reflections, meaning making, and internal dialogs were happening. Some psychoanalysts label this level the domain of "intrapsychic autonomy" (Ewing, 1991). A high socio-cultural level of functioning required that individuals follow the rules of the familial-hierarchical etiquette of obedience. As Roland discovered, the major conflicts that his clients brought to his treatment room were based on a strong suppression of thoughts and feelings, and especially the feelings of individual identity, autonomous strivings, and unique creativity, at the personal level, and for the sake of the demands for submission and unquestionable respect for elders and superiors at the socio-cultural level. These facts indicated that Indians have internal, private lives filled with needs for individuation, autonomy, and personal identity that may come into a sharp conflict with hierarchical-collectivistic ideology of their culture.

But to fully understand the specific Indian utilization of the human need for autonomy, as Roland commented, one has to acknowledge the importance of nourishing their spiritual selves. He understood the spiritual self as an experiential striving to "be merged with the god, goddess, or incarnation ... and in turn through the merger [one] expects the reciprocity of divine bliss" (Roland, 1988, p. 295). As he further mentioned, this "religious experience enables the person to become increasingly individuated, differentiated, and separated from the intensely emotional, familial involvements" (Roland, p. 296). In India, human autonomy is, first of all, spiritual autonomy, autonomy to worship gods, to reflect on their lives, and freedom to follow their divine teachings. Indian culture allows and facilitates individual's increasing involvement in the realization of the spiritual self, through which a person acquires relative independence of others in the fulfillment of their ideals, personal growth, esteem, and other essential autonomy-related capabilities (Shweder, Much, Mahapatra, & Park, 2003). Thus, we may say that, based on Roland's account, psychological autonomy is practiced in Indian society in two forms: through the individualized self, similar to the individualized self of Westerners, and through the spiritual self. Through the individualized self, which is mostly related to real life events and accomplishments, Indians acknowledge, reflect, and develop their personal proclivities, self-determination, emotional autonomy, and inner world of personal experience, whereas through the spiritual self, which binds them with the divine world of the sacredness, they are able to deepen their independence from others in the gratification of their spiritual needs and the realization of their karma.

Psychological/cultural anthropologist Ewing (1991) extended the same line of arguments about the relevance of psychological autonomy to the study of Pakistani women within the context of their extended families. She started her investigation with the same thesis that Western social scientists routinely treat South Asian cultures as emphasizing "hierarchy and community" and valuing "interdependence" "rather than individuality and autonomy" (Ewing, 1991, p. 132). She also correctly admitted that this denial of psychological autonomy is nothing but confusion, which is based on the failure to clearly differentiate among the cultural concepts of personality, "behavioral patterns that are shaped by social expectations", and the intrapsychic organization of a person's inner world of private thoughts, motivations, and feelings (Ewing, 1991, p. 132). With regard to autonomy she found it useful to differentiate *interpersonal autonomy* from *intrapsychic autonomy*. Summarizing her conceptualization of these concepts, they can be defined the following way. Intrapsychic autonomy is related to the existence of ego boundaries and the ability to separate the external and internal sources of need fulfillment and self-esteem. An intrapsychic autonomous person is less dependent on the environment in organizing and managing his or her behavior, and takes responsibility for his or her own actions and life. Interpersonal autonomy is definitionally, though not functionally, distinct from the intrapsychic one. This form of autonomy characterizes the mode of social relationships among members of a family or a community. The basic tenets of interpersonal autonomy include the cultivation of personal individuality, having a high demand for privacy, demonstrating relative independence from others in satisfying one's needs, and striving for self-sufficiency. Ewing's major point is that Pakistani women lack interpersonal autonomy, but their psychological health depends on the presence of intrapsychic autonomy, because it provides a healthy outlet for their psychological need for autonomy. Based on the analysis of several cases, she concluded that "there is considerable evidence to suggest that in many South Asian families, individual family members do in fact act in an autonomous fashion intrapsychically, though they operate within a highly 'engaged' interpersonal network of family relations and expectations. Despite a high degree of interpersonal engagement, South Asians often display a considerable ability to maintain their own perspective and remain attuned to their own needs and to the needs of others while accepting the demands for conformity within the family" (Ewing, p. 139).

These accounts of autonomy in the South Asian context convey several important ideas for this book's arguments. First, that it is crucially important to differentiate the socio-cultural ideologies of personhood and interpersonal relations that direct people's behavior on the social level from the persons' intrapsychological realm of their private reflections, personal needs, goals, and feelings. This internal world is the space for personal and motivational autonomy where people make decisions about their own actions and life course, where they contemplate the societal prescriptions for actions and decide whether to follow them or not. Second, there are conceptual confusions regarding various levels of human autonomy manifestations and the theoretical differentiation of various forms of autonomy from related concepts, such as interdependence, independence and individualism, collectivism, and others. These confusions require more elaborated conceptual framing of the concept of psychological autonomy. But probably the most important conclusion is that the members of these restrictive and hierarchical cultures possess this undeniable capability and need for personal autonomy. Cultures, in our case the Indian one, may be less restrictive to the personal autonomy of its members during their more mature ages and may provide a special domain for its unrestricted exercise, such as private spirituality. The individual's psychological autonomy may be in conflict with the dominant social prescriptions in these Eastern cultures, just as they are often so within Western societies (see, e.g., Kasser, Cohn, Kanner, & Ryan, 2007). As a result of this conflict, if human autonomy is either undeveloped or strongly suppressed, then mental health problems could emerge. This conclusion means that psychological autonomy is universally essential for people's mental health and ultimately for their happiness and the good life.

Happiness, Human Autonomy, and Self-Determination in Modern Psychology

Modern psychology has always been split on the issues of human autonomy, freedom, and happiness, directly or indirectly. We identify three major trends of thoughts on this issue. One trend, which is comprised of Skinnerian (Skinner, 1971) as well as modern cognitive psychologists (Bargh, 2004; Wegner, 2002, 2008), has tried to follow the demand of scientific determinism to find the ultimate causes of human behavior by precluding consideration of subjective experience and the intentional nature of human reasoning as determinant of action. In other words, according to this position, real determining causes of human behavior should be independent of the consciousness of acting individuals and should explain both consciousness and behavior. The idea of human happiness and the directions for a good life have never been an issue within this trend of psychological thinking. The second trend is represented by a variety of theories that could be linked to a postmodernist, social constructionist movement wherein people's psychological processes and states have been presented as social constructions, as texts, or sets of discourses (Benson, 2001; Burr, 2003; Gergen, 1997; Harré, 1993). These socio-cultural constructions or scripts are always relative, fluid, and fundamentally not essentialistic and, as a result, they completely depend on their social cultural interpretation. And the third trend that has been strongly devoted to the investigation and understanding of the conditions for people's happy and harmonious lives, including people's autonomy, agency, and freedom, is represented by humanistic psychoanalysis (Fromm, 1947, 1976; Horney, 1950), humanistic psychology (Maslow, 1968; Rogers, 1961, 1977), existential psychology (Frankl, 1971, 1988; May, 1981, 1961), phenomenological and hermeneutic psychology (Pfänder, 1908; Ricoeur, 1950; Sugarman & Martin,

2004), and self-determination theory (Ryan & Deci, 2004; Ryan & Deci, 2006; Ryan et al., 2008). The representatives of this trend, although very diverse and different in their philosophical and empirical backgrounds, find the determinants of good lives for humans and their well-being in autonomous human consciousness, as well as in people's ability to reflect on their life conditions, both internal and external, and, based on this ability, to be relatively independent builders of their own destiny, happiness, and harmonious lives.

A Deterministic Trend in Modern Psychology

We find it appropriate to start this short review with the Skinnerian account of people's freedom and autonomy (Skinner, 1971). In his book *Beyond Dignity and Freedom,* Skinner very explicitly expressed views that have shaped discussions of this issue for decades. In this book, Skinner fought against any conception of "an inner or autonomous man." To him this conception is similar to a medieval homunculus, which metaphorically represents a power of individual consciousness to reflect on and guide one's own behavior. This "autonomous man" was created, according to Skinner, as an explanatory metaphor because of scholars' ignorance about the real and objective causes of behavior. These real causes of human behavior can only be discovered by a scientific (meaning modeled from the natural sciences) analysis of behavior. Together with the "autonomous man," Skinner tried to refute people's attributes such as purposes, intentions, plans, and states of mind, portraying them as mentalistic constructions that should be scientifically explained instead of being used as explanatory categories *per se*. The main idea of the Skinnerian scientific analysis of behavior is to search for the real causes of both the human mental states and behavior, via contingencies of reinforcement. By replacing the "autonomous man" with a set of externally crafted contingencies of reinforcement (although he admitted that a man himself may be a creator of these contingencies), behavioral scientists were expected to be able to develop "a technology of behavior" that would change and control people's behavior for the better. So, the ultimate purpose of the Skinnerian scientific analysis of behavior is not people's good and moral lives, not their happiness, but the opportunity to control people and change their behavior in desired directions.

These very ideas are still pervasive and strong in modern cognitive psychology. Incredibly similar arguments against human self-determination and autonomy can be found in works of modern cognitive psychologists such as Bargh (1999, 2000) and Wegner (2002, 2008, 1999). Bargh, for instance, explicitly stated that "...the contemporary cognitive perspective, in spirit as well as in practice, seeks to account for psychological phenomena in terms of deterministic mechanisms" (1999, p. 463). And further he explained these "deterministic mechanisms" using a similar logic to Skinner. Bargh used the opinion of Neisser from his "Cognitive Psychology" book who called the explanation of the "problem of the executive" by referring to a "homunculus or 'little person in the head'" non-scientific. And further, Bargh used the opinion that Barsalou expressed in his 1993 review of cognitive psychology "in which he [Barsalou] too calls free will a homunculus, noting that, most cognitive psychologists believe that the fundamental laws of the physical world determine human behavior completely," (Bargh, 1999, p. 463). Bargh's own thesis is that "most of a person's everyday life is determined not by their conscious intentions and deliberate choices, but by mental processes that are put into motion by features of environment and that operate outside of conscious awareness and guidance" (p. 462). (We are curious whether he wrote this and his other publications driven not by "conscious intentions and deliberate choices", but by the directions of the "features of environment", while being consciously unaware of what he was doing and lacking rational guidance.) Bargh's final verdict is that "free will (together with autonomy and self-determination) is un-natural" (2008) and is not worth the special attention of scientists.

The similar position, that human consciousness and related to it self-determination and free will are epiphenomena of actual causal forces of human behavior and consciousness itself, was expressed by Wegner (1999). He stated that "... will is not a psychological force that causes action. Rather, as a perception that results from interpretation, it is a conscious experience that may only map rather weakly, or perhaps not at all, into the actual causal relationships between the person's cognition and action" (p. 481). In his book *The Illusion of Conscious Will* (2002), Wegner elaborated these and related ideas, that self-determination is an illusion or rather a reflection and interpretation by the individual mind of a real causal dynamic streaming from the environment and the brain. For a critical analysis of these ideas see Libet (1999), Mele (2009), Modell (2008), and Sternberg (2010). Thus, we may say that Skinner, with his anti-autonomy ideas, is well and alive in the works of modern psychologists. What is important for us here is that by removing self-determination and autonomy from the realm of the actual causal powers of humans' lives, these post-Skinnerian psychologists create more problems for human and social sciences than they solve. If we accept this position, the issues of people's happiness and good lives, self-development, responsibility, creativity and innovations, culture creation and change, and many other problems will remain unresolved, because all of them depend on people's self-determination, imagination, and ability for autonomous functioning, which are impossible to study and understand from the position of the post-Skinnerian determinism, where they are ruled out *a priori*.

Social Constructionism in Modern Psychology and the Question of Human Agency and Happiness

Because of the high complexity of the concept of social constructionism (SC) in modern philosophy and the social sciences, we will limit our analysis only to those versions of social constructionism that exist in modern psychology (Burr, 2002, 2003; Gergen, 1985, 1997; Harré, 1983, 1993), and that are analyzed and reviewed in the works of Polkinghorne (2001), Raskin (2002), and Schwandt (2000).

1 Introduction

The fundamental generic form of social constructionism states that everything that comprises humanness in humans, their selves, motives, goals, values, emotions, and thoughts, is socially constructed, meaning that these psychological states and processes are the results of negotiations, interactions, and conversations among the members of the community in which they happen to be born. Psychological processes, according to this position, are inherently social and public, and social interactions, conversations, and discourses are responsible for the emergence of the "psychological." Only through analysis of these social interaction-level processes can psychologists study and understand psychological phenomena.

Two classifications of various forms of social constructionism (SC) are useful for our analysis. The first was provided by Schawndt (2000), who differentiated between a "weak" or "ordinary sense" constructionism and a "strong" social constructionism; the second was presented by Burr (2003) by differentiating "micro" and "macro" forms of social constructionism. According to Schawnd, weak SC is implicitly or explicitly embedded into both ordinary and scientific thinking of modern people through the ideas that a researcher, with the help of a scientific community, actively constructs knowledge by generating data through theory-driven observations. These observations are guided by particular conceptual frameworks that demand paying attention to and select specific elements of a phenomenon at issue and then shape the generated data as a representation of both a specific theoretical point of view as well as an aspect of the reality under investigation. This form of social constructionism is known as "scientific perspectivism" (Giere, 2006), which has become a cornerstone of the post-positivistic movement (Polkinghorne, 1983). Weak SC does not deny the existence of real social and psychological worlds, but highlights an active, selective, and perspectival nature of our quest for understanding and explaining them. Shwandt (2000) characterized the strong or radical form of SC as the following. Based on Wittgenstein's idea of language games, radical constructionists state that representations of the world have nothing to do with the real world itself because they are constructed within and depend upon the language games and forms of life of a particular socio-cultural-linguistic community. As a result of this dependence, radical constructionists argue that "all statements of the true, the rational, and the good are the products of various particular communities of interpreters and thus to be regarded with suspicion", and that "...it is only within and with reference to a particular form of life that the meaning of an action can be described and deciphered" (Schwandt, 2000, p. 200). Polkinghorn (2001) worded this thesis of postmodernism in the following way: "people's understanding of the world, others, and themselves are a function of their different culturally given interpretative schemes, and their thoughts and actions always are mediated and constructed through the lens of these schemes" (p. 89). Polkinghorne also claimed that social constructionists deny the existence of the personal self. For them, "the concept of self is held to be a fictional creation of Western grammar and cognitive schemes" (p. 88). If self, as a center of experience and actions from the point of view of an experiencing and acting individual, disappears, then there is no place for self-determination or self-regulation and consequently no place for human autonomy. According to strong SC, if psychologists are willing to talk about these concepts, they should be "removed from the head and placed within the sphere of social discourse" (Gergen, 1985, p. 271).

As stated by Burr (2003), micro SC "sees social construction taking place within everyday discourse between people in interaction" (p. 21). This means that interpersonal linguistic interactions are responsible for the construction of personal identities, selves, and other psychological attributes of interacting people. On the other hand, "macro social constructionism acknowledges the constructive power of language, but sees this as derived from, or at least related to, material or social structures, social relations, and institutionalized practices" (p. 22). The representatives of this form of SC seriously consider "the constructive force of culturally available discourses" (p. 203). For the followers of Foucault within this approach, the concept of power is at the heart of their analysis of social reality. In cultural and social anthropology, which have gone through the interpretavist turn headed by Geertz (1998), macro SC exists under the terms of the "cultural relativism" (Hatch, 1983) and/or "cultural determinism" of psychological states and processes. In the social sciences this approach was labeled a "standard social science model" (Tooby & Cosmides, 1992), which assumes a complete dependence of psychological characteristics of people on social institutions, social arrangements, and roles. The common feature of these approaches is that a person is treated as a derivate of social, cultural, linguistic/discursive structures and as a result "the individual and self are seen as illusion or at best constructions over which we have little control" (Burr, 2003, p. 183). With regard to human flourishing, social constructionist/feminist social scientists stated, "We maintain that the bounded, autonomous self that strides through a positive life is an illusion, as the notion that human flourishing and happiness are readily available to all" (Becker & Marecek, 2008a, p. 1767). Thus, social constructionism, with its denial of the essentialistic and a cultural understanding of person and self found in mainstream psychology, swings to another extreme proposing that all psychological features are public and social and should be treated as functions of cultural or interpersonal practices and discourses.

What do all these systems of thinking have to do with the topic of this book – human happiness and autonomy? There are several serious implications to consider. First, as within the "deterministic approach"' in cognitive psychology, self, self-determination, and self-development have been declared to be illusions and have been emptied of their deeply psychological, existential and, finally, human content by replacing them with social discourses and cultural ideologies. Social constructionism of all forms denies the existence of "our intra-psychic make-up that forms the basis of our actions" (Burr, 2003, p. 24), including our values, moral imperatives, desires, wants, hopes, and "our continuous sense of self" (Archer, 2000, p. 3), and, as a result, our agency, autonomy, and self-determination. "Macro social constructionism tends toward the 'death of the subject' where the person can be conceptualized only as the outcome of discursive and societal structures" (Burr, p. 23). Thus, within constructionistic accounts, a person has been transformed into a puppet of social and conversational public forces that leaves no space for his or her own internal world, psychological privacy, self-change, or self-development. It is fair to say that many social constructionists are struggling to put human agency into the context of social constructions. Burr commented that the micro social constructionism "implicitly affords us personal agency" (p. 23). Kenwood (1996) stated directly that "... it is precisely *agency* – indeed, *voluntary* agency – that puts the 'construction' into 'constructionism.' Without the capacity to choose among informed alternatives, that is, without the possibility of acting otherwise, people could not meaningfully be said to 'construct' anything at all" (p. 534). Obviously SC needs human autonomous agency, but for them it is the mystical agency of a discourse-user, which has no explanatory power within this paradigm.

The issue of happiness and the good life is also a problematic topic for social constructionists. The major representatives of this movement have hardly ever addressed it in a direct manner, but we have still been capable of tracing this topic through the works of critical cultural psychologists, who at some point turn their attention to the analysis of the mainstream positive psychology.[3] We extracted two major ideas that some of the authors of that issue (see footnote 3) and corresponding publications have made with regard to human happiness. The first idea, that the thesis that happiness and the good life are achievable by individual efforts, is "narrow and ethnocentric" because it is built on the Western/American ideology of individualism, and, thus, is not universal, *a priori* biased and is wrong. The second idea is that real happiness can only come from the ideology of collectivism and from a submergence of an individual to his or her collectivity. These scholars suggest that we should dissolve the personal autonomous self together with its ability for reflection and self-determination in sociality, and this depsychologization and deindividuation of humans is presented as a standard of the good life for the majority of the world's population (Becker & Marecek, 2008a, 2008b; Christopher & Hickinbottom, 2008). These authors argue that if people are unhappy, it is because they are submerged in a bad sociality; to make them happy, this sociality must be changed. Individual efforts of reflection, self-improvement, and self-development are rejected from the start as narrow-minded and futile efforts informed by the wrong and ethnocentric ideology of individualism. Thus, as in the more explicit forms of SC, these critical psychologists deny the experiencing and reflective self, and they deem as peripheral the inner psychological world, where autonomous and private thoughts and reflections unfold. There seems to be no place for human happiness and psychological freedom here; this is only slavery in a social cage.

But there is still a question to ask: Are people's eudaimonic happiness and the good life strongly culturally relative, or despite socio-cultural influences are they universal across cultures? Many scholars argue that there are near universal foundation for people's good lives across nations and cultures (Harrison, 2000; Hatch, 1983; Nussbaum, 2000). We agree with Nussbaum (2000) that there are universal "human capabilities, that is, what people are actually able to do and to be [which is] informed by an intuitive idea of a life that is worthy of the dignity of the human being" (p. 5). Thus, the good life is the life that allows people to

---

[3]See a special issue of the journal *Theory & Psychology* "Thinking through positive psychology" 2008, Vol. 8(5).

exercise their capabilities, where being agents and thinking for themselves is a central one. A similar idea is expressed by SDT researchers regarding the existence of human basic psychological needs – needs for autonomy competence and relatedness — the satisfaction of which lies at the basis of psychological health, growth, and development across cultures (Ryan & Deci, 2000a). This existence of fundamental human capabilities and psychological needs that build the psychological background of a decent human life, which the Greeks' labeled eudaimonia, provides a counter-relativistic basis for understanding people's well-being and a life of high quality across different cultures (Hatch, 1983). Indeed, this capabilities and psychological needs approach gives us the opportunity to establish relatively universal and objective criteria for evaluating people's wellness and goodness of life and to avoid radical cultural relativism: the ability to exercise humans' capabilities and satisfy psychological fundamental needs are the standards to evaluate their social and cultural environments and establish nearly universal criteria of people's flourishing.

The Humanistic Trend in Modern Psychology

Humanism in the social and human sciences generally means that human beings, their dignity, well-being, and flourishing are considered to be yardsticks for evaluating societies, cultures, and various political and ideological constructions (Hatch, 1983). "The humanistic movement in psychology has emphasized the search for a philosophical and scientific understanding of human existence that does justice to the highest reaches of human achievement and potential" (Moss, 2001, p. 5).

In the context of this book the following aspects of humanistic psychology are important to highlight. One is fundamentally concerned with people's flourishing, personal growth and mature development, with those qualities of people's lives that relate to people's self-actualization, optimal functioning, and happiness (Maslow, 1971; May, 1953, 1981). For Rogers (1961), for example, the concept of becoming "the fully functioning person" constitutes the essence of living the good life. This is how Rogers defined it: "The good life ... is the process of movement in a direction which the human organism selects when it is inwardly free to move in any direction, and the general qualities of this selected direction appear to have a certain universality" (Rogers, 1961, p. 187). Along with such characteristics as having openness to experience, trust in one's organism, living in the present, a high congruence among awareness, experience, and communication, and some others (see Rogers, 1961, p. 107), the fully functioning person, according to Rogers, has the feeling of "the most complete and absolute freedom" (Rogers, p. 193) to make his or her own choices, "... to become himself or to hide behind a façade; to move forward or to retrogress; to behave in ways which are destructive of self and others; or in ways which are enhancing; quite literally free to live or die, in both the physiological and psychological meaning of those terms" (Rogers, p. 192). Thus, psychological freedom in Rogers's theorizing appears to be the attribute of both 'the good life' and the person who lives this life through full and complete functioning. In a similar vein, Maslow (1971) defined the goal of human growth as "the psychological health" that he equated with "productiveness," "self-actualization," "authenticity," "full-humanness," and some other qualities (p. 226). He understood self-actualization, a core concept in his theory, as the "acceptance and expression of the inner core or self, i.e., actualization of … latent capacities and potentialities, 'full functioning,' availability of the human and personal essence" (Maslow, 1971, p. 227). You do not need to stretch your imagination too much to see the similarities between these humanistic understandings of the good life and the ideas of eudaimonia and happiness that follow in this volume.

Many humanistic psychologists believe that people's motivation is a crucial aspect of their lives that contributes to people's optimal functioning and eudaimonic happiness. In this context, human autonomy together with motivation toward "self-actualization," "being-motivation," "meta-motivation," and "meta-needs" are continually present in the theorizing of humanistic psychologists. A psychologically healthy individual, according to Maslow (1971), transcends "the deficiency-needs" and is motivated by the "being-needs"; satisfaction of these needs leads to authenticity, nondefensive perception of reality, constructive relationships with other people, and creativity. Psychological autonomy, which he equates with the motivation of the "being-needs," allows fully functioning individuals not only to be free in pursuing their potentialities and needs, but also to merge easily with a larger social whole. Maslow, drawing from Angyal (1941), called this amalgamation with a social whole "a state of homonomy." He argued that only through full homonomy, when a person experiences oneself as an organic part of a large social community, may a healthy individual reach full autonomy. This means that, for Maslow, autonomy has nothing to do with encapsulated selfishness and egotism. This is the same idea that we want to entertain in this book. Almost all humanistic psychologists have spoken about human autonomy and psychological freedom as a fundamental condition for growth and maturity. May (1953/1973), for example, provided the following interpretation of psychological freedom. "Freedom is man's capacity to take a hand in his own development. It is our capacity to mold ourselves. Freedom is the other side of consciousness of self: if we were not able to be aware of ourselves, we would be pushed along by instinct or the automatic march of history" (p. 160). This understanding of freedom is very close to the definition of autonomy given by the Stoic philosophers, Spinoza, and Kant. The authors of this volume endorse such an understanding also.

A humanistic approach to human functioning is inevitably concerned with the social conditions that promote or thwart the development of humans' healthy motivation as well as their ultimate happiness, flourishing, and the good life. For Rogers (1961), interpersonal relations between a client and a therapist, and among people in general, are the most important condition for clients to experience change and for people to thrive. Based on his summary of "helping relationships" we may conclude that only in relationships that are saturated with trust, respect, an understanding of other people's needs and attitudes, and support for the freedom to make one's own choices can clients experience the security and comfort to remove their defensiveness; similarly, given these conditions, ordinary people become empowered to pursue their own happiness in the most unrestricted and uncompromised way. This type of relationship has been identified by SDT researchers as *autonomy supportive* (Ryan & Deci, 2000b).

Humanistic psychologists have always been interested in examining the complex relations of a fully functioning healthy person with his or her socio-cultural environment as well as the conditions in such an environment that facilitate or hinder the actualization of people's capacities and characteristics. This interest corresponds with our concern to establish theoretical and empirical bases for understanding those conditions in distal social environment that universally provide support and facilitation of human psychological autonomy and people's flourishing. In this context we want to quote Maslow: "... a society or a culture can be either growth-fostering or growth-inhibiting.... The 'better' culture gratifies all basic human needs and permits self-actualization. The 'poor' cultures do not" (1971, p. 233). He also clearly articulated dialectical relationships between an emergent autonomous person and culture: culture is a condition without which the actualization of humanness is impossible, but finally people must be relatively independent from culture to become who they are. May (1953/1973) conveyed a very similar idea: "... our social and economic ideal be *that society which gives the maximum opportunity for each person in it to realize himself, to develop and use his potentialities and to labor as a human being of dignity giving to and receiving from fellow men.* The good society is, thus, the one which gives the greatest freedom to its people – freedom ... as the opportunity to realize ever greater human values. It follows that collectivism, as in fascism and communism, is the denial of these values, and must be opposed at all costs" (p. 160).

Ultimately, the topics of this volume are these three constituents: (1) fundamental concern with people's health, eudaimonic happiness, and optimal functioning across different domains, (2) an emphasis on people's healthy motivation as a condition for this functioning and wellness to take place, and (3) the role social contexts plays in the unfolding of these two ingredients. Human autonomy and self-determination are considered to be fundamental factors that allow these three components to interact in the most optimal way. The findings presented in this book, unlike much of orthodox humanistic theorizing, are supported by empirical evidence, and yet in general are in a full concordance with the insights and conclusions of the psychologists of humanism.

A Short Review of the Chapters

Part I A Theoretical Context of Human Autonomy and People's Flourishing

The book starts with the chapter "Positive Psychology and Self-Determination Theory: A Natural Marriage" by Kennon Sheldon and Richard Ryan. The goal of this chapter is to situate self-determination theory within the context of modern positive psychology, which is the main framework for this book series. The chapter discusses both the positive psychology movement and the self-determination theory, arguing that self-determination theory is a prototypical example of a positive psychology theory. Self-determination theory provides an integrated and scientifically supported framework for understanding people's optimal functioning, while also addressing "negative" conditions that can get in the way of this process. Accusations that positive psychology is overly individualistic are considered from the lens of self-determination theory, which has already faced and answered such challenges. The authors suggest that the positive psychology movement can utilize self-determination theory as a general framework within which to conduct many types of well-being research.

In the third chapter, "A Self-Determination Theory Perspective on Social, Institutional, Cultural, and Economic Supports for Autonomy and Their Importance for Well-Being" Richard Ryan and Edward Deci discuss modern conceptions of happiness, including hedonic and eudaimonic perspectives. They distinguish happiness as a symptom rather than *sine qua non* of well-being, and they relate the latter to the human capability for autonomous self-regulation. Using a self-determination framework they define autonomy and detail its essential functional role in allowing individuals within any culture to satisfy basic psychological needs for competence and relatedness, and thus to attain psychological well-being and happiness. The chapter also highlights how capacities for autonomous self-regulation, although evolved and "natural" to all humans, are dependent on both proximal (e.g., familial, interpersonal) and distal (political, cultural, economic) supports, and how need thwarting aspects of social environments can undermine autonomy and wellness.

In the fourth chapter of the first part of the book, "Dialectical Relationships Among Human Autonomy, the Brain, and Culture," Valery Chirkov examines relationships among human psychological autonomy, the brain, and culture. Human autonomy is presented as an evolved natural property of the *Homo sapiens* species that has dialectical relations with people's socio-cultural environments and is a universal and necessary condition for people' optimal functioning. The human brain and culture are required for this capacity to evolve and be developed. The author states that human autonomy is not a social construction and not an illusion: It is a real psychological power behind people's lives and actions but it requires a socio-symbolic context to emerge. Autonomous people can overcome their dependency on cultural norms and prescriptions by reflecting on social and cultural influences and acting either with or against them. Human autonomy is a universal condition for people to grow, flourish, and be happy. In this chapter the author also identifies and discusses socio-cultural conditions that promote and facilitate human autonomy. He labels them the culture of horizontality vs. the culture of verticality. The chapter ends with a review of the cross-cultural research in self-determination and autonomous motivation that supports many of the stated propositions.

Part II Human Autonomy Across Cultures and Domains of Life: Health, Education, Interpersonal Relationships, and Work

In the fifth chapter, "The Role of Autonomy in Promoting Healthy Dyadic, Familial, and Parenting Relationships Across Cultures," C. Raymond Knee and Ahmet Uysal explain how autonomy facilitates closeness and healthy interpersonal relationships. Based on rich empirical material, they demonstrate that among couples, relationship autonomy and need fulfillment are associated with numerous positive processes that facilitate and strengthen people's ties, such as a deeper understanding of each other and a more constructive approach to conflict management and resolution; among families, parental autonomy support is associated with various indicators of positive internalization, children's self-development, and the relational health and well-being of both parents and children. The authors come to the conclusion that autonomy is important for healthy and optimally functioning personal relationships. Despite the few cross-cultural studies on this topic the authors justifiably infer that this conclusion may be extended to non-Western countries.

In the sixth chapter "Do Social Institutions Necessarily Suppress Individuals' Need for Autonomy? The Possibility of Schools as Autonomy Promoting Contexts Across the Globe," Johnmarshall Reeve and Avi Assor discuss the organization of education across the globe with regard to how autonomy promoting these organizations are. Recognizing that some social institutions attain seemingly harmonious functioning by suppressing individuals' autonomy, the first half of the chapter argues that these hierarchical institutions do not have to be autonomy suppressive. The second half of the chapter illustrates how schools can function as autonomy-promoting cultural institutions, even when embedded within hierarchical societies that contrast social hierarchy against individual autonomy. The authors state that to be truly autonomy-promoting, schools should be designed in ways that (a) allow students to shape important aspects of the school and support students' attempts to form authentic and direction-giving values, goals, and interests, and (b) offer frequently recurring opportunities for students to experience autonomy during learning activities. The authors offer numerous examples of these two key features of autonomy-promoting schools from different countries. Finally they ask the question "How feasible is it to bring about autonomy-supportive schools around the world?" The authors answer that although such schools are quite feasible in egalitarian countries with autonomy-conductive social norms, they are unlikely cultural products in hierarchical countries with control-conducive social norms.

In the seventh chapter "Physical Wellness, Health Care, and Personal Autonomy," Geoffrey Williams, Pedro Teixeira, Eliana Carraca, and Ken Resnicow review the self-determination theory perspective and current empirical evidence linking personal autonomy with physical well-being within and across cultures. Their main thesis is that a clear understanding of the relation between autonomy and physical well-being is relevant in all cultures. They provide two reasons for this. First, as SDT predicts, evidence suggests that higher levels of personal autonomy universally result in better physical well-being, and, second, recent developments in biomedical ethics and informed decision making have elevated respect for patient autonomy to be the explicit, highest level goal of health care. The authors emphasize that together empirical evidence and these ethical mandates foretell an increasing emphasis on the role personal autonomy should play in the delivery of health care. In this chapter, they have systematically reviewed the literature for studies that report the quantitative relations between different measures of personal autonomy and physical health and autonomy and health-related behaviors. They discovered that most studies occur within single cultures, and find consistent, positive relations between personal autonomy, or its change, and physical health. They discuss these findings, their limitations and suggest future research that can more fully establish and explore the causal linkages between personal autonomy and physical well-being.

In the eighth chapter "Autonomy in the Workplace: An Essential Ingredient to Employee Engagement and Well-Being in Every Culture," Marylène Gagné and Devasheesh Bhave address the role workers' autonomy plays in the lives of modern organizations. They summarize an impressive amount of management research which has investigated this problem from a wide variety of different perspectives. In their review they specifically focus on evidence in the area of job design and management practices showing how various management choices and policies affect worker autonomy. Organizational research guided by self-determination theory is also described and shown to provide a theoretical background within which to integrate different perspectives of this line of the analysis. Throughout this discussion, they also evaluate the cross-cultural applicability of research and practice with regard to enhancing workers, autonomy, engagement, and empowerment.

Part III. Human Autonomy in Modern Economy, Democracy Development, and Sustainability

In the ninth chapter, "Capitalism and Autonomy," Tim Kasser states that the means by which a culture organizes itself economically has important implications for people's experience of autonomy. Despite claims that freedom is maximized under the form of neo-liberal, laissez-fair capitalism which is practiced in many Anglo nations, several types of evidence suggest that the values, ideologies, and institutions of such economic systems can diminish people's feelings of self-determination. For example, new analyses presented in this chapter show that, compared to citizens living in wealthy nations that place more restrictions on the activity of the "free market," citizens living in "economically free" wealthy nations more highly value power and hierarchy, and view autonomy and self-direction as less important. Other research reviewed here shows that some of the personal beliefs, behaviors, and laws central to the smooth functioning of laissez-faire, consumer capitalism do not provide people with optimal experiences of freedom and autonomy. This analysis thus demonstrates the potential usefulness of self-determination theory for understanding economic systems in particular and cultural systems in general.

In the tenth chapter, "Economy, People's Personal Autonomy, and Well-Being," Maurizio Pugno argues that the concept of personal autonomy helps explain the gap between economic growth and people's well-being, which is the phenomenon that although we keep getting richer, we do not get happier. The arguments, based on a variety of specific evidence drawn from psychology, especially self-determination theory, and from economics and sociology, run as follows. First, people's well-being has been negatively affected by the deterioration of their autonomy, which is a basic psychological need, and by the compensatory need for financial success and status. Secondly, some important factors that appear to promote economic growth in advanced countries, and especially in the US, also hamper the development of people's personal autonomy. Conventional explanations of the income/well-being gap based on social comparison, rising expectations, and deteriorated social relationships can thus be integrated and strengthened.

In the eleventh chapter, "The Development of Conceptions of Personal Autonomy, Rights, and Democracy and Their Relation to Psychological Well-Being," Charles C. Helwig and Justin McNeil demonstrate that children in a variety of cultural contexts have been shown to develop concerns with personal autonomy and rights, and these conceptions not only place limits on the forms of social organization seen as legitimate but also have relevance for children's psychological well-being. Although many current psychological theories relegate freedoms, rights, and democracy to products of Western intellectual traditions or cultural settings, a body of new and emerging psychological evidence, conducted in a variety of cultural settings, both Eastern and Western, and from a variety of theoretical perspectives, including self-determination theory, suggests otherwise. Areas of personal jurisdiction, choice, and participation are claimed by children and adolescents themselves as they develop explicit conceptions of their own autonomy and reflect on the different types of social rules and structures that they experience in their daily lives. These conceptions of autonomy and democracy have been shown to have functional significance for the realization of individuals' psychological well-being in diverse cultural settings.

In the twelfth and final chapter "Personal Autonomy and Environmental Sustainability", Luc G. Pelletier et al. discuss personal autonomy in the context of environmental sustainability, which is becoming an ever more important challenge for people around the world. This challenge is related to the increasing concern about how we can meet the needs of the present without compromising the ability of future generations to meet their needs. The authors argue that to achieve sustainability, people must not only attempt to reconcile growing concerns about a full spectrum of environmental issues with socio-economic issues and societal quality of life issues but they also have to achieve a substantial shift in values, attitudes, and behaviors so that pro-environmental behaviors are sustained and become a part of people's lifestyles. In their chapter, the authors examine how self-determination theory can provide an effective theoretical framework to guide research and interventions on pro-environmental behavior and sustainable development. Their analysis of recent research shows that, like the internalization of activities in other life domains, conditions that respect people's needs for autonomy, competence, and relatedness, as well as their desire to be effective in dealing with the challenges of the ecological situation, allow them to gradually internalize socially valued PEBs and make them personally endorsed activities. In conclusion, they state that the achievement of sustainability also provides a unique context to advance our knowledge on how SDT can guide research on the impact of government policies, on the influence of media, and on how people deal with the internal conflicts that result from simultaneously being aware of environmental issues, socio-economic issues, and societal quality of life issues.

Together these chapters provide considerable evidence for the multiple linkages between autonomous functioning and the well-being and integrity of individuals, groups, nations, and the planet as a whole. They also highlight the social and political obstacles, as well as the needed facilitating conditions, to supporting individuals in their natural tendencies toward the optimization of health, wellness, and community. As we look ahead to the future of humanity, it is clear that the decisions we make concerning how we organize ourselves and how we pursue "the good life" will heavily impact the whole planet. In that regard we hope the perspectives offered herein facilitate deeper inquiries into the social conditions that can best ensure our collective safe passage and happiness.

References

Ali, S. M., & Haq, R. U. (2006). Women's autonomy and happiness: The case of Pakistan. *Pakistan Development Review, 45*, 121–136.

Angyal, A. (1941). *Foundations for a science of personality*. New York: Pergamon Press.

Archer, M. S. (2000). *Being human: The problem of agency*. Cambridge: Cambridge University Press.

Bargh, J. A. (2004). Being here now: Is consciousness necessary for human freedom? In J. Greenberg, S. L. Koole, & T. Pyszczynski (Eds.), *Handbook of experimental existential psychology* (pp. 385–397). New York: The Guilford Press.

Bargh, J. A. (2008). Free will is un-natural. In J. Baer, J. C. Kaufman & R. F. Baumeister (Eds.), *Are we free? Psychology and free will.* (pp. 128–154). Oxford: Oxford University Press.

Bargh, J. A., & Chartrand, T. L. (1999). The unbearable automaticity of being. *American Psychologist, 54*(7), 462–479.

Bargh, J. A., & Ferguson, M. J. (2000). Beyond behaviorism: On the automaticity of higher mental processes. *Psychological Bulletin, 126*(6), 925–945.

Becker, D., & Marecek, J. (2008a). Dreaming the American dream: Individualism and positive psychology. *Social and Personality Psychology Compass, 2*(5), 1768–1780.

Becker, D., & Marecek, J. (2008b). Positive psychology: History in the remaking? *Theory and Psychology, 18*(5), 591–604.

Benson, C. (2001). *The cultural psychology of self: Place, morality and art in human worlds*. London: Routledge.

Burr, V. (2002). *The person in social psychology*. East Sussex: Psychology Press.

Burr, V. (2003). *Social constructionism* (2nd ed.). London, New York: Routledge.

Chan, J. (2002). Moral autonomy, civil liberties, and Confucianism. *Philosophy East and West, 52*(3), 281–310.

Cheng, C.-Y. (2004). A theory of Confucian selfhood: Self-cultivation and free will in Confucian philosophy. In K.-I. Shun & D. B. Wong (Eds.), *Confucian ethics: A comparative study of self, autonomy, and community* (pp. 124–142). New York: Cambridge University Press.

Chong, K.-C. (2003). Autonomy in the analects. In K. Chong, S. Tan, & C. L. Ten (Eds.), *The moral circle and the self: Chinese and western approaches* (pp. 269–282). Chicago: Open Court.

Christopher, J. C., & Hickinbottom, S. (2008). Positive psychology, ethnocentrism, and the disguised ideology of individualism. *Theory and Psychology, 18*(5), 563–589.

Deci, E. L., & Ryan, R. M. (Eds.). (2002). *Handbook of self-determination research*. Rochester, NY: The University of Rochester Press.

de Heer, C. (1969). *Makar, eudaimon, olbios, eutychia: A study of the semantic field denoting happiness in Ancient Greek to the end of the fifth century B.C.* Amsterdam: Adolf M. Hakkert.

Devine, J., Camfield, L., & Gough, I. (2008). Autonomy or dependence-or both? Perspectives from Bangladesh. *Journal of Happiness Studies, 9*, 105–138.

Dumont, L. (1985). A modified view of our origins: The Christian beginnings of modern individualism. In M. Carrithers, S. Collins, & S. Lukes (Eds.), *The category of the person: Anthropology, philosophy, history* (pp. 93–122). Cambridge: Cambridge University Press.

Elvin, M. (1985). Between the earth and haven: Conceptions of the self in China. In M. Carrithers, S. Collins, & S. Lukes (Eds.), *The category of the person: Anthropology, philosophy, history* (pp. 156–189). Cambridge: Cambridge University Press.

Engstrom, A., & Whiting, J. (Eds.). (1996). *Aristotle, Kant, and the Stoics: Rethinking happiness and duty*. Cambridge: Cambridge University Press.

Ewing, K. P. (1991). Can psychoanalytic theories explain the Pakistani woman? Intrapsychic autonomy and interpersonal engagement in the extended family. *Ethos, 19*(2), 131–160.

Frankl, V. (1971). *Man's search for meaning: An introduction to logotherapy*. New York: Poket Books.

Frankl, V. (1988). *The will to meaning: Foundation and applications of logotherapy* (5th ed.). New York: Plume.

Fromm, E. (1947/1990). *Man for himself: An inquiry into the psychology of ethics*. New York: Henry Holt and Company.

Fromm, E. (1976). *To have or to be?* New York: Continuum.

Geertz, C. (1998). *Interpretation of cultures*. New York: Basic Book, Inc.

Gergen, K. J. (1985). The social constructionist movement in modern psychology. *American Psychologist, 40*(3), 266–275.

Gergen, K. J. (1997). Social psychology as social construction: The emerging vision. In C. McGarty & A. Haslam (Eds.), *The message of social psychology: Perspectives on mind in society*. Oxford: Blackwell.

Giere, R. N. (2006). *Scientific perspectivism*. Chicago: The University of Chicago Press.

Grolnick, W. S., Ryan, R. M., & Deci, E. L. (1997). Internalization within the family: The self-determination theory perspective. In J. E. Grusec & L. Kuczynski (Eds.), *Parenting and children's internalization of values* (pp. 135–161). New York: Wiley.

Guyer, P. (2000). *Kant on freedom, law, and happiness*. Cambridge: Cambridge University Press.

Harrison, L. E. (2000). Why culture matters? In L. E. Harrison & S. P. Huntington (Eds.), *Culture matters: How values shape human progress* (pp. xvii–xxxiv). New York: Basic Books.

Harré, R. (1983). *Personal being: A theory for individual psychology*. Oxford: Blackwell.

Harré, R. (1993). *Social being* (2nd ed.). Oxford: Blackwell.

Hatch, E. (1983). *Culture and morality: The relativity of values in anthropology*. New York: Columbia University Press.

Hollis, M. (1985). Of masks and men. In M. Carrithers, S. Collins, & S. Lukes (Eds.), *The category of the person: Anthropology, philosophy, history* (pp. 217–233). Cambridge: Cambridge University Press.

Horney, K. (1950). *Neurosis and human growth*. New York: Norton.

Kenwood, C. (1996). Does volition need social constructionism? *Theory & psychology, 6*(3), 533–538.

Kasser, T., Cohn, S., Kanner, A. D., & Ryan, R. M. (2007). Some costs of American corporate capitalism: A psychological exploration of value and goal conflict. *Psychological Inquiry, 18*, 1–22.

Libet, B. (1999). Do we have free will? In B. Libet, A. Freeman, & K. Sutherland (Eds.), *The volitional brain: Towards a neuroscience of free will* (pp. 45–57). Thorverton: Imprint Academic.
Lukes, S. (1973). *Individualism*. New York: Harper Row.
Maslow, A. (1968). *Toward a psychology of being* (2nd ed.). Princeton, NJ: Van Nostrand.
Maslow, A. (1971). Some basic propositions of a growth and self-actualization psychology. In E. A. Southwell & M. Merbaum (Eds.), *Personality: Readings in theory and research* (pp. 221–234). Belmont, CA: Broke/Cole.
May, H. (2010). *Aristotle's ethics: Moral development and human nature*. London: Continuum.
May, R. (1953/1973). *Man's search for himself* (1st ed.). New York: Norton.
May, R. (Ed.). (1961). *Existential psychology*. New York: Random House.
May, R. (1981). *Freedom and destiny* (1st ed.). New York: Norton.
McMahon, D. M. (2004). From the happiness of virtue to the virtue of happiness: 400 B.C.–A.D. 1780. *Daedalus, 133*(2), 5–17.
McMahon, D. M. (2006). *Happiness: A history*. New York: Grove Press.
Mele, A. R. (2009). *Effective intentions: The power of conscious will*. Oxford: Oxford University Press.
Mines, M. (1988). Conceptualizing the person: Hierarchical society and individual autonomy in India. *American Anthropologist, 90*(3), 568–579.
Modell, A. (2008). The agency of the self and the brain's illusion. In R. Frie (Ed.), *Psychological agency: Theory, practice, and culture* (pp. 35–49). Cambridge, MA: MIT Press.
Moss, D. (2001). The roots and genealogy of humanistic psychology. In K. J. Schneider, J. F. T. Bugental, & J. F. Pierson (Eds.), *The handbook of humanistic psychology: Leading edges in theory, research, and practice* (pp. 5–20). Thousand Oaks, CA: Sage Publications.
Nussbaum, M. (2000). *Woman and human development: The capabilities approach*. Cambridge: Cambridge University Press.
Pfänder, A. (1908/1967). *Phenomenology of willing and motivation and other phaenomenologia* (H. Spiegelberg, Trans.). Evanston, IL: Northwestern University Press.
Polkinghorne, D. (1983). *Methodology for the human sciences: Systems of inquiry*. Albany, NY: State University of New York Press.
Polkinghorne, D. (2001). The self in humanistic psychology. In K. J. Schneider, J. F. T. Bugental, & J. F. Pierson (Eds.), *The handbook of humanistic psychology: Leading edges in theory, research, and practice* (pp. 81–99). Thousand Oaks, CA: Sage Publications.
Raskin, J. D. (2002). Constructivism in psychology: Personal construct psychology, radical constructivism, and social constructionism. In J. D. Raskin & S. K. Bridges (Eds.), *Studies in meaning: Exploring constructivist psychology* (pp. 1–25). New York: Pace University Press.
Ricoeur, P. (1950/1966). *Freedom and nature: The voluntary and the involuntary*. Evanston, IL: Northwestern University Press.
Rogers, C. (1961). *On becoming a person: A therapist's view of psychotherapy*. Boston: Houghton Mifflin Company.
Rogers, C. (1977). *Carl Rogers on personal power*. New York: Delacorte Press.
Roland, A. (1988). *In search of self in India and Japan: Toward a cross-cultural psychology*. Princeton, NJ: Princeton University Press.
Ryan, R. M., & Deci, E. L. (2000a). The darker and brighter sides of human existence: Basic psychological needs as a unifying concept. *Psychological Inquiry, 11*(4), 319–338.
Ryan, R. M., & Deci, E. L. (2000b). Self-determination theory and the facilitation of intrinsic motivation, social development, and well-being. *American Psychologist, 55*(1), 68–78.
Ryan, R. M., & Deci, E. L. (2004). Autonomy is no illusion: Self-determination theory and the empirical study of authenticity, awareness, and will. In J. Greenberg, S. L. Koole, & T. Pyszczynski (Eds.), *Handbook of experimental existential psychology*. New York: The Guilford Press.

Ryan, R. M., & Deci, E. (2006). Self-regulation and the problem of human autonomy: Does psychology need choice, self-determination, and will? *Journal of Personality, 71*(6), 1557–1585.

Ryan, R. M., Huta, V., & Deci, E. L. (2008). Living well: A self-determination theory perspective on eudaimonia. *Journal of Happiness Studies, 9*, 139–170.

Ryff, C. D., & Singer, B. H. (2008). Know thyself and become what you are: A eudaimonic approach to psychological well-being. *Journal of Happiness Studies, 9*, 13–39.

Sanderson, A. (1985). Purity and power among the Brahmans of Kashmir. In M. Carrithers, S. Collins & S. Lukes (Eds.), *The category of the person: Anthropology, philosophy, history* (pp. 190–216). Cambridge, UK: Cambridge University Press.

Schwandt, T. A. (2000). Three epistemological stances for qualitative inquiry: Interpretavism, hermeneutics, and social constructionism. In N. K. Denzin & Y. S. Lincoln (Eds.), *Handbook of qualitative research* (2nd ed., pp. 189–213). Thousand Oaks, CA: Sage.

Shweder, R. A., Much, N. C., Mahapatra, M., & Park, L. (2003). The big three of morality (autonomy, community, and divinity) and the big three explanations of suffering. In R. A. Sweder (Ed.), *Why do men barbecue? Recipes for cultural psychology* (pp. 74–133). Cambridge, MA: Harvard University Press.

Singer, M. (1972). Industrial leadership, the Hindu ethic, and the spirit of socialism. In M. Singer (Ed.), *When a great tradition modernizes: An anthropological approach to Indian civilization*. New York: Praeger Publishers.

Skinner, B. F. (1971). *Beyond freedom and dignity*. New York: Knopf.

Spinoza, B. (2000). *Ethics* (G. H. R. Parkinson, Trans.). Oxford: Oxford University Press.

Sternberg, E. J. (2010). *My brain made me do it: The rise of neuroscience and the threat to moral responsibility*. Amherst, NY: Prometheus Books.

Strange, S. K., & Zupko, J. (2004). *Stoicism: Traditions and transformations*. Cambridge: Cambridge University Press.

Sugarman, J., & Martin, J. (2004). Toward an alternative psychology. In B. D. Slife, J. S. Reber, & F. C. Richardson (Eds.), *Critical thinking about psychology: Hidden assumptions and plausible alternatives* (pp. 251–266). Washington, DC: American Psychological Association.

Tooby, J., & Cosmides, L. (1992). The psychological foundations of culture. In J. H. Barkow, L. Cosmides, & J. Tooby (Eds.), *The adapted mind: Evolutionary psychology and the generation of culture* (pp. 19–136). New York: Oxford University Press.

Uyl, D. D. (2003). Autonomous autonomy: Spinoza on autonomy, perfectionism, and politics. In E. F. Paul, F. D. Miller, & J. Paul (Eds.), *Autonomy* (pp. 30–69). Cambridge: Cambridge University Press.

Wallis, K. C., & Poulton, J. L. (2001). *Internalization: The origin and construction of internal reality*. Buckingan: Open University Press.

Waterman, A. S., Schwartz, S. J., & Conti, R. (2008). The implications of two conception of happiness (hedonic enjoyment and eudaimonia) for the understanding of intrinsic motivation. *Journal of Happiness Studies, 9*, 41–79.

Wegner, D. M. (2002). *The illusion of conscious will*. Cambridge, MA: Bradford Books, The MIT Press.

Wegner, D. M. (2008). Self is magic. In J. Baer, J. C. Kaufman, & R. F. Baumeister (Eds.), *Are we free? Psychology and free will* (pp. 226–247). Oxford: Oxford University Press.

Wegner, D. M., & Wheatley, T. (1999). Apparent mental causation: Sources of the experience of will. *American Psychologist, 5*(7), 480–492.

Wong, D. (2008). Chinese ethics. In E. N. Zalta (Ed.), *Stanford encyclopedia of philosophy*. Available from http://plato.stanford.edu/entries/ethics-chinese

Yu, J. (2009). *The ethics of Confucius and Aristotle: Mirrors of virtue*. London: Routledge.

Part I
A Theoretical Context of Human Autonomy, People's Well-Being, and Happiness

Chapter 2
Positive Psychology and Self-Determination Theory: A Natural Interface

Kennon M. Sheldon and Richard M. Ryan

This book, which applies self-determination theory (SDT) to understand how positive social and environmental change may be promoted around the world, is part of a whole series of books on positive psychology (PP). A natural question is, "how does SDT relate to PP?" Is SDT an example of PP? Does SDT supply something essential to PP, something that other "positive" theories do not?

In this chapter we will address these questions, showing that SDT is a prototypical example of a theory within the broader field of PP because SDT is designed to explain optimal motivation thereby explaining a host of positive outcomes including well-being, performance, resilience, and personal growth. However, we will also show that SDT goes beyond most PP theories because it also provides a dialectical account of the "negative" factors and processes which can get in the way of peoples' optimal functioning. This account is important, because several commentators have decried the seemingly one-sided focus of PP, PP's failure to address how negative psychological, interpersonal, and cultural processes operate, and PP's failure to address how negative events such as oppression, confusion, or rejection can serve as challenges that lead to more positive individual functioning in the long run (Lazarus, 2003; Ryff, 2003; Young-Eisendrath, 2003). SDT also provides a universalist or trans-cultural account of optimal human functioning, based on evolutionary-psychological or adaptationist reasoning. Thus, SDT shows at least one way in which PP can supply constructs that cut across cultures and affect wellness in all humans. Below we consider PP and SDT in more detail.

Positive Psychology

What is PP? It is a conceptual movement in both the research and applied arms of the psychological community which seeks to rectify the "negative" biases of traditional psychology so that a full accounting of human nature and behavior can emerge. Prior negative biases include assumptions that humans are by nature prone to be

---

K.M. Sheldon (✉)
Department of Psychology, University of Missouri, Columbia, MO 65211, USA
e-mail: SheldonK@missouri.edu

selfish and self-centered more than to be prosocial and other-centered; assumptions that humans are prone to errors and mistakes more than to successes and accuracies; assumptions that humans are prone to cowardice and corruption more than to courage and elevation; and assumptions that humans are prone to selfish competition more than to mutually beneficial cooperation (Sheldon & King, 2001). Put differently, because psychologists seek objectivity and are wary of self-serving biases which might cloud their thought, there has been a predominant tendency to view humans in unflattering or cynical terms, as creatures beset by problems, deficiencies, and self-serving motives. This tendency to view people and their experience negatively or with suspicion began with Freud but continued to characterize the theorizing of many major schools of thought during the twentieth century, including psychodynamic, behavioral, evolutionary, and clinical perspectives.

Of course, many humanist thinkers and writers in the past, including romantics such as Rousseau and Keats, educators such as Dewey and Piaget, and psychologists such as Rogers, Maslow, and May, have focused on the positive aspects of human nature. However these positive perspectives have tended to be drowned out in "hard core" and grant-funded research psychology by the more pessimistic and cynical assumptions, in large part because many humanists rejected the notion that humans could and should be studied by quantitative methods (Seligman & Csikszentmihalyi, 2000). This left the field to those who were willing and able to experimentally test their ideas—the skeptical scientists. Another influence on the negative bias devolves from the fact that psychological research has often focused on finding the breakdown points in peoples' social, emotional, and cognitive functioning. Of course, studying when and how a system breaks down is an important way to understand the underlying functioning of that system. But understanding how a system adapts and evolves may be just as important. Many times, the latter understanding can be increased just by adding another assessment point, subsequent to the original breakdown.

Thus PP, in contrast to much prior research, is about uncovering the features of human nature that *work*—understanding what goes right, how adaptive systems function, and why the average person does well, such that most people live lives of integrity and contentment (Sheldon & King, 2001). These questions certainly existed in the research literature prior to PP, but they were often marginalized. PP has provided an umbrella for such inquiries as well as a forum for like-minded researchers to meet and collaborate with one another.

Importantly, PP has the potential to go beyond prior humanistic theorizing about human nature because of its willingness to "get its hands dirty" in the muck of quantitative data collection and interpretation. One of the core ideas of PP is to put even the most humanistic of ideas to empirical test, and meet the most rigorous standards and the most exacting levels of peer review. PP topics have, accordingly, been increasingly funded by agencies such as NIMH and NSF. Thus positive psychological perspectives are not just Pollyanna-style illusions, unsupported by quantitative data; they aim at reliability, and warrant serious consideration and application. Finally, PP is not a religion, although it sometimes seems that some people think of it that way. Instead it is a direction or avenue of thought, whose claims and conclusions can be challenged and overthrown, just as can be any scientific theory or paradigm.

Self-Determination Theory

What is SDT? Although other chapters will answer this question in greater detail, suffice it here to say that SDT, which dates back several decades (e.g., Deci & Ryan, 1985, 1991, 2000; Deci, 1971), is an organismic-dialectic theory of human motivation that makes positive starting assumptions about default human nature—namely, that people are naturally inclined to learn, to grow, to assimilate important cultural values, and to connect and contribute to others. These "positive" assumptions are surely consistent with PP's focus on the often overlooked admirable characteristics of human nature (Keltner, 2009). Indeed, the importance of starting with this assumption can hardly be overstated: It is easier to bring about optimal states if these need merely to be facilitated and encouraged within an already inclined human nature than if they need to be somehow grafted onto a negative or resistant human nature.

Importantly, SDT does not ignore that individuals can behave in "bad" ways (e.g., selfish, cruel, dishonest) just as easily as they can behave in "good" ways (prosocial, open, vital, and connected). However rather than seeing negative traits as central characteristics of human nature, SDT sees them as an outcome of need frustrating conditions, in development and in the current context. Again, SDT suggests that under typical conditions of nurturance and support humans are more inclined toward growth and relatedness, explaining why such functioning is predominant much more often than not. At the same time the theory suggests that non-supportive, need thwarting conditions can result in compromised functioning and development, as well as many of the more negative attributes so often attributed to "human nature."

What is the data to support SDT's claim that there is a predominantly or originally positive human nature, which can be demonstrated and enhanced through scientific means? This is a complex question with no simple answers. However, one type of supportive evidence was recently provided by Sheldon, Arndt, and Houser-Marko (2003), who sought to demonstrate the existence of an "organismic valuing process" which enables people (potentially) to detect what is foreign and alien, versus what is congruent, and to use this information to choose and move toward healthier modes of living. Of course, this does not always happen, but we suggest it happens more often than not. Specifically, Sheldon et al. (2003) showed that when people shift in their values, they tend to shift in "intrinsic" directions (i.e., toward community, intimacy, and growth), and away from "extrinsic" goals such as money, image, and appearance. Sheldon et al. interpreted this as indicative of a built-in propensity to shift in healthy directions when given the opportunity to reconsider one's earlier choices. The intrinsic shift effect occurred at multiple time scales and was not reducible to mere social desirability or self-presentational concerns. Sheldon et al. (2004) found a similar intrinsic shift effect over the 4-year college career; seniors had become less materialistic and image-conscious than their freshmen selves, a fact which explained their increased well-being over the 4 years of college.

Weinstein and Ryan (2010) recently studied everyday helping behaviors, and showed how SDT can explain such "positive inclinations" in human nature, and how they can be [3]naturally[2] motivated. Using both experimental and experience-sampling methods, they demonstrated that when people were autonomously helping others they experienced personal autonomy, and feeling of competence and relatedness, which in turn enhanced their well-being. When pressured to help, however, they experienced not only lower autonomy, but less connection and efficacy as well. That is, although helping had no external reward, it was inherently satisfying when done volitionally. Moreover this research also showed that the recipients of help, even when naïve to helpers[1] motives, benefited more when helpers were autonomous.

Let us return to the question of what constitutes adequate, versus inadequate, contextual support for positive outcomes. SDT addresses this crucial question primarily by focusing on authority–subordinate relations, in which one person (i.e., a parent, teacher, boss, or coach) has power over another (i.e., a child, student, employee, or athlete; Deci & Ryan, 1985). Of course, such power inequalities characterize a large percentage of the role-relationships in which people find themselves. Over the last three decades SDT has demonstrated the crucial importance of authority autonomy-supportiveness (versus controllingness), for a wide variety of outcomes including subordinate's performance, motivational internalization, emotional tone, and personal growth. This research indicates that when authorities support choice and encourage self-regulation within their subordinates those subordinates are more likely to thrive, perform well, and develop to the maximal extent. Supporting autonomy can be difficult to do, and indeed there are dynamics in which the very need for autonomy generates a threat to authorities to which they respond by controlling the subordinate. Yet this tends to backfire and thus paradoxically, controllers may manage best by controlling least.

As we will show below, the SDT analysis (and its detailed supportive research base) has important implications for many positive psychological interventions and areas, such as life-coaching, well-being therapy, mentoring, leadership, and even community organizing. SDT can be used to examine how any program, administered by one person to a second person, can be delivered in order to maximize the second person's acceptance and benefit from that program. SDT also has important implications for understanding the positive effects of successful programs. Consider this question: How do we know a program is working? One answer is because it is meeting peoples' needs. According to SDT, properly designed action-contexts meet or enhance peoples' basic psychological needs and allow people to fully internalize the motivation to engage in that context; as a result, they learn, thrive, and grow to the maximal extent in that context. Thus, SDT provides an integrated temporal path model specifying both distal context-level antecedents and proximal individual-level mediators, as a means of understanding the production of optimal outcomes, at both individual and contextual levels. We hope to show that SDT can provide a rich and integrated causal account of the entire suite of positive processes that PP hopes to promote.

SDT in Application: An Empirical Example

Sheldon and Krieger (2007) presented data which well illustrate this integrated causal sequence. These researchers sought to apply SDT to explain the declining well-being and increased mental health problems experienced by law students during the course of law school, problems which were first documented in the 1980s by Benjamin and colleagues (Benjamin, Kaszniak, Sales, & Shanfield, 1986). Based on Krieger's experience and research as a clinical law professor (Krieger, 1998), Sheldon and Krieger (2004) predicted and found sharp declines in student intrinsic motivation during the first year at a traditional law school, changes which helped explain students' increasing depression and distress. Students also evidenced declining prosocial values and increasing image and appearance values during the first year. These findings suggested that legal education as currently practiced may undermine or coarsen student motivation, and be in need of some modification.

Sheldon and Krieger (2007) extended these findings by following two samples of students through all 3 years of law school, one sample from a school with a more traditional model of legal education, and one from a more progressively oriented school. The traditional program emphasizes faculty scholarship, intellectual status, and student competition, and offers relatively little practical training in being a lawyer. The progressive program emphasizes egalitarian student–faculty and student–student relations and offers much hands-on experience in learning to be a lawyer.

Figure 2.1 contains the full temporal path model that was supported by the data. Although students at the two schools started out equal in Law School Aptitude Test (LSAT) scores, motivation, and well-being, by the middle of the

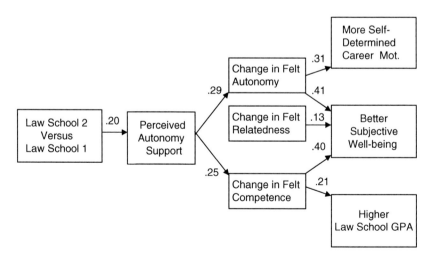

Fig. 2.1 Parameter estimates for the path model. *Note*: All coefficients significant at the 0.01 level except relatedness to well-being ($p < 0.05$). All downstream variables residualized to remove the effects of race, age, gender, prior job experience, loan balances, and the Year 1 versions of the variable (where appropriate)

second year significant school-level differences were observed in the perceived autonomy-supportiveness (versus controllingness) of each school's faculty, as assessed by the Learning Climate Questionnaire (Black & Deci, 2000). These differences in turn predicted reduced autonomy and competence need-satisfaction in the traditional school students near the end of the third year. Relatedness need-satisfaction was not affected by faculty autonomy-support, presumably because students meet relatedness needs outside of school and student–faculty relations. In the final step of the model, reductions in autonomy need-satisfaction from Year 1 to 3 uniquely predicted reduced intrinsic and self-determined motivation for the first law job after graduation, and also reduced subjective well-being in general. Reductions in competence need-satisfaction also predicted reduced subjective well-being, and uniquely predicted poorer academic performance. Thus, this study provided strong new support for SDT's basic causal model, given its temporal length, its applied importance, and the informative mix of between-group and within-group processes observed.

Implications

Several further observations should be made concerning this data. First, significant mediation occurred at every step. Thus, the school-level or between-school differences in need-satisfaction (and in the three outcomes) were mediated by the school-level mean differences in faculty autonomy-support (versus controllingness), and the autonomy-support to outcome effects were mediated by changes in need-satisfaction. This means that differences in the rated controllingness of the faculty at the two schools could completely explain the differential effects of the two school contexts upon their students. This supports the SDT strategy of focusing primarily on autonomy-supportiveness (vs. controllingness) as the crucial social-contextual variable.

Second, the observed results could not be explained by demographic differences between students at the two schools (such as their initial age, gender composition, or job experience, or their final loan balances). For example, although older students felt more controlled by faculty within both samples, and although students at the more progressive school were older, age differences between the schools could not explain the school-level autonomy-support difference. This supports the quasi-experimental design of the study and boosts the inference that actual differences in the learning climate that students encounter upon arriving at the school can explain the differential outcomes.

Third, students at *both* law schools experienced persistent significant declines in motivation and well-being over the 3 years, just less so at the more progressive school. This suggests that the more progressive school had not solved all problems, but at least was making some headway! One limitation of this study is that we do not yet know if graduate or professional students of other kinds also experience problems. Perhaps the stress, low pay, and servitude of extended student-hood drags down graduate students everywhere—be it history, art, nursing, biology, medicine, or psychology

Fourth, the findings went beyond mere self-report outcomes (i.e., job motivation, well-being, need-satisfaction). Sheldon and Krieger (2007) were able to obtain multi-state bar exam data for the two schools (the multi-state section is taken by all US examinees), and showed that students graduating from the more progressive program score significantly higher on this exam. This was especially noteworthy because the two entering classes in our study were identical (as noted before) in undergraduate GPA and in LSAT scores. This tells us that the students at the more traditional school under-achieved, a fact which should get the attention of Deans, administrators, and regents alike! Alternatively, the students at the more progressive school over-achieved—either way, the difference is important.

It is also important to point out that SDT propositions have been supported by rigorous experimental research, and not just by correlational data as in the Sheldon and Krieger (2007) example. Dozens of studies have experimentally manipulated contextual autonomy-supportiveness (versus controllingness), finding strong causal effects of this difference. Also, a few experimental studies have begun to simultaneously manipulate all three of the needs specified by SDT, not just autonomy. As one example, Sheldon and Filak (2008) conducted a $2 \times 2 \times 2$ factorial experiment in which participants' autonomy, competence, and relatedness needs were either supported or denied by the experiment and experimenter, in the context of learning to play the game "Boggle," in which one tries to find as many words as possible within a letter grid. Sheldon and Filak (2008) found that all three factors had independent effects on participant's mood, motivation, and objective performance in playing the game. Thus, participants who received supports for all three needs performed best in the task, and enjoyed it the most. There were no significant interactions between three needs, further supporting the claim that each is singularly important. Again, this is one of the few studies manipulating all three needs at once; most SDT research focuses primarily on autonomy-support as the most important variable for defusing unequal power relations and promoting full engagement by subordinates, as in the Sheldon and Krieger (2007) study. Thus, autonomy support receives further consideration below.

Relevance of the SDT Analysis for PP Theorists and Practitioners I: Supporting Autonomy

We believe the SDT analysis has important implications for many positive psychological interventions and areas, such as life-coaching, well-being therapy, mentoring, leadership, and even community organizing. It appears vital that the administrators of such programs attend carefully to the experience of those enrolled in the program. Are enrollees enabled to feel that their perspectives are acknowledged and respected, that self-regulation and self-direction within the context are fostered, and that meaningful choices and options are provided? If these qualities are present, it may almost not matter which type or content of program is administered—peoples' natural problem-solving and happiness-finding abilities will be engaged. In this vein, Sheldon, Joiner, and Williams (2003) argued that autonomy-support is a *mode*, that can be employed to improve the effectiveness of *any* therapy or treatment program (be it interpersonal, dynamic, cognitive-behavioral, or even electro-shock). If it is delivered in a controlling way, the program will likely fail, or produce weaker or non-lasting results; if it is delivered in an autonomy-supportive way, it has a better chance of producing the desired effects. Again, SDT is a dialectical theory of motivation which tries to explain how motivation can be undermined or coarsened as well as how motivation can be enhanced and elevated. Although people are engaged in a life-long quest to become more self-determining and self-regulating, many factors can derail this somewhat fragile process. SDT provides means for understanding both negative and positive influences upon the process.

Might we surmise that, compared to a traditional law professor, a "positive psychology" coach or practitioner would intuitively understand the importance of being autonomy-supportive rather than controlling, or the importance of focusing on intrinsic motivation rather than inducements, so that that these problems do not arise in his or her practice? Perhaps—but in our experience, even progressively and positively oriented practitioners can be over-controlling! The practitioner has the power, the responsibility, and the need to be effective, for his or her own reasons; this can make it very difficult to step back so that the client's own self-regulatory propensities can (often slowly) come to the fore. Often the client may feel hesitant, looking for reasons not to invest full effort; an overly assertive practitioner may cue precisely such reactance-based withdrawal. Or, the client may feel weak, dependent, and desirous of strong structure and control; this also can pull controlling behavior from the practitioner which is non-optimal in the long run.

In discussing these complex interpersonal dynamics, Sheldon et al. (2003) suggested that autonomy-support is a difficult skill that can take a lifetime to develop. Being a mentor who fully supports the self-determination of one's charges takes respect, patience, self-reflection, and genuine caring, and in an important sense, autonomy support may represent the very essence of good teaching and nurturing. Thus, just because a practitioner identifies him or herself as a positive psychologist (rather than some other kind of psychologist), does not mean that he or she has already mastered this skill! Parenting provides a good example—parents all know how difficult it can be to encourage responsibility and self-direction in a child, especially when we become impatient or disappointed and seek easier or more expedient routes to the results we want. Those are the times when we can be most controlling, or say the most hurtful things, to the ultimate detriment of our children.

Of course structure and discipline can be very helpful, but again, only if they are delivered in an autonomy-supportive mode (Sheldon et al., 2003). In fact a long tradition of research within SDT has differentiated structure vs. non-structure (providing inputs that promote competence or not), from autonomy versus control (which concerns whether those inputs are experienced as interesting and valued, or as forced and resented; Grolnick & Ryan, 1989; Jang, Reeve & Deci, in press). Structure *and* autonomy-support may sound paradoxical, but discipline and structure can be internalized and integrated by those adopting it, or simply externally regulated or pressured from the outside, with quite different consequences for long-term persistence, performance and wellness.

Relevance of the SDT Analysis for PP Theorists and Practitioners II: Assessing and Supporting Needs

Another implication of these findings for PP arises from the demonstrated importance of psychological need-satisfaction. SDT likens the psychological needs to the biological needs of a plant. Just as a plant will thrive given adequate sun, soil, and water, a human self will thrive to the extent its psychological needs are met (i.e., it will feel and do well). Conversely, just as a plant will wither without proper nutrients, so will a human self (i.e., it will feel and do poorly; Ryan, 1995). In the Sheldon and Krieger (2007) data, 3-year changes in autonomy and competence need-satisfaction, explainable by the particular school the student attended, completely explained the negative effects of a controlling learning climate upon the outcomes. The traditional school did not meet its students' needs as well, and students suffered as a result (i.e., they "withered").

Thus, we argue that any helping, training, supporting, teaching, coaching, or counseling context, "positive" psychology or otherwise, will serve its clients better if it attends to clients' levels of need-satisfaction. This might involve regular assessments or discussions to detect positive or negative trends in clients' need-satisfaction, and the development of interventions, when necessary, to better tailor mentoring styles and practices to meet student needs. For example, tweaking a grading system (i.e., turning it into a mastery rather than a performance based system, or eliminating a mandatory curve) might revive competence needs; relaxing a stringent but irrational program requirement might revive autonomy needs; and encouraging student–faculty mixers might revive relatedness needs. All of these processes can be measured and modified, as a basis for understanding and improving the effects of interventions.

In sum, via its concepts of self-determined motivation, psychological needs, and contextual autonomy-support, SDT supplies significant conceptual and practical leverage for gaining new process understanding of why some programs work better (or worse) than others. The SDT approach supplies a comparative framework that could be applied not only to training and educational institutions, but to all human organizations from companies to cultures.

Cross-Cultural Application of SDT

The importance of the latter point is worth further consideration. As was discussed in the first chapter, important challenges to SDT have come from cultural relativists who do not accept the universal importance of felt autonomy. Their argument is that autonomy is only emphasized or trained in certain cultures, particularly westernized or individualistically oriented cultures. In collectivist or more traditional cultures, autonomy is de-emphasized so that the group and social norms become the more important determinants of behavior. Based on an underlying expectancy value perspective, cultural relativists also assume therefore that autonomy would not be associated with well-being in collectivist cultures (as it would in western cultures). That is, if autonomy is not a universal need then differential associations should be found, which will indicate that autonomy is a locally conditioned preference only.

A significant strength of SDT is that rather than ignoring this critique, researchers have instead empirically examined the issue. Dozens of studies now demonstrate that autonomy, defined and measured in the way prescribed by SDT, is predictive of individual health and thriving in every culture examined. For example, Sheldon et al. (2004) showed that the felt self-determination of personal goals predicted multiple indicators of well-being, to an equal extent in Turkey, China, South Korea, Taiwan, and the USA. Feeling that one identifies and enjoys one's goals, rather than feeling pressured or compelled to do them, predicts better emotional tone in any context. Cultural relativists often have "independence" in mind when they critique autonomy, defined as a "go it alone and damn the consequences" mentality. SDT agrees that such an independent or reactive interpersonal orientation is likely to be problematic, both for individuals and their societies. There are also other corrosive forms of modern individualism, such as narcissism, materialism, and excessive status-seeking, that some theorists link with excessive autonomy and permissiveness. However, much data now show that true autonomy—defined as feelings of self-ownership, feelings of internally endorsing (rather than resisting) one's behavior, and feelings of following one's own developing interests—is not the same as independence, narcissism, materialism, hedonism, and the like. Furthermore, *true* autonomy, *does* predict happiness and well-being in every cultural context examined so far.

Thus, we suggest SDT can offer PP significant leverage for understanding the common processes that produce positive thriving in any person and culture, by virtue of basic human nature. In other words, SDT's ultimately biological perspective, based on the negentropic and self-organizational capabilities of life itself, provides an important anchor for PP as it also seeks to develop proper understanding of human variety and diversity. Obviously, for complete understanding it is essential to know how people are the same as well as how they differ across cultural, political, and economic settings. Consideration of basic human nature might also help researchers avoid cultural or historical biases and myopias. If SDT is correct, satisfaction of the basic psychological needs will remain demonstrably important for people in any context, culture, or era. What may vary across contexts, cultures, and eras is *how* the needs are satisfied, *how much* they are satisfied, and how much satisfaction or dissatisfaction *affects* different types of outcomes. These are important topics of contemporary research.

We hope this chapter has succeeded in its goal, of briefly introducing and comparing positive psychology and self-determination theory, and showing that the two approaches have a "natural marriage." We have argued that SDT can bring a variety of important assets to this marriage: An empirically grounded but broadly focused theory of basic human nature that sees humans as inherently active and health-seeking, until contextual and interpersonal conditions fail to support these predispositions; an empirically backed theory of how program providers, counselors, teachers, coaches, parents, and managers can best engage the growth and creative capabilities of their subordinates; an empirically backed means of assessing the effectiveness of a program or contextual design, by examining its effects on basic need-satisfaction; and finally, a theoretical perspective that data suggest is equally applicable in any context or culture. PP also brings important assets to the Interface, from the SDT perspective: a potential forum in which the SDT message and research findings can receive wider, and more widely funded, attention.

In sum, Self-determination theory provides a basic meta-theory and formal set of mini-theories that can be readily applied to empirical investigations within positive psychology. Nearly any positive psychology construct, intervention, or process, that is, can be examined for its relations with autonomy, and with basic psychological need-satisfactions more generally. Reciprocally, as research in PP unfolds on topics such as gratitude, forgiveness, emotional intelligence training, or resilience focused counseling, SDT research should be attempt to see how these phenomena relate to its need-satisfaction models, and SDT researchers should strive to inform and refine PP interventions using its motivational toolkits. SDT might, in this limited sense, provide a common framework or "lingua franca" concerning positive change and its internalization, whose skeleton can be further filled out by the fast growing body of PP research.

References

Benjamin, G. A. H., Kasvniak, A., Sales, B., & Shanfield, S. B. (1986). The role of legal education in producing psychological distress among law students and lawyers. *America Bar Foundation Research Journal, 23*, 225–252.

Black, A. E., & Deci, E. L. (2000). The effects of instructors' autonomy support and students' autonomous motivation on learning organic chemistry: A self-determination theory perspective. *Science Education, 84*, 740–756.

Deci, E. L. (1971). Effects of externally mediated rewards on intrinsic motivation. *Journal of Personality and Social Psychology, 18*, 105–116.

Deci, E. L., & Ryan, R. M. (1985). *Intrinsic motivation and self-determination in human behavior*. New York: Plenum.

Deci, E. L., & Ryan, R. M. (1991). A motivational approach to self: Integration in personality. In R. Dienstbier (Ed.), *Nebraska symposium on motivation*: Vol. 38. *Perspectives on motivation* (pp. 237–288). Lincoln, NE: University of Nebraska Press.

Deci, E. L., & Ryan, R. M. (2000). The "what" and "why" of goal pursuits: Human needs and the self-determination of behavior. *Psychological Inquiry, 11*, 227–268.

Keltner, D. (2009). *Born to be good: The science of a meaningful life*. New York: Norton.

Krieger, L. S. (1998). What we're not telling law students – and lawyers – that they really need to know: Some thoughts-in-acting toward revitalizing the profession from its roots. *Journal of Law and Health, 13*, 1–48.

Lazarus, R. S. (2003). The lazarus manifesto for positive psychology and psychology in general. *Psychological Inquiry, 14*, 173–189.

Ryan, R. M. (1995). Psychological needs and the facilitation of integrative processes. *Journal of Personality, 63*, 397–427.
Ryff, C. D. (2003). Corners of myopia in the positive psychology parade. *Psychological Inquiry, 14*, 153–159.
Seligman, M. E. P., & Csikszentmihalyi, M. (2000). Positive psychology: An introduction. *American Psychologist, 55*, 5–14.
Sheldon, K. M., Arndt, J., & Houser-Marko, L. (2003). In search of the organismic valuing process: The human tendency to move towards beneficial goal choices. *Journal of Personality, 71*, 835–869.
Sheldon, K. M., Elliot, A. J., Ryan, R. M., Chirkov, V., Kim, Y., Wu, C., et al. (2004). Self-concordance and subjective well-being in four cultures. *Journal of Cross-Cultural Psychology, 35*, 209–233.
Sheldon, K. M., & Filak, V. (2008). Manipulating autonomy, competence, and relatedness in a game-learning context: New evidence that all three needs matter. *British Journal of Social Psychology, 47*, 267–283.
Sheldon, K. M., Joiner, T., & Williams, G. (2003). *Self-determination theory in the clinic: Motivating physical and mental health.* London: Yale University Press.
Sheldon, K. M., & King, L. K. (2001). Why positive psychology is necessary. *American Psychologist, 56*, 216–217.
Sheldon, K. M., & Krieger, L. (2004). Does law school undermine law students? Examining changes in goals, values, and well-being. *Behavioral Sciences and the Law, 22*, 261–286.
Sheldon, K. M., & Krieger, L. K. (2007). Understanding the negative effects of legal education on law students: A longitudinal test and extension of self-determination theory. *Personality and Social Psychology Bulletin, 33*, 883–897.
Young-Eisendrath, P. (2003). Response to lazarus. *Psychological Inquiry, 14*, 170–172.

Chapter 3
A Self-Determination Theory Perspective on Social, Institutional, Cultural, and Economic Supports for Autonomy and Their Importance for Well-Being

Richard M. Ryan and Edward L. Deci

Around the globe today people struggle both for freedom and for the good life. They fight for freedom from oppressive external controls, and they struggle to be able to express and autonomously pursue their abiding cultural, spiritual, and personal values. Everywhere, too, people also seek the good life. They work to realize culturally sculpted aspirations and life goals that can to a greater or lesser extent fulfill their promise for fostering happiness and well-being.

In this chapter we apply a *self-determination theory* (SDT; Deci & Ryan, 1985; Ryan & Deci, 2000a, b) framework to explore two main questions. First, why, and to what extent, is the promotion of autonomy necessary for the attainment of well-being? Second, concerning visions of the good life, why are some lifestyles and aspirations more wellness producing than others? In the first of these questions we explore the importance of volition in the behaviors people undertake. In the second, we consider not the "why," but the "what," of people's behavior. In doing so, we explore the contents of the goals or aspirations to which people allocate behavioral resources, and relative yield of these goals in terms of happiness and well-being.

To anticipate our conclusions, people's autonomous functioning and their attainment of wellness are indeed deeply connected. *Autonomous self-regulation* is central in allowing the individual to choose and most fully develop preferred ways of being, and in doing so to satisfy basic psychological needs which in turn lead to vitality and happiness. That is, when autonomous, people typically optimize the satisfaction of their basic psychological needs, often through behaviors that have larger social benefits. Thus, SDT suggests a link between autonomy and need fulfillment, the feelings of wellness that derive from need fulfillment, and the productivity and cultural enrichments autonomy-supportive environments so frequently yield.

Although autonomy is functionally important to wellness, the life goals and lifestyles people pursue also differ in their capacity to produce happiness and well-being. Our findings show that pursuit of some culturally constructed visions of the "good life" yields, in a relatively direct way, the fundamental psychological need

---

R.M. Ryan (✉)
Department of Clinical and Social Sciences in Psychology, University of Rochester, Rochester, NY 14627, USA
e-mail: ryan@psych.rochester.edu

satisfactions that SDT hypothesizes underlie wellness. In contrast other life goals distract from, or even thwart basic need satisfactions, and therefore fail to support well-being. The evidence we review, in fact, gives strong credence to some well-known "secrets of happiness" based on goals for intimate relationships, contributing to community, and pursuing personal growth, and it dispels some popular myths that the road to happiness entails garnering wealth, image, or fame.

Finally, when we look at social contextual effects we find that controlling environments, whether they are familial, institutional, cultural, economic, or political, interfere with wellness and happiness by undermining autonomous functioning. In contrast, support for autonomy is associated with individual thriving, and national quality of life.

Happiness and Well-Being Debated

Well-being and happiness: what defines them and what brings them about are perennially debated topics, ones that have engaged many of the world's great minds. Without unveiling a ready list of quotes to prove it, many of our most revered figures, both secular and non-secular, have grappled with the happiness issue, and seem to agree on some essentials. For many—and here we include Jesus, Confucius, Buddha, and Aristotle, among others—happiness is not fostered by selfishness or over-consumption; it is instead fostered by reflective, purposive living in accord with deeply held social values. In terms of contents it is typically said to lie in such things as personal growth, loving relationships, and giving to one's community rather than the pursuit of vanity and image, riches and power, and other such worldly ideals. Such are the well-known secrets of happiness according to those deemed our most wise.

Despite the weightiness of these figures, there are clearly other opinions. According to many contemporary cultural icons, from the USA's Donald Trump to today's global Hip-Hop stars, the key to happiness is the *psychology of more*: more money, more fame, more attractiveness. This image of the good life is continuously reinforced by the media and advertising industry. They deliver this sermon: Without having more and more one cannot be successful or happy. Furthermore, the values corresponding to this message—namely, that money, image, and fame are among the most important aims in life—are being widely internalized and practiced. For example, a 2007 Pew research poll found that eight of ten US "gen-nexters" (young adults) reported that being wealthy is the top or second most important life goal in their peer group. More of these young adults would rather be a celebrity's assistant than a federal judge or a Harvard professor. In short, many in this generation (and in their parents' before them) have accepted this idea of the good life. Around the globe the message is similarly sinking in: consumerism is the new way forward.

Whatever one thinks about these opposing views of happiness or their implications for the future, both sides of the debate represent *opinions*. That is, Aristotle may have reasoned correctly that those who live a *eudaimonic life* (i.e., his good life of moderation, self-actualization, and reflective action) have the highest well-being and are also the most likely to experience happiness. Yet, it might also be the case that the "Donald Trump message" of finding the good life through wealth, consumption, and image is more on target in today's increasingly capitalistic, competitive, and materialistic world. For us, however, which of these views fulfills its promise is an empirical question, not a matter of opinion.

Self-determination theory (SDT; Deci & Ryan, 1985; Ryan & Deci, 2000b) is a research-based theory of motivation and personality development that has also focused on happiness and well-being. As an empirical approach, SDT is interested in getting evidence-based answers to questions about what makes people not only motivated, but also what makes them thrive or flourish. It offers testable hypotheses about what produces and sustains people's fullest, healthiest functioning and psychological wellness. In our research we look at wellness with an array of outcomes, including subjective well-being, or happiness, as well as freedom from stress, anxiety, and depressive symptoms, and experiencing vitality and integration in functioning. But more importantly, the SDT framework allows one to go beyond the compiling of outcomes, to an understanding of why and how social and cultural conditions support or thwart happiness and wellness. In this chapter we examine the theory and its assumptions, and we review some representative empirical findings supporting its approach to wellness.

Happiness and Wellness Defined

Defining well-being and happiness seems clear enough—doesn't everyone know what it is? Yet the study of happiness and well-being is anything but straightforward. In fact, something of a row got started when Kahneman, Diener, and Schwarz (1999) introduced their "science of well-being" by defining wellness in strictly hedonic terms. Somehow the stark and bold definition of well-being as merely the *presence of positive affect and the absence of negative affect* rekindled the need of many scholars to articulate a fuller conception of wellness, not just as happy feelings, but also as a fully functioning human being (e.g., Deci & Ryan, 2008; Ryan & Deci, 2001; Ryff & Singer, 2008; Waterman, Schwartz, & Conti, 2008). Many of these rekindled conceptions draw heavily from Aristotle's eudaimonic perspective in which happiness is defined not in terms of feeling states, but in terms of a way of living in which one's human capacities are fully employed and realized (Ryan, Huta, & Deci, 2008).

SDT has been vigorously involved in this discussion, (see, e.g., Kashdan, Biswas-Diener, & King, 2008; Ryan & Huta, 2009). In contradistinction to purely hedonic approaches, SDT distinguishes happiness, which is a subjective experience of positive versus negative mood, from wellness, which concerns *full and vital functioning*. In the SDT view one can identify many means to happiness, only some of which would be considered healthy or indicative of wellness (Huta & Ryan, in press). Conversely within SDT the capacity to be unhappy, for example to be sad or distressed after a loss, and to allow authentic feelings to be in awareness, can often be more indicative of wellness than an incongruent demeanor of happiness. SDT thus specifically embraces the idea that wellness is not equivalent to happiness, positive affect, or an absence of negative affect. Wellness instead is open, engaged, and healthy functioning. This full functioning conduces to happiness but does not guarantee it (Ryan & Deci, 2001), whereas happiness may be evident when people either are or are not living well.

Basic Needs Underlying Wellness

Just as there are specific needs underlying physical health, psychological wellness also requires specific supports and nutriments. A focus of SDT is thus on facilitating satisfaction of the *basic psychological needs* that lead to vitality and wellness, where needs are defined as the necessary nutriments for thriving. According to SDT there are three broad categories of such nutriments: supports for autonomy, for competence, and for relatedness. Specifically, SDT suggests that people are most active, thriving, and fully functioning in contexts where they can experience competence, relatedness, and autonomy. As all three are considered basic psychological needs, the neglect or thwarting of any is expected to lead to impoverished functioning and ill-being. This prediction holds not only at the general (cross-domain or time) level, but also within domains, and even within brief time periods.

For example, recently Ryan, Bernstein, and Brown (2010) followed the daily moods and vitality levels of adult workers across their weekly lives. The mood patterns in these adults showed a very robust weekend effect, with rising positive affect and subjective vitality, and lower negative affect, and fewer physical symptoms reported on weekends. The data further showed that the weekend mood effects were fully mediated by the lower experiences of autonomy and relatedness people feel on workdays. Because most workers don't feel much autonomy on their jobs or connection to their work groups, they experience lower happiness. The study proved evidence that on everyday-basis fluctuations in basic psychological need satisfactions substantially account for relative happiness, and even feelings of physical health.

A complementary study by Baard, Deci, and Ryan (2004) showed that employees of banking firms who experienced greater satisfaction of the needs for autonomy, competence, and relatedness while at work also displayed both better performance and greater psychological wellness on the job than those who experienced lesser satisfaction of the basic needs.

The relation between basic psychological need satisfaction and well-being has also been documented in other life domains, and with regard to outcomes from relationship quality to psychopathology. We point to just a few examples. La Guardia, Ryan, Couchman, and Deci (2000) found that individuals were more securely attached and evidenced more relational well-being within those close relationships where they experienced greater satisfaction of the three psychological needs. Stated differently, satisfaction of each of the needs for autonomy, competence, and relatedness within a relationship contributed independently to the overall quality of that relationship. Patrick, Knee, Canevello, and Lonsbary (2007) similarly documented the important links between need satisfaction and well-being in close relationships. Further, in two studies of exercise, Wilson, Longley, Muon, Rodgers, and Murray (2006) found that need satisfaction was positively associated with well-being and also that changes in need satisfaction over time were also associated with changes in well-being. Chirkov, Ryan, & Willness (2005) found that basic need satisfaction predicted not only the well being but also the cultural integration (versus cultural estrangement) of both Brazilians and Canadians. Finally, Ryan, Deci, Grolnick, and La Guardia (2006) reviewed substantial research showing that thwarting of the basic psychological needs plays an important role in the development of many psychopathologies ranging for example from rigid character disorders to depression.

Autonomy as a Key to Wellness

SDT asserts not only that basic psychological need satisfactions are associated with well-being, but also the theory highlights how autonomy is particularly relevant to thriving. In this section we discuss the central role played by autonomy, or true self-regulation, for living in a healthy, full-functioning way. Autonomy we argue is central for allowing individuals to grow, and to choose and develop preferred ways of being, which lead to both vitality and happiness. When autonomous, persons are most likely to optimize satisfaction of the psychological needs. Thus, SDT suggests a link from autonomy to need fulfillment, and to the feelings of happiness that derive from need fulfillment.

Autonomy is first and foremost a characteristic of actions. To the extent an action is autonomous it is characterized by feeling volitional or self-endorsed. When people are acting autonomously they are fully behind their own actions—they feel choiceful and integrated in behaving. Accordingly, not all intentional actions are autonomous. Many in fact are motivated by external controls and are experienced as heteronomously motivated. SDT in fact sees motivation as a differentiated phenomenon: There are different types of motivation that vary in their relative autonomy.

In terms of the most general types, SDT distinguishes *intrinsic motivation*, which is characterized by behavior that is motivated by its inherent satisfactions, and *extrinsic motivation*, which is evident in behaviors that are instrumental or done for consequences separable from the activity itself (Ryan & Deci, 2000a). Within the category of extrinsic motivations, SDT makes further differentiations based on the phenomenal source of motivation. These span from externally regulated actions (i.e., actions perceived to be controlled by others) that feel non-autonomous, all the way up to integrated motivations that are experienced as stemming from the actor's most central and important values. We specify four types of extrinsic motivation and emphasize that a person could potentially experience intrinsic motivation and each of the four extrinsic motivations while doing a particular behavior.

Intrinsic motivation. When intrinsically motivated, people engage their environments out of interest and for the sheer enjoyment and challenge in acting. This interested engagement is accompanied by an experience of volition, because when intrinsically motivated people are acting with full willingness. Indeed, any factors in the environment that detract from a sense of volition or choice also undermine intrinsic motivation (Deci & Ryan, 1985). Thus, in line with SDT, research has shown that intrinsic motivation is supported by meaningful choice (Patall, Cooper, & Robinson, 2008) and opportunities to experience competence (Vallerand & Reid, 1984), but it is also readily undermined by controlling rewards and other pressures and inducements (Deci, Koestner, & Ryan, 1999).

Intrinsic motivation is especially important in the promotion of intellectual and social development. In early development children learn by playing and exploring, activities that are invariantly intrinsically motivated. Such behaviors do not need to be reinforced or rewarded to occur, but they do require certain social supports or contexts. When children have nurturing environments characterized by autonomy support and non-intrusive parental involvement they are more likely to be robustly intrinsically motivated, whereas deprivations of either autonomy or relatedness inhibit this import inner resource (Grolnick & Seal, 2008). Despite its robust relationships with growth and learning, unfortunately few schools capitalize enough on this inner resource, instead attempting to promote development through external controls and evaluations. Yet when educators do harness intrinsic motivation the results in terms of persistence at and quality of learning can be profound (Ryan & Deci, 2000a).

With increasing age people typically spend less time engaged in playful activities, in part because of socialization and the increasing responsibilities that come with social development. Nonetheless, intrinsic motivation remains an important source of both learning and vitality throughout the lifespan. In pursuing intrinsically motivated activities, people experience intrinsic need satisfaction, and restoration from ego-depletion due to external control (Ryan & Deci, 2008a). When intrinsically motivated people also tend to experience positive affect and enjoyment making this kind of free pursuit important to overall happiness.

Extrinsic motivation. Technically the term "extrinsic motivation" refers to doing an activity to obtain an outcome separate from the behavior itself (Ryan & Deci, 2000a). Originally, some theorists (e.g., de Charms, 1968; Harter, 1981) viewed extrinsic motivation in opposition to intrinsic motivation and, thus extrinsic motivation was thought to be invariantly non-autonomous, whereas intrinsic motivation was considered autonomous. SDT argues, however, that although it is true that intrinsic motivation is autonomous, extrinsic motivations can vary in the degree to which they are volitional (Ryan & Connell, 1989), with some being highly autonomous and others being highly controlled. More specifically, SDT distinguishes four types of extrinsic motivation that fall along an underlying continuum of autonomy.

The least autonomous type of extrinsic motivation is *external regulation*, in which the behavior is done to obtain external rewards or to avoid punishments. For example, a worker may produce items efficiently to obtain offered incentives or to avoid the threat of job loss. Such efficient work would likely be perceived as being regulated by an external source and thus as being controlled. A somewhat more autonomous form of extrinsic motivation is *introjected regulation*, in which the reason for the behavior lies in internal (rather than external) contingencies. In introjection a person may act in order to avoid feelings of disapproval or guilt, or, on the "approach side" of introjection, to feel more approval and/or self-esteem. For example, a young musician may practice to avoid feeling guilty for not having done so. Although introjection-based behaviors emanate from dynamic forces inside the person (rather than the proximal social environment), introjected regulation still has the phenomenal feel of forces acting on the self, as the person feels compelled by "shoulds," by projected evaluations, or by the imagined opinions of others. Thus, like external regulation, behaviors motivated by introjects are experienced as relatively non-autonomous.

A yet more autonomous form of extrinsic motivation is labeled *identified regulation*. A person is identified with the regulation of action to the extent that the motives or reasons for acting are personally valued and self-endorsed. There is thus a feeling of ownership and willingness in identified regulation not found in introjection or external regulation. Accordingly, such behaviors are self-congruent and experienced as relatively autonomous. It is noteworthy here that a person can identify with obligations or duties, which even though they may originate "outside" the self can be more or less self-endorsed and truly volitionally undertaken. The final, most autonomous form of extrinsic motivation is *integrated regulation*, in which one identifies with the regulation of the behavior. The identification is then experienced as authentically congruent, including in relation to other aspects of the person's motivations and practices. When integrated, people are mindfully behind their actions and are volitional and wholehearted in carrying them out. Accordingly they display the highest quality of action.

The importance of considering the degree of internalization and integration of identities, values, and even self-concepts cannot be overstated. In connecting with family and culture people adopt various identifications and behavioral "repertoires" concerning school, morality, religion, politics, health, and all other salient issues and domains. The individual adopts or internalizes these to various degrees and works to integrate them. According to SDT, the less integrated a given identification the less fully functioning the individual will be when enacting it, and the more defensiveness will be required to maintain the identification. SDT further assumes that under typical, "good-enough" conditions people actively attempt to internalize and integrate socially endorsed values, identities, and regulations (Ryan, 1995). These norms, rules, and values will be more fully integrated to the self, and therefore more relatively autonomous, to the extent that: (a) these rules and values are transmitted in an autonomy supportive rather than controlling way; and (b) the rules, norms, or values are themselves not antithetical to basic need fulfillment. In other words, both the process and the content of socialization bear on the readiness of individuals to internalize the regulation of any given behavior.

Internalization is also important with respect to organizational authority and political adherence. The very concept of *legitimacy* is, on the psychological side, an issue of internalization. When authorities or their regulations are seen by their constituents as not legitimate, this means they are not internalized: They are not backed by the self of the individuals subjected to them. External regulation in the form of force or direct control does not in itself convey legitimacy, and indeed, the appearance of excessive external control can often undermine perceived legitimacy (Bartlett, 2009). In fact, socialization that relies on less coercion is predicted by SDT to facilitate greater internalization, other things being equal. Reciprocally the less-value individuals experience in a regulation the more controlling authorities must become in order to engender compliance. We see this dynamic often in coercive organizations and regimes.

It is also important to see internalization in its complexity. Within the SDT model, underlying most behaviors are multiple forms of regulation. For example, a behavior may be both valued for its outcomes and enjoyable to do, in which case the person might be motivated by both identified regulations and intrinsic motivation. This is often the case in sport (e.g., Pelletier, Fortier, Vallerand, & Brière, 2001; Reid, Vallerand, Poulin Crocker, & Farrell, 2009), but also for some individuals in domains such as work, school, and community activities. Other behaviors, such as certain prosocial acts, might be both based in introjections (one feels one should do it) and identified regulations (one experiences personal value in doing it). Since each of these different underlying forms of regulation has distinct properties, knowing the configuration and relative strength of each can be important, as well as the overall *relative autonomy* of behavior, when all motives are considered (Ryan & Connell, 1989).

Correlates of relative autonomy. The relative autonomy with which extrinsic motivation is regulated is, according to SDT, differentially associated with full functioning and organismic wellness. The reasons for this are clear: as people more willingly pursue activities they do so with more energy, exhibit more vitality, and have more positive experience. They also tend to perform better and get greater competence satisfaction. Finally, because of people's basic need for relatedness, autonomously pursued activities are often relational, connecting people more deeply with each other. The empirical evidence supporting this claim that relative autonomy predicts both need satisfaction and wellness across settings and cultures is extensive. In what follows we simply illustrate with a few examples.

There is a vast literature applying SDT to education (see Niemiec & Ryan, 2009). In part this reflects the importance of autonomy in a domain where learning is the central goal, because there cannot be quality learning without true volition. Accordingly, autonomous self-regulation has been shown to promote greater conceptual learning (e.g., Benware & Deci,1984; Grolnick & Ryan, 1987), performance (e.g., Black & Deci, 2000), and behavioral adjustment (e.g., Grolnick, Ryan, & Deci, 1991). Autonomous self-regulation has also been associated with lower dropout from school (Vallerand & Bissonnette, 1992). The positive role of autonomy support in schools has been identified across a broad array of cultures (Chirkov, 2009).

In the realm of health care it is similarly the case that many health outcomes are dependent on the patient's willingness to engage in changes. In line with this, autonomous self-regulation for health-behavior change has been shown to be a central predictor of outcomes (see Ryan, Williams, Patrick, & Deci, 2009). For example, more autonomous motivations for smoking cessation predicted smokers' likelihood of maintaining long-term tobacco abstinence (Williams, Niemiec, Patrick, Ryan, & Deci, 2009). Among patients with diabetes, Williams et al. (2009) found that autonomous self-regulation for medication use predicted higher perceived competence, greater medication adherence, and improved physiological outcomes.

In the work domain, it is clear that every manager would like employees who were identified with the values of work and interested in a job well done. Managerial autonomy support appears to foster greater need satisfaction, including satisfaction of the autonomy need, and is associated with both greater work engagement and positive experience (Baard et al., 2004; Gagne & Deci, 2005). Interestingly, autonomous self-regulation among unemployed individuals has been associated with greater well-being and job-search intensity (Vansteenkiste, Lens, Dewitte, De Witte, & Deci, 2004).

In the study of ill-being, disturbances of autonomy are highly salient. In fact environments that actively thwart the development of autonomy are implicated in a number of psychopathologies such as borderline personality disorders (e.g., Ryan, 2005). Additionally, in various disorders autonomous regulation is functionally disrupted, leading to compromised outcomes and ill-being (Ryan et al., 2006). Accordingly, recent research on psychotherapy suggests that support for autonomy is critical in ameliorating psychological distress, from depression to impulsive disorders (Ryan & Deci, 2008b; Ryan, Lynch, Vansteenkiste, & Deci, in press; Zuroff et al., 2007).

Although we could more extensively review additional domains, such as sport and exercise (e.g., Pelletier et al., 2001; Standage & Ryan, in press), political engagement (Koestner, Losier, Vallerand, & Carducci, 1996), religion (e.g., Ryan, Rigby, & King, 1993), volunteer work (Gagne, 2003; Weinstein & Ryan, 2010), and other areas of interest, our point is merely to illustrate that autonomy is indeed critical to full functioning and wellness in and across contexts. The findings show that autonomous self-regulation is associated with increased behavioral persistence; improved task performance; and greater psychological, physical, and social wellness. Thus, the relative autonomy with which behavior is regulated appears to be an important antecedent of "the good life" and the happiness that derives from it.

Autonomy and Relatedness: Their Dynamic Interplay

Thus far we have argued that autonomy is functionally critical for healthy development, fulfilling engagement, and a satisfying life. However, for many scholars the very concept of autonomy as a fundamental need is an anathema. In particular, many psychologists view autonomy as being antithetical to the value of relatedness—that is, to the need for being connected with others (e.g., Jordan, 1997; Markus, Kitayama, & Heiman, 1996). This disparity comes about in part because the concept of autonomy is conflated with that of independence, selfishness, or individualism. From the SDT perspective, autonomy is not synonymous with any of these concepts, but instead is defined as volition, willingness, and endorsement.

SDT research has shown, for example, that in close friendships, feeling a sense of autonomy is essential for a high-quality relationship, and further that experiencing mutuality of autonomy support is related to relational and personal well-being (Deci, La Guardia, Moller, Scheiner, & Ryan, 2006). Similarly, La Guardia et al. (2000) found that the degree to which one experienced satisfaction of the autonomy need within one's closest relationships predicted the quality of those relationships. Of course, if one were to interpret autonomy to mean selfishness and independence—that is, if autonomy were understood to mean doing whatever one feels like doing regardless of one's partner—autonomy would not enhance the relational quality, for people need to feel satisfaction of both the relatedness need and the autonomy need to flourish within the relationship. Simply stated, autonomy, as we define it, is not antagonistic to relatedness, for there is a synergy in the satisfaction of these two needs. In fact people often feel highly autonomous when engaging in behaviors done for their partners (Gaine & La Guardia, 2009). Acting in a way that thwarts either a sense of autonomy or relatedness, however, will result in decrements in interpersonal relational quality and well-being.

Similarly, some have argued that autonomy, while important in western cultures, is not important in eastern cultures where collectivism rather than individualism is the stronger cultural value (e.g., Markus et al., 1996). Yet, SDT argues that one can be autonomous either when acting for a collective or when acting individualistically. Further of course, one could be controlled when acting in the service of either a collective or oneself. In support of this viewpoint, Chirkov, Ryan, Kaplan, and Kim (2003) found that in both eastern and western cultures (viz., South Korea, Russia, Turkey, and the US) people who reported behaving more autonomously also reported greater psychological well-being, an effect that was not moderated by cultural context. Since then many studies have found similar results.

It is critical then to see the importance of autonomy support across cultural contexts. For example Jang, Reeve, Ryan, and Kim (2009) recently showed how teacher autonomy support enhanced, and teacher controllingness diminished, psychological need satisfaction of Korean high school students, resulting in both more negative academic and well-being outcomes. Here, in a collectivistic setting, autonomy support retains its positive functions in facilitating internalization, need satisfaction and wellness.

This and other research indicates that the autonomy and relatedness needs go hand-in-hand for optimal functioning in relationships and in general regardless of one's culture. Indeed, if the two needs are pitted against each other, as they are when one offers conditional regard, the consequences are negative for the recipient of the regard (e.g., Assor, Roth, & Deci, 2004). It is also interesting to note that, when people feel autonomous, they will often also feel relatedness for they experience the psychological freedom that allows them to pursue meaningful connections with others.

Differential Aspirations: Intrinsic and Extrinsic Life Goals

Focusing on the relative autonomy of goals is content-free as a prescription for happiness. That is, to suggest that the affordance of autonomy leads to happiness is to suggest that when given an opportunity to self-regulate people tend to optimize need satisfactions and move in a direction of wellness and integrity. Indeed, SDT is based on the assumption that support for autonomy conduces to wellness, implying such a trust in the organismic process.

At the same time, this process-oriented approach concerning "why" people are pursing some outcome does not preclude an "on average" analysis of the contents of those desired outcomes—that is, of "what" individuals are pursuing. It is no doubt the case that some goals or aims are more and some are less conducive to wellness and happiness. Indeed, it also turns out to be the case that when people are acting more autonomously they are more likely to pursue some types of goals rather than others. Accordingly, in recent years within SDT there has been an active focus on different types of goal contents and their impacts on well-being.

Beginning in the early 1990s Kasser and Ryan (e.g., 1993, 1996) began examining the aspirations people had for their futures and the relations of these life goals to wellness. For example, Kasser and Ryan (1996) surveyed both college students and urban adults concerning their life goals and identified two distinct goal complexes. The first factor, labeled *extrinsic aspirations,* included values for wealth, fame, and an appealing image, whereas the second, labeled *intrinsic aspirations,* included values for personal growth, close relationships, community contribution, and physical health. The structural distinction between the intrinsic and extrinsic aspirations has since been observed in multiple studies, including one that surveyed samples from 15 cultures throughout the world (Grouzet et al., 2005). As noted earlier, the extrinsic aspirations tend to be those associated with the consumer-oriented, self-centered values that are frequently heralded in modern culture, whereas the intrinsic goals focus on personal development, generative activities, and connections with others, better reflecting a eudaimonic lifestyle Aristotle might have advocated (Ryan et al., 2008). Therefore, it is important to ascertain whether the pursuit and attainment of intrinsic (relative to extrinsic) aspirations differentially predict full functioning and happiness.

In their early study Kasser and Ryan (1996) found that those who placed strong importance on intrinsic (relative to extrinsic) aspirations reported higher well-being and lower ill-being in both college students and adults. Subsequently Ryan et al. (1999) found similar results in both the US and Russian samples. Sheldon et al. (2004) showed this pattern across four cultural groups. Vansteenkiste, Neyrinck, Niemiec, Soenens, de Witte, and Van den Broeck (2007) reported that adult employees in Belgium who held an extrinsic (relative to intrinsic) work value orientation evidenced less work-related satisfaction, dedication, and vitality, and more work-family conflict, emotional exhaustion, and turn-over intentions. The deleterious consequences of holding an extrinsic (relative to intrinsic) work value orientation were mediated by need satisfaction experienced at work. In the exercise domain, Sebire, Standage, and Vansteenkiste (2009) showed that intrinsic (relative to extrinsic) goals predicted cognitive, affective, and behavioral outcomes through their associations with autonomy, competence, and relatedness. These studies exemplify the growing body of evidence supporting the differential impact of intrinsic versus extrinsic aspirations on happiness and well-being outcomes. Sadly, in fact, evidence amassed over the last seven decades points to a cultural trend within the USA toward more extrinsic goals, which in turn has been linked to increased rates of mental distress and psychopathology (Twenge et al., 2010). The question is how far the extrinsic virus of consumption and self-focus will spread over these next historically and environmentally critical decades.

Attainment of life goals. Other research in SDT has examined how *attaining* intrinsic (relative to extrinsic) aspirations (as opposed to just pursuing them) affects life outcomes, including happiness. In contrast to most expectancy-value theories, which suggest that attainment of all valued goals is beneficial to well-being (e.g., Locke & Latham, 1990) regardless of their contents, SDT has a more differentiated prediction. Specifically we suggest that the attainment of intrinsic goals enhances wellness, whereas the attainment of extrinsic goals typically does not. That is, because of their differential associations with the basic psychological needs, SDT asserts that attainment of intrinsic aspirations is likely to promote wellness, whereas attainment of extrinsic aspirations is unlikely to benefit well-being, and may at times contribute to ill-being.

A number of studies have provided support for these hypotheses. Kasser and Ryan (2001) found that attaining intrinsic (relative to extrinsic) aspirations was positively associated with higher psychological health and quality of interpersonal relationships. Similar results were also obtained in the Russian and US samples reported by Ryan et al. (1999). In a sample of senior citizens, Van Hiel and Vansteenkiste (2009) reported that attainment of intrinsic aspirations was associated with higher ego-integrity and death acceptance, whereas attainment of extrinsic aspirations was associated with more despair. Niemiec, Ryan, and Deci (2009) used a longitudinal design to examine young adults' goal attainment from 1 to 2 years post-college, an important period marked by transition into adult identities and lifestyles. Results showed that whereas the attainment of intrinsic aspirations promoted psychological health, the attainment of extrinsic aspirations was unrelated to well-being and was positively associated with indicators of ill-being. In line with SDT, the benefits of attaining intrinsic aspirations for psychological health were mediated by satisfaction of the basic psychological needs.

In sum, research from SDT indicates that greater valuing of intrinsic relative to extrinsic life goals is associated with enhancement of psychological wellness, including traditional indicators of happiness. In addition, whereas the attainment of intrinsic goals enhances wellness, attainments of extrinsic goals contribute little to wellness once people are above poverty levels. Importantly, such associations have been observed in numerous contexts, lending credibility to the postulate that basic need satisfaction, which more readily accrues from the pursuit and attainment of intrinsic aspirations, is a universal component of optimal functioning and wellness. Thus, which "good life" people choose to pursue matters, as not all aspirations are equally likely to foster need satisfaction and happiness.

Social Contexts, Need Satisfaction, Autonomy, and Intrinsic Aspirations

Thus far, we have argued and reviewed supportive research concerning: (1) a strong relation between satisfaction of the basic needs for autonomy, competence, and relatedness and people's experiences of full functioning and well-being; (2) autonomous self-regulation (including both intrinsic motivation and well-internalized extrinsic motivation) being a reliable predictor of need satisfaction, effective performance, and eudaimonic living; and (3) the pursuit and attainment of intrinsic goals being more likely when people are autonomously motivated and being associated with greater well-being than the pursuit and attainment of extrinsic goals.

We turn now to the role of social contexts in this network of relations. We have argued that when people feel satisfaction of the basic psychological needs they will maintain their intrinsic motivation, internalization extrinsic motivation, and pursue and attain intrinsic goals. Accordingly, SDT has proposed that interpersonal contexts that support satisfaction of the three basic psychological needs represent an optimal context for promoting psychological wellness and effective functioning. In fact, it is likely that more research has addressed the effects of social contexts on motivation, performance, and well-being than any other component of the theory. Accordingly, we will be able to review only a very small percentage of that work.

Considerable research has examined the effects of autonomy-supportive versus controlling social contexts on a range of mediating and outcome variables. For example, the first of these studies (Deci, Schwartz, Sheinman, & Ryan, 1981) found that when classroom teachers of elementary students were more autonomy supportive the students were more intrinsically motivated, perceived themselves to be more competent at their schoolwork, and had higher self-esteem. Similarly, when managers were more autonomy supportive, their employees were more trusting of the organization and were more satisfied with various aspects of their work lives (Deci, Connell, & Ryan, 1989). Parents who were judged by observers to be more autonomy supportive had children who were more autonomous in doing their schoolwork and were rated as more competent by their late-elementary-school teachers (Grolnick & Ryan, 1989). A study by Pelletier et al. (2001) of elite Canadian swimmers showed that those whose coaches were more autonomy supportive were more autonomously motivated and persisted at their sport longer than those whose coaches were less autonomous.

Similarly, studies have shown that autonomy supportive socializing contexts also lead people to develop more intrinsic life goals. For example, Kasser, Ryan, Zax, and Sameroff (1995) found that when mothers of 4-year old children were authoritarian and cold (i.e., were low in autonomy support) their children tended to place much stronger importance on extrinsic aspiration than on intrinsic aspirations when they were in their late teens. Williams, Cox, Hedberg, and Deci (2000) found that teenagers who experienced their parents as being more autonomy-supportive had more intrinsic goals and were less likely to engage in high-risk behaviors such as using tobacco and alcohol and having early sexual intercourse. Finally, Sheldon and Kasser (2008) found that college students who experienced psychological threats tended to become more focused on extrinsic life goals.

The studies of social contextual influences, only a few of which we have mentioned, have been both developmental and social psychological in nature. That is, some of them have examined the effects of socializing contexts on the development of individual differences both with regard to domain-specific autonomy and intrinsic aspirations, as well as on well-being and other positive outcomes. Other studies have examined how autonomy-promoting factors in the immediate social environment facilitate the states of autonomy and wellness. In reviewing most of these studies we have spoken of autonomy-supportive versus controlling contexts, yet some of the studies have been formulated more broadly in terms of need-supportive versus need-thwarting environmental factors. Thus, some studies have found that support for, rather than thwarting of, the autonomy, competence, and relatedness needs promotes autonomous motivation and well-being (e.g., Jang et al., 2009; La Guardia et al., 2000; Niemiec et al., 2006). It turns out that typically when an environment is autonomy supportive, it tends also to support the competence and relatedness needs, so some of the studies of autonomy support have been de facto studies of need support. This makes sense because authority figures who support autonomy will, because they consider the individual's internal frame of reference, often also provide active support for competence and relatedness or will at least allow the target individuals to pursue their own competence and relatedness satisfaction.

The various studies of need support we have reviewed examined the impacts of relatively proximal factors in the lives of the target participants—parents of children, teachers of students, managers of employees, and physicians of patients, for example. SDT is, however, also concerned with the influence of more distal influences shaped by institutional, cultural, and economic factors. For example, school-district policies affect the motivation and well-being of students in the district, and top-level corporate officers affect the lives of employees who are many levels below them and who may live thousands of miles away. Similarly, insurance company regulations affect the motivation and experiences of individual patients, in part by affecting the behavior of health care professionals but perhaps in other more direct ways as well.

At an even more distal, societal level, economic and political structures can affect the motivation and well-being of individuals within the society, again, either directly or mediated through other more proximal influences. SDT maintains that at each level of proximity, the effects of environmental influences can be analyzed in terms of the degree to which they tend to support versus thwart need satisfaction.

For example, the American corporate capitalist system of economics involves the owners of capital (and their surrogates) using incentives to control individuals' behavior. The advertising industry emphasizes extrinsic goals, such as accumulating material goods and developing an image that will attract attention and recognition. Consequently this economic system does, through these and numerous other pathways, set forth controlling influences that negatively affect the autonomy of individuals within the culture (Kasser, Cohn, Kanner, & Ryan, 2007). In addition some of these influences, which emphasize individualism, competition, and sometimes selfishness, are likely to have the functional significance of thwarting people's relatedness as well, further yielding negative effects on their psychological health and well-being (e.g., Kasser et al., 2007). At the same time that the capitalist system has strong controlling and even amotivating elements, it simultaneously provides substantial opportunities for exercising initiative and autonomy for those with skills and/or resources. Unlike central planning economies there is more latitude in choosing careers and locations to live (Deci et al., 2001). Entrepreneurs have opportunities for a wide range of activities that are potentially lucrative and at the same time allow for the experiences of autonomy and competence satisfaction. Thus, for different individuals the system can be experienced differently, providing far more or far less support for their basic needs. Yet it is also important to keep in mind that an abundance of research has shown that tangible rewards do tend on average to be experienced as controlling and thus undermining of autonomy (Deci et al., 1999). Thus it is not surprising that within the capitalist system many people lack autonomy on an everyday basis, a pattern which experiential data from average workers has been supporting (e.g., Ryan et al., 2010).

Other economic systems can be similarly analyzed in terms of supports versus thwarts for basic needs. Political systems can also be so analyzed, as can laws that exist within them. A democratic political system, for example, certainly allows greater support for autonomy than does a totalitarian one (e.g., Downie, Koestner, & Chua, 2007), yet small pockets of great wealth within a democratic system, as is the case in the US, can wield undue control and influence over others in the system, leaving many people feeling amotivated and helpless in relation to politics and the resulting policies.

Our aim here is not to do a comprehensive analysis of economic or political systems, but instead to point out that contextual effects on people's basic psychological needs are a function of multiple interacting levels of influence. Political freedoms, economic opportunities and security (which affords freedoms), and institutional dynamics all impact a person's autonomy, and his or her capacity to fulfill basic needs.

Summary

The SDT approach to understanding happiness distinguishes between happiness that is viewed solely as the relative presence of positive affect and the relative absence of negative affect however those experiences are attained, and happiness that typically results from the experience of what has been called full functioning—that is, of using one's capacities in an open, interested, and committed way, with a full sense of endorsement and concurrence.

Autonomy, or true self-regulation, and intrinsic goals are critical elements for the SDT approach to full functioning and to the happiness typically associated with it. When people act autonomously, rather than being controlled or amotivated, they act with a sense of choice, are more mindful, think flexibly, and express their values and interests. Such actions provide basic need satisfaction that results in psychological health and well-being at both the state level and the more-enduring person level. Further, pursuing and attaining intrinsic goals such as personal development, relationships, community, and health, rather than extrinsic goals such as material goods, fame, and image have been found to be associated with greater need satisfaction and enhanced wellness.

To be autonomous, to act from one's intrinsic interests and from internalized values and regulations are inherent human processes. Remarkably, these integrative and need fulfilling tendencies lead people to connect with each other, and to identify with people outside themselves and close kin. Autonomy is in this sense a key to true community. Yet these natural processes require nutriments and supports, both proximal and distal, to function effectively. As we know from evolutionary psychology our human nature is contingent; what our genes provide is not a set of specific behaviors but a capacity to develop certain behaviors and sensibilities under specifiable environmental conditions (Wilson, 1996). SDT specifically argues that for people to manifest intrinsic motivation, healthy internalization, and need satisfying life-goals they require social and cultural supports for the satisfaction of their basic psychological needs. The availability of such supports is affected by social contexts ranging in proximity from individual relationships to ambient cultural structures, to economic and political systems. These all influence motivation and wellness by representing either supports for or obstacles to satisfaction of these basic psychological needs. In short, human thriving, full functioning, and the happiness that entails psychological freedom and the life well-lived result when people act more autonomously, pursue more intrinsic goals, and experience satisfaction of their basic psychological needs for autonomy, competence, and relatedness.

References

Assor, A., Roth, G., & Deci, E. L. (2004). The emotional costs of parents' conditional regard: A self-determination theory analysis. *Journal of Personality, 72*, 47–88.

Baard, P. P., Deci, E. L., & Ryan, R. M. (2004). Intrinsic need satisfaction: A motivational basis of performance and well-being in two work settings. *Journal of Applied Social Psychology, 34*, 2045–2068.

Bartlett, K. T. (2009). Making good on good intentions: The critical role of motivation in reducing implicit workplace discrimination. *Virginia Law Review, 95*, 1893–1972.

Benware, C., & Deci, E. L. (1984). Quality of learning with an active versus passive motivational set. *American Educational Research Journal, 21*, 755–765.

Black, A. E., & Deci, E. L. (2000). The effects of student self-regulation and instructor autonomy support on learning in a college-level natural science course: A self-determination theory perspective. *Science Education, 84*, 740–756.

Chirkov, V. I. (2009). A cross-cultural analysis of autonomy in education: A self-determination theory perspective. *Theory and Research in Education, 7*, 253–262.

Chirkov, V. I., Ryan, R. M., Kim, Y., & Kaplan, U. (2003). Differentiating autonomy from individualism and independence: A self-determination theory perspective on internalization of cultural orientations and well-being. *Journal of Personality and Social Psychology, 84*, 97–110.

Chirkov, V. I., Ryan, R. M., & Willness, C. (2005). Cultural context and psychological needs in Canada and Brazil: Testing a self-determination approach to the internalization of cultural practices, identity, and well-being. *Journal of Cross-Cultural Psychology, 36*, 423–443.

de Charms, R. (1968). *Personal causation: The internal affective determinants of behavior.* New York: Academic Press.

Deci, E. L., Connell, J. P., & Ryan, R. M. (1989). Self-determination in a work organization. *Journal of Applied Psychology, 74*, 580–590.

Deci, E. L., Koestner, R., & Ryan, R. M. (1999). A meta-analytic review of experiments examining the effects of extrinsic rewards on intrinsic motivation. *Psychological Bulletin, 125*, 627–668.

Deci, E. L., La Guardia, J. G., Moller, A. C., Scheiner, M. J., & Ryan, R. M. (2006). On the benefits of giving as well as receiving autonomy support: Mutuality in close friendships. *Personality and Social Psychology Bulletin, 32*, 313–327.

Deci, E. L., & Ryan, R. M. (1985). *Intrinsic motivation and self-determination in human behavior.* New York: Plenum.

Deci, E. L., & Ryan, R. M. (2008). Hedonia, eudaimonia, and well-being: An introduction. *Journal of Happiness Studies, 9*, 1–11.

Deci, E. L., Ryan, R. M., Gagné, M., Leone, D. R., Usunov, J., & Kornazheva, B. P. (2001). Need satisfaction, motivation, and well-being in the work organizations of a former eastern bloc country. *Personality and Social Psychology Bulletin, 27*, 930–942.

Deci, E. L., Schwartz, A. J., Sheinman, L., & Ryan, R. M. (1981). An instrument to assess adults' orientations toward control versus autonomy with children: Reflections on intrinsic motivation and perceived competence. *Journal of Educational Psychology, 73*, 642–650.

Downie, M., Koestner, R., & Chua, S. N. (2007). Political support for self-determination, wealth, and national subjective well-being. *Motivation & Emotion, 31*, 188–194.

Gagné, M. (2003). The role of autonomy support and autonomy orientation in prosocial behavior engagement. *Motivation and Emotion, 27*, 199–223.

Gagné, M., & Deci, E. L. (2005). Self-determination theory and work motivation. *Journal of Organizational Behavior, 26*, 331–362.

Gaine, G. S., & La Guardia, J. G. (2009). The unique contributions of motivations to maintain a relationship and motivations toward relational activities to relationship well-being. *Motivation and Emotion, 33*, 184–202.

Grolnick, W. S., & Ryan, R. M. (1987). Autonomy in children's learning: An experimental and individual difference investigation. *Journal of Personality and Social Psychology, 52*, 890–898.

Grolnick, W. S., & Ryan, R. M. (1989). Parent styles associated with children's self-regulation and competence in school. *Journal of Educational Psychology, 81*, 143–154.

Grolnick, W. S., Ryan, R. M., & Deci, E. L. (1991). The inner resources for school achievement: Motivational mediators of children's perceptions of their parents. *Journal of Educational Psychology, 83*, 508–517.

Grolnick, W. S., & Seal, K. (2008). *Pressured parents, stressed-out kids: Dealing with competition while raising a successful child.* Amherst, NY: Prometheus Press.

Grouzet, F. M., Kasser, T., Ahuvia, A., Dols, J. M. F., Kim, Y., Lau, S., et al. (2005). The structure of goals across 15 cultures *Journal of Personality and Social Psychology, 89*, 800–816.

Harter, S. (1981). A new self-report scale of intrinsic versus extrinsic orientation in the classroom: Motivational and informational components *Developmental Psychology, 17*, 300–312.

Huta, V., & Ryan, R. M. (in press). Pursuing pleasure or virtue: The differential and overlapping well-being benefits of hedonic and eudaimonic motives. *Journal of Happiness Studies.*

Jang, H., Reeve, J., Ryan, R. M., & Kim, A. (2009). Can self-determination theory explain what underlies the productive, satisfying learning experiences of collectivistically oriented Korean students? *Journal of Educational Psychology, 101*, 644–661.

Jordan, J. V. (1997). Do you believe that the concepts of self and autonomy are useful in understanding women? In J. V.Jordan (Ed.), *Women's growth in diversity: More writings from the stone center* (pp. 29–32). New York: Guilford.

Kahneman, D., Diener, E., & Schwarz, N. (Eds.). (1999). *Well-being: The foundations of hedonic psychology.* New York: Russell Sage Foundation.

Kashdan, T. B., Biswas-Diener, R., & King, L. A. (2008). Reconsidering happiness: The costs of distinguishing between hedonics and eudaimonia. *The Journal of Positive Psychology, 3,* 219–233.

Kasser, T., Cohn, S., Kanner, A. D., & Ryan, R. M. (2007). Some costs of American corporate capitalism: A psychological exploration of value and goal conflicts. *Psychological Inquiry, 18,* 1–22.

Kasser, T., & Ryan, R. M. (1993). A dark side of the American dream: Correlates of financial success as a central life aspiration. *Journal of Personality and Social Psychology, 65,* 410–422.

Kasser, T., & Ryan, R. M. (1996). Further examining the American dream: Differential correlates of intrinsic and extrinsic goals. *Personality and Social Psychology Bulletin, 22,* 80–87.

Kasser, T., & Ryan, R. M. (2001). Be careful what you wish for: Optimal functioning and the relative attainment of intrinsic and extrinsic goals. In P. Schmuck & K. M. Sheldon (Eds.), *Life goals and well-being: Towards a positive psychology of human striving* (pp. 115–129). Goettingen: Hogrefe & Huber Publishers.

Kasser, T., Ryan, R. M., Zax, M., & Sameroff, A. J. (1995). The relations of maternal and social environments to late adolescents' materialistic and prosocial values. *Developmental Psychology, 31,* 907–914.

Koestner, R., Losier, G. F., Vallerand, R. J., & Carducci, D. (1996). Identified and introjected forms of political internalization: Extending self-determination theory. *Journal of Personality and Social Psychology, 70,* 1025–1036.

La Guardia, J. G., Ryan, R. M., Couchman, C. E., & Deci, E. L. (2000). Within-person variation in security of attachment: A self-determination theory perspective on attachment, need fulfillment, and well-being. *Journal of Personality and Social Psychology, 79,* 367–384.

Locke, E. A., & Latham, G. P. (1990). *A theory of goal setting and task performance.* Englewood Cliffs, NJ: Prentice-Hall.

Markus, H. R., Kitayama, S., & Heiman, R. J. (1996). Culture and basic psychological principles. In E. T. Higgins & A. W. Kruglanski (Eds.), *Social psychology: Handbook of basic principles* (pp. 857–913). New York: Guilford.

Niemiec, C. P., Lynch, M. F., Vansteenkiste, M., Bernstein, J., Deci, E. L., & Ryan, R. M. (2006). The antecedents and consequences of autonomous self-regulation for college: A self-determination theory perspective on socialization. *Journal of Adolescence, 29,* 761–775.

Niemiec, C. P., & Ryan, R. M. (2009). Autonomy, competence, and relatedness in the classroom: Applying self-determination theory to educational practice. *Theory and Research in Education, 7,* 133–144.

Niemiec, C. P., Ryan, R. M., & Deci, E. L. (2009). The path taken: Consequences of attaining intrinsic and extrinsic aspirations in post-college life. *Journal of Research in Personality, 43,* 291–306.

Patall, E. A., Cooper, H., & Robinson, J. C. (2008). The effects of choice on intrinsic motivation and related outcomes: A meta-analysis of research findings. *Psychological Bulletin, 134,* 270–300.

Patrick, H., Knee, C. R., Canevello, A., & Lonsbary, C. (2007). The role of need fulfillment in relationship functioning and well-being: A self-determination theory perspective. *Journal of Personality and Social Psychology, 92,* 434–457.

Pelletier, L. G., Fortier, M. S., Vallerand, R. J., & Brière, N. M. (2001). Associations among perceived autonomy support, forms of self-regulation, and persistence: A prospective study. *Motivation and Emotion, 25,* 279–306.

Reid, G., Vallerand, R. J., Poulin, C., Crocker, P., & Farrell, R. (2009). The development and validation of the pictorial motivation scale in physical activity. *Motivation and Emotion, 33,* 161–172.

Ryan, R. M. (1995). Psychological needs and the facilitation of integrative processes. *Journal of Personality, 63*, 397–427.
Ryan, R. M. (2005). The developmental line of autonomy in the etiology, dynamics, and treatment of borderline personality disorders. *Development and Psychopathology, 17*, 987–1006.
Ryan, R. M., Bernstein, J. H., & Brown, K. W. (2010). Weekends, work, and well-being: Psychological need satisfactions and day of the week effects on mood, vitality, and physical symptoms. *Journal of Social and Clinical Psychology, 29*, 95–122.
Ryan, R. M., Chirkov, V. I., Little, T. D., Sheldon, K. M., Timoshina, E., & Deci, E. L. (1999). The American dream in Russia: Extrinsic aspirations and well-being in two cultures. *Personality and Social Psychology Bulletin, 25*, 1509–1524.
Ryan, R. M., & Connell, J. P. (1989). Perceived locus of causality and internalization: Examining reasons for acting in two domains. *Journal of Personality and Social Psychology, 57*, 749–761.
Ryan, R. M., & Deci, E. L. (2000a). Intrinsic and extrinsic motivations: Classic definitions and new directions. *Contemporary Educational Psychology, 25*, 54–67.
Ryan, R. M., & Deci, E. L. (2000b). Self-determination theory and the facilitation of intrinsic motivation, social development, and well-being. *American Psychologist, 55*, 68–78.
Ryan, R. M., & Deci, E. L. (2001). On happiness and human potentials: A review of research on hedonic and eudaimonic well-being. In S. Fiske (Ed.), *Annual Review of Psychology* (Vol. 52, pp. 141–166). Palo Alto, CA: Annual Reviews, Inc.
Ryan, R. M., & Deci, E. L. (2008a). From ego depletion to vitality: Theory and findings concerning the facilitation of energy available to the self. *Social and Personality Psychology Compass, 2*, 702–717.
Ryan, R. M., & Deci, E. L. (2008b). A self-determination approach to psychotherapy: The motivational basis for effective change. *Canadian Psychology, 49*, 186–193.
Ryan, R. M., Deci, E. L., Grolnick, W. S., & La Guardia, J. G. (2006). The significance of autonomy and autonomy support in psychological development and psychopathology. In D. Cicchetti & D. J. Cohen (Eds.), *Developmental psychopathology* (pp. 795–849). Hoboken, NJ: Wiley.
Ryan, R. M., & Huta, V. (2009). Wellness as healthy functioning or wellness as happiness: The importance of eudaimonic thinking. *The Journal of Positive Psychology, 4*, 202–204.
Ryan, R. M., Huta, V., & Deci, E. L. (2008). Living well: A self-determination theory perspective on eudaimonia. *Journal of Happiness Studies, 9*, 139–170.
Ryan, R. M., Lynch, M. F., Vansteenkiste, M., & Deci, E. L. (in press). Motivation and autonomy in counseling, psychotherapy, and behavior change: A look at theory and practice. *The Counseling Psychologist*.
Ryan, R. M., Rigby, S., & King, K. (1993). Two types of religious internalization and their relations to religious orientations and mental health. *Journal of Personality and Social Psychology, 65*, 586–596.
Ryan, R. M., Williams, G. C., Patrick, H., & Deci, E. L. (2009). Self-determination theory and physical activity: The dynamics of motivation in development and wellness. *Hellenic Journal of Psychology, 6*, 107–124.
Ryff, C. D., & Singer, B. H. (2008). Know thyself and become what you are: A eudaimonic approach to psychological well-being. *Journal of Happiness Studies, 9*, 13–39.
Sebire, S. J., Standage, M., & Vansteenkiste, M. (2009). Examining intrinsic versus extrinsic exercise goals: Cognitive, affective, and behavioral outcomes. *Journal of Sport and Exercise Psychology, 31*, 189–210.
Sheldon, K. M., Elliot, A. J., Ryan, R. M., Chirkov, V. I., Kim, Y., Wu, C., et al. (2004). Self-concordance and subjective well-being in four cultures. *Journal of Cross-Cultural Psychology, 35*, 209–223.
Sheldon, K. M., & Kasser, T. (2008). Psychological threat and extrinsic goal striving. *Motivation and Emotion, 32*, 37–45.
Standage, M., & Ryan, R. M. (in press). Self-determination theory and exercise motivation: Facilitating self-regulatory processes to support and maintain health and well-being. In

G. C. Roberts & D. C. Treasure (Eds.), *Motivation in sport and exercise* (Vol. 3). Champaign, IL: Human Kinetics.

Twenge, J., Gentile, B., DeWall, C. N., Ma, D., Lacefield, K., & Schurtz, D. R. (2010). Birth cohort increases in psychopathology among young Americans, 1938–2007: A cross-temporal meta-analysis of the MMPI. *Clinical Psychology Review, 30*, 145–154.

Vallerand, R. J., & Bissonnette, R. (1992). Intrinsic, extrinsic, and amotivational styles as predictors of behavior: A prospective study. *Journal of Personality, 60*, 599–620.

Vallerand, R. J., & Reid, G. (1984). On the causal effects of perceived competence on intrinsic motivation: A test of cognitive evaluation theory. *Journal of Sport Psychology, 6*, 94–102.

Van Hiel, A., & Vansteenkiste, M. (2009). Ambitions full filled? The effects of intrinsic and extrinsic goal attainment on older adults' ego-integrity and death attitudes. *International Journal of Aging and Human Development, 68*, 27–51.

Vansteenkiste, M., Lens, W., Dewitte, S., De Witte, H., & Deci, E. L. (2004). The "why" and "why not" of job search behavior: Their relation to searching, unemployment experience, and well-being. *European Journal of Social Psychology, 34*, 345–363.

Vansteenkiste, M., Neyrinck, B., Niemiec, C. P., Soenens, B., de Witte, H., & Van den Broeck, A. (2007). On the relations among work value orientations, psychological need satisfaction, and job outcomes: A self-determination theory approach. *Journal of Occupational and Organizational Psychology, 80*, 251–277.

Waterman, A. S., Schwartz, S. J., & Conti, R. (2008). The implications of two conceptions of happiness (hedonic enjoyment and eudaimonia) for the understanding of intrinsic motivation. *Journal of Happiness Studies, 9*, 41–79.

Weinstein, N., & Ryan, R. M. (2010). When helping helps: Autonomous motivation for prosocial behavior and its influence on well-being for the helper and recipient. *Journal of Personality and Social Psychology, 98*, 222–244.

Williams, G. C., Cox, E. M., Hedberg, V., & Deci, E. L. (2000). Extrinsic life goals and health risk behaviors in adolescents. *Journal of Applied Social Psychology, 30*, 1756–1771.

Williams, G. C., Niemiec, C. P., Patrick, H., Ryan, R. M., & Deci, E. L. (2009). The importance of supporting autonomy and perceived competence in facilitating long-term tobacco abstinence. *Annals of Behavioral Medicine, 37*, 215–324.

Williams, G. C., Patrick, H., Niemiec, C. P., Williams, L. K., Devine, G., Lafata, J. E., et al. (2009). Reducing the health risks of diabetes: How self-determination theory may help improve medication adherence and quality of life. *Diabetes Educator, 35*, 484–492.

Wilson, E. O. (1996). *In search of nature*. Washington, DC: Island Press.

Wilson, P. M., Longley, K., Muon, S., Rodgers, W. M., & Murray, T. C. (2006). Examining the contributions of perceived psychological need satisfaction to well-being in exercise. *Journal of Applied Biobehavioral Research, 11*, 243–264.

Zuroff, D. C., Koestner, R., Moskowitz, D. S., McBride, C., Marshall, M., & Bagby, M. (2007). Autonomous motivation for therapy: A new common factor in brief treatments for depression. *Psychotherapy Research, 17*, 137–147.

Chapter 4
Dialectical Relationships Among Human Autonomy, the Brain, and Culture

Valery I. Chirkov

The objective of all the chapters in this volume is to demonstrate that human autonomy, when it is successfully executed in the different domains of people's lives, works nearly universally in promoting people's optimal functioning, healthy living, and well-being. This chapter will address debates about the cultural universality vs. cultural relativity of human autonomy by considering autonomy's relations with psychological well-being in different cultural contexts. The main thesis that will be defended is that human autonomy is an evolved natural property of *Homo sapiens* that has dialectical relations with people's socio-cultural environments and is a universal and necessary condition for people to be come fully functioning individuals. To defend this thesis, first, a relevant conceptual framework will be outlined. Then, based on brain research and evolutionary and system-theories, I will argue that human autonomy is a natural tendency that requires a brain of human-scale complexity to emerge. Within the same line of arguments I will show that the existence of human autonomy and self-determination does not violate the principle of determinism. After that I will address the dialectical relations between human autonomy and culture and highlight the factors and conditions that either facilitate or hinder the functioning of autonomous people within a society. This chapter will conclude with a review of empirical studies based on SDT propositions that support many of the arguments stated in the first part of the chapter.

One of the reasons for writing this chapter is my strong belief that the thesis that human autonomy is an illusion is not only mistaken, but is also dangerous for the further development of our civilization. This is because this thesis moves one of the fundamental conditions for people's humanness and well-being into the domain of relativity, social negotiation, and linguistic construction, leaving people without solid grounding for their search for better lives. For me these are not purely academic arguments; rather, these are disputes about the very essence of human beings and the future of humanity.

V.I. Chirkov (✉)
Department of Psychology, University of Saskatchewan, Saskatoon, SK, Canada S7N 5A5
e-mail: v.chirkov@usask.ca

The Nature of the Arguments Around Human Autonomy and Happiness

Scholars who critique the idea of autonomy as an evolved natural human capacity represent several perspectives in the current psychological and social sciences (See the review in the Introduction). One of these perspectives follows the requirements of scientific determinism that states that mental phenomena, including consciousness, free will, autonomy, rational intentionality, and related mental processes, cannot be the determining forces of human behaviour because they themselves have their own determinants that ultimately explain the causal power of these high-level mental capacities (for a more detailed discussion of this position see Baer, Kaufman, & Baumeister, 2008). This position logically leads to the statements that self-determination and self-governance are 'illusions' (Wegner, 2002) and even 'unnatural' (Bargh, 2008) phenomena that should be avoided as the object of scientific psychological research if scientists want to understand the real causal determinants of people's behaviours, thoughts, and feelings. Being too busy with finding the ultimate determinants of mental states and behaviour, the representatives of this 'deterministic' position have never addressed the questions of the relationships between the nature of people's feelings of self-determination and their psychological well-being, optimal functioning, and happiness.

Another perspective on the issue of human autonomy and happiness can be labeled here as 'cultural relativism'. Representatives of this standpoint attack the idea of human autonomy as a universal natural capability of human beings by stating that human autonomy, just as all other capabilities of human beings, is dependent for its existence on the linguistic and symbolic tools provided by cultural communities. Based on this correct thesis they draw the controversial conclusion that the nature of human autonomy is culturally constructed, meaning that autonomy only exists to the extent that people in a particular community believe in it, and negotiate its existence. Hence, autonomy exists as far as there are corresponding rules and grammars of the communities' linguistic and cultural 'games'. According to this relativist position, human autonomy is not a natural evolved capacity but a constructed socio-cultural entity that is based on negotiations and agreements among the members of a cultural community. In this case, the relationships between autonomy and well-being within a society depend on the constructed value of autonomy in that society. If people's personal values and practices, including autonomy, fit the values structure of a society, then people experience high well-being; conversely, the misfit of individuals' and societal values regarding autonomy will lower individuals' well-being. The opposition to cultural relativism is often labelled 'cultural universalism'. Supporters of the universalist position state that autonomy is a human capacity that brings people feelings of complete lives, deep eudaimonic happiness and high psychological well-being in any cultural community regardless of the value that it has within the ideologies of these societies.

The point of view presented in this chapter tries to reconcile these perspectives by emphasizing the dialectical nature of the relationships between human autonomy, the brain and culture. The phenomena of human autonomy and self-determination sound indeterministic and unscientific only if the scholars use the idea of a centuries-old mechanistic, 'bottom-up' Cartesian determinism. It is stated here that in order to understand the deterministic power of self-governance, researchers should use a systems-theory-based notion of systemic emergent properties and the idea of 'top-down' causation of these properties on the components of the systems. It is also argued that neither the relativist nor the universalist position reflects the complexity of the relations between autonomous individuals and their cultural communities. These relations are dialectical, meaning that culture is absolutely necessary for human autonomy to develop from potentiality to actuality; but, when autonomy has been fully developed, an autonomous person can reflect on the cultural influences and prescriptions and either endorse or reject them, thus becoming relatively independent of socio-cultural influences. With regard to people's happiness and well-being, this argument leads to the statement that as soon as people have developed and started exercising their autonomous agency, they will experience eudaimonic happiness, the happiness of being rational, self-governed, and fully functioning human beings. Experiencing this kind of happiness does not depend on the ideology and value of autonomy within a community.

A Conceptual Framework

Philosophers, social scientists, and psychologists use various concepts to describe the phenomenon which this book is devoted to: *autonomy* (Paul, Miller, & Paul, 2003; Ryan, Deci, Grolnick, & La Guardia, 2006; Taylor, 2005), *freedom and free will* (Baer et al., 2008; Dennett, 1986, 2003; Pink, 1996), *agency* (Martin, Sugerman, & Thompson, 2003; Mele, 2005; Taylor, 1985), *psychological* and *autonomous agency* (Frie, 2008; Mele, 2001) and *self-determination* (Deci & Ryan, 2002). An elaborated analysis of these concepts indicates that they all refer to the same very complex psychological and socio-cultural phenomenon, each highlighting different aspects of it.

Following the conceptual framework of the SDT (Ryan & Deci, 2004; Ryan et al., 2006) and expanding it by using the works of philosophers, including the interpretations of the Stoics (Cooper, 2003), Spinoza (Uyl, 2003) and Kant (Guyer, 2003), as well as social scientists and the psychologists mentioned above, the following conceptual network can be suggested. *Human psychological autonomy*,[1] which should be differentiated from *biological* (Varela, 1979) and *political* autonomy, can be divided into at least two forms: *personal autonomy* and *motivational autonomy*. *Personal autonomy*[2] is a condition of people's lives when they are self-ruled,

---

[1] From Ancient Greek αὐτονομία (autonomia), from αὐτόνομος (autonomos) 'having its own laws', from αὐτός (autos-'self') + νόμος (nomos-'law'). (Concise Oxford English Dictionary, Soanes & Stevenson, 2008).

[2] Philosophers have also labeled this form of autonomy *global* or *dispositional autonomy* (Oshana, 2003).

self-directed, and self-governed[3] by self-generated or freely internalized rules and norms, that become their laws regarding the choices of the ends and directions of their lives. The 'laws' of personal autonomy include moral norms, personal life-goals and ways of life, and personal philosophies. These laws are built on the awareness of one's own needs and capacities, on the consideration of the needs, goals, and personal autonomy of other people, as well as of the needs and goals of communities and societies; they are governed by reflective and rational reasoning. In order to rule one's life, these laws should be developed in a self-determined manner based on the adequate knowledge of how the world works, followed by reflections on one's own capacities, internal pressures from sensual and biological desires as well as the demands and expectations of other people. When these 'laws' are fully developed, the person must care about them. People are considered to be personally autonomous if they use these 'laws' to govern their lives and if they stay true to them regardless of their social disapproval or life hardships.

Motivational autonomy[4] is a particular case of the self-regulation of people's actions and behaviours in specific contexts and situations, which is "characterized by an open processing of possibilities and a matching of these with sensibilities, needs and known constraints" (Ryan et al., 2006, p. 797). It is usually an act of self-directedness when the agents experience authority over and ownership of their specific behaviours: academic, work, physical exercises, health maintaining, etc. (Ryan et al., 2006). Typically, personally autonomous individuals govern their behaviours through autonomous motivation, but not always. Personally non-autonomous individuals may also have episodes of motivational autonomy in their activities but commonly this is not the case. Motivational autonomy is also built on reflection and rational reasoning with regard to different pressures both internal – biological urges, psychological wants and desires – and external – the demands and expectations of other people regarding this particular behaviour. "Autonomy concerns how various urges, pushes, desires, primes, habits, goals, and needs from the brain, the body and the context are orchestrated within the individual" (Ryan & Deci, 2004, p. 450). A special form of behavior motivation is represented by the concept of *intrinsic motivation*, which is built on the emotions of curiosity, enjoyment and interest toward a particular activity (Deci & Ryan, 1985). It is not appropriate to label intrinsic motivation as autonomous, because it is not based on reflections and rational considerations of different constrains and options. But both of them – autonomous and intrinsic motivation – are self-determined, because they

---

[3] 'Self' in this case is understood as a centre of experience, reasoning, and acting from the perspective of a functioning person (Gallagher, 2000; May, 1961). A more through definition of self (perspectival) is provided by Martin et al (2009) which I fully endorse: "This is a self understood as an embodied first-person perspective (an 'I'), the worldly experience of which enable a constantly evolving self-understanding (a 'me') with sufficient stability and coherence to permit generally effective personal functioning in the biophysical and sociocultural world in which it develops" (p. 110).

[4] Philosophers label this form of autonomy *local autonomy* (Oshana, 2003); SDT psychologists call it *autonomous motivation*.

both emanate from a person's self, but through different psychological mechanisms. Both personal and motivational autonomy can be conceptualized as a continuum from autonomous to heteronomous or controlled forms of regulations (Ryan & Deci, 2000b). SDT considers human autonomy in both forms as a fundamental psychological need (Ryan & Deci, 2000a) because, when fully exercised, it brings to people feelings of deep satisfaction and eudaimonic pleasure that is incomparable with the pleasure of gratified sensual or bodily desires. Together with this eudaimonic pleasure comes deep happiness and full satisfaction with one's life. Psychological autonomy is a human potentiality that can become an actual power under directed education and training within certain social conditions.

Both forms of autonomy provide a basis for *freedom of choice and actions*, which is a person's ability, as Locke worded it, "to think, or not to think; to move, or not to move, according to the preference or direction of his own mind" (from Guyer, 2003, p. 71). *Agency*, in a conventional sense, is the ability to act (Guyer, 2003, p. 74). Although some scholars (Martin et al., 2003) equate this concept with the presented understanding of autonomy,[5] I will follow the conventional understanding of this term – agency as an ability to act. The reason for this is that agency, as a person's capacity to initiate a particular behaviour, may stem from either autonomous or heteronomous sources, and therefore agency could be *autonomous* or *heteronomous* (Ryan et al., 2006). This means that a person's ability to act can be governed either by his or her own self-generated laws, or it can be based on heteronomous internal or external forces. *Self-determination* is a general term that can be applied to different aspects of human functioning, when they refer to self-initiation, self-direction, and self-guidance of one's actions. It may mean a self-determined reasoning that creates personal laws for one's behaviour or an ability to live according one's own laws (being a self-determined master of one's own life-goals and choices) or being a one's own source of particular behaviours (self-determined motivation).

Evolutionary and Biological Basis of Human Autonomy

From an ontological point of view, psychological autonomy, self-determination, and the feeling of freedom are experiential subjective phenomena to which researchers have access only through phenomenological descriptions (Ryan & Deci, 2004; Ryan et al., 2006). On the other hand, they are real psychological phenomena that exist independently of our own and other people's beliefs or opinions about them, and, thus, they can be the objects of an empirical scientific analysis. This fact of the subjective and experiential nature of autonomy and self-determination makes

---

[5]"... Human agency is the deliberate, reflective activity of a human being in framing, choosing, and executing his or her actions in a way that is not fully determined by factors and conditions other than his or her own understanding and reasoning. Such other factors and conditions include external constrains and coercions, as well as intentional constrains over which the person has no conscious control." (Martin et al., 2003, p. 82).

the exploration of their biological and neurophysiological natures a very complex and sophisticated endeavour. A new discipline – 'neurophenomenology'[6] (Varela, Thomson, & Rosch, 1991) – has emerged to study the neurophysiological basis of these and related mental phenomena (David, Newen, & Vogeley, 2008; Libet, Freeman, & Sutherland, 1999; Schwabe & Blanke, 2007).

The proposition that autonomy exists as a real psychological capability implies that it has evolved during evolution and that the human biological make-up should support it. That is why it is not surprising that scholars have been trying to find these evolutionary and biological roots of human autonomy and freedom (Dennett, 2003; Libet et al., 1999; Ryan, Kuhl, & Deci, 1997; Varela, 1979; Waller, 1998). Dennett (2003) stated that an increase of the degrees of freedom of living creatures has accompanied every step of their evolution: from bacteria to plants, to animals, and, finally, to human beings. However, human freedom is fundamentally different from animal freedom: although animals can enjoy many more degrees of freedom than plants – birds may fly whenever they want – it is only human freedom that is based on a language-shaped ability for conscious and rational reflection on the ends and means of one's everyday actions and life, including one's own death. It is logical to assume that this evolved psychological autonomy – when human beings are able to reflect on their desires and urges, postpone them, and generate options for acting by rationally evaluating these options before their execution – has brought humans survival advantages that are incomparable in their benefits to the ones that animals have.

Our body, including our brain, is equipped to exercise autonomy, free will, and self-determination (Libet et al., 1999). 'Is equipped' does not mean a direct and hard-wired neurophysiological determination of autonomy – there is no a centre for autonomy in our brain; instead it means that the human brain is capable of producing symbolic mental representations which, as I show later, lie at the basis of human autonomy and self-determination. The emergence of psychological autonomy is a result of systemic organismic processes and is a fundamental characteristic of the human species (Juarrero, 1999; Martin et al., 2003; Murphy & Brown, 2007; Ryan et al., 1997). Our ability to have and to exercise autonomous agency is inherited in our evolutionary based biological make-up as a potentiality, and it does not automatically, click on when a child is born. It develops through the physical and linguistic interactions of an active human organism, which is equipped with the specialized brain, with its social and symbolic environments (Martin, 2008). In order to understand the organization of the biological and neurophysiological basis of autonomy, scientists should stop contemplating this capability in terms of mechanistic determinism and should instead use systemic, organismic, and dialectical thinking.

---

[6]Neuromenological is an academic discipline that mixes neuroscience and phenomenological observation; this is also a science that studies the neurophysiological basis of human's different states of consciousness.

The Systems and Organismic Approach to Autonomy as an Emergent Property

The thesis that will be presented in this section can be formulated in the following way. Human autonomy and self-determination are real psychological powers of the conscious mind. They are emergent systemic qualities of a complex hierarchical system of the human body embedded into physical and socio-cultural worlds. The existence of these psychological powers does not contradict the idea of determinism, as long as this idea is substantially upgraded from the centuries-old Cartesian-Newtonian bottom-up mechanistic determinism to the modern conception of the top-down determinism in complex hierarchical organismic systems (Juarrero, 1999; McDonough, 1997; Murphy & Brown, 2007; Sheldon, 2004).

According to the systems approach, humans' brains, bodies, actions, and whole lives could be represented as the systems that are made up of nested low-level sub-systems that function through constant interactions with these systems' environments: physical, social, and symbolic. When these systems are in place and functioning, new properties, including mental ones, emerge (Murphy & Stoeger, 2007). These emergent mental phenomena demonstrate new causal powers that are not exhibited by the constituents of these systems and cannot be deduced from the laws pertaining to them (Murphy & Brown, 2007; Murphy & Stoeger, 2007; Sperry, 1991). Some systems theorists have also called these properties the 'holistic' properties (Murphy, et al., 2007, p. 80). "The existence and relative autonomy of holistic properties and of a kind of top-down influence over the properties and dynamics of systems constituents remain both the key defining character and the most criticized claim of arguments for emergence" (Murphy, et al., 2007, p. 80). People's consciousness, rationality, and autonomous agency are examples of these emergent holistic mental phenomena (Juarrero, 1999). One of the fundamental capacities of these mental properties is their ability to exert a top-down or downward causation on the components of the system that produced them: emotions, desires, behaviours, and thoughts. In the case of psychological autonomous agency, this downward causation represents the self-determination of human behaviour. This self-determination should not be interpreted as a mystical and undeterministic 'divine' power, or as an unscientific 'homunculus', but as a biologically-based natural human capacity to exercise the power of downward causation. This downward self-determinism of high-level systems is exerted through the constraints that the systems impose on their parts by changing the probability of the components' behavior. These constraints are not external material or energetic forces that coerce the systems and their parts to change, but intra-systemic relational properties that limit or close off alternatives for the components' behavior based on the states of other components, the history of the previous states of the systems, and because of the context in which the systems are embedded (Juarrero, 1999; Murphy, et al., 2007). In the case of human psychological autonomy this self-determination means that a mindful person who functions in physical and socio-symbolic environments, and who can be considered as a high-level system, acquires the emergent property to impose limits on this system's components: emotions, primary desires, images, thoughts, and actions. This property is a basis of human autonomy. Thus, self-determination and autonomy are real and powerful forces and should be studied as any other psychological phenomena. "...We are not merely products of environment plus biology, but are causal players in our own right, and this in such a way as (potentially) to be the most significant creator of ourselves. We are (somewhat) autonomous, self-directed shapers of our own future character and behaviour" (Murphy, et al., 2007, p. 86).

It is important to note that, according to Juarrero (1999), the higher-level neuro-socio- psychological systems, which produce emergent properties, have more degrees of freedom and greater repertoires of actions than any of their constituent components. This means that a person who exercises autonomous agency and self-determination has an increased capability not only of constraining various emotional reactions and motivational urges (which are the components of the low-level regulatory systems) that he or she considers inappropriate, but also of making choices that would not have been available if this person were guided only by these emotions and motivations. Therefore, such systems become self-maintaining and relatively stable constructions with a dramatic increase of qualitatively new alternatives and options on a systemic level. This systemic autonomy and self-regulation manifests in people's orientation toward their future and in their ability to impose constraints on those interfering forces that may prevent their movement along this orientation. Consequently, autonomous human beings have the capability not only of constraining their emotions and thoughts that do not meet the requirements of a current situation, but they also acquire an increased opportunity to develop new and creative ways of dealing with various circumstances that arise in life. It is logical to expect that such systems will have a higher level of durability and stability over time that, in psychological language, could be translated as high psychological strength, positive well-being, and better mental health.

Applying the evolutionary principle to human actions, Murphy and Brown (2007, pp. 110–131) suggested the following hierarchy of the regulation of the behaviours of living beings. (1) *Reflexive regulation behaviour* is based on the mechanisms of various visceral reflexes. In humans, this form of behaviour is represented in the homeostatic responses of the autonomous nervous system, or in the stable patterns of repetitive movements, such as walking, running, and similar habitual skills; (2) *Unreflective adaptable behaviour* regulation is based on trial-and-error learning and learning by imitation. In human beings, this type of behaviour is difficult to disentangle from a chain of purposeful actions in which they are typically embedded. An example of this is learning to ride a bicycle, where verbal instructions could do very little above the pure trial-and-error way of acquiring a new feeling of the balancing a body over a swinging base. There is a sub-category of this behaviour known as '*post-reflective – automatic' behaviour*, the actions that were reflective at the beginning of their learning (driving, for example) eventually become automatic. Some modern psychologists (Bargh & Ferguson, 2000; Bargh, 2008) have recently embossed these types of behaviours on their shields as they fight against a more adequate understanding of reflective and deliberate freedom of rational thinking; (3) *Reflective adaptive regulation of actions* represents an exclusively human form of behavioural adaptation. All its forms, both non-symbolic, which may also found in some animals, and symbolic "are mediated by…some form of neural/mental representation of the situation and possibilities for action" (Murphy et al., 2007, p. 120).

The most relevant for our analysis are *symbolic reflective actions,* which are regulated by language-based mental representations of external and internal states of affairs. An important property of these symbolic representations is their ability to reflect relations among other similar representations as well as among lower-level mental representations. This capacity to signify relations and the relational properties of the world allows human beings to construct abstract concepts and associations among them; this power of abstraction gives people freedom from their immediate environment and biological states. Consequently, this freedom from the immediacy of a particular situation constitutes, according to Murphy and Brown (2007), the first emancipating property of symbolic representations. The second one is their ability to represent the minds of other individuals and, through developing the mental representations of social relationships, to open unlimited opportunities for social communication. The third emancipating attribute of humans' symbolic representations is their capacity to construct probable scenarios of potential actions and, as a result, to mentally play out various alternatives of behaviours before executing them. The fourth feature of these representations is their capability to symbolize the process of a person's own mental activity, including emotional, motivational, and cognitive processes, and make them the objects of one's attention, reflective understanding, and contemplation. Thus, through the emergence of symbolic representations, human beings acquire the ability to not only be aware of their environment and mentally distance themselves from it, but also to reflect upon the pattern of one's own reactions to this environment and distance oneself from them as well. With these symbolic representations in place, people's autonomy and self-determination acquire their foundation and substantiation. As philosopher Deacon stated, "symbolic analysis is the basis for a remarkable new level of self-determination that human beings alone have stumbled upon. The ability to use virtual reference to build up elaborate internal models of possible futures, and to hold these complex visions in mind with the force of the mnemonic glue of symbolic inference and descriptive shorthand, gives us unprecedented capacity to generate independent adaptive behaviours" (Deacon, 1997, p. 434). Thus, the emergence of symbolic representations in the human species, as a new regulative medium, constitutes a fundamental evolutionary break-through that makes human autonomy and self-determination possible. The two fundamental constituents of emergent autonomy are the human brain and socio-cultural environment, which I will analyze in the following sections.

The Brain, Frontal Lobes, and Human Autonomy

The neurophysiological evidence regarding the biological basis of human autonomy came from studies of humans' volitional acts and of the processes of decision making while choosing different courses of actions (Libet et al., 1999). After evaluating several accounts of the neurophysiological correlates of human volition and freedom of will (David et al., 2008; Farrer & Frith, 2002; Koechlin, Ody, & Kouneiher, 2003; Libet et al., 1999; Spence & Frith, 1999), the following synopsis can be provided. According to these neuroscientists, several areas of the frontal lobes together with various sub-cortical structures are associated with deciding when to act, which actions to perform, and the feeling of ownership of these actions. These areas include, but are not limited to, the Dorsolateral Prefrontal Cortex (DLPFC) with its connections with another cortical area – the Posterior Parietal Cortex (PPC) – together with their involvement with subcortical structures, such as the anterior cingulae, the supplementary motor aria (SMA) and the basal ganglia. According to Fuster (2002), the prefrontal lobes execute four main functions: (1) they conduct the temporal integration of behaviour with regard to biological and cognitive goals; (2) they organize working memory, that allows one to manipulate the information that is directly involved in the execution of a volitional action; (3) they prepare the organism for an action by creating a preparatory set; and, finally (4) they execute an inhibitory control over the internal and external impulses that may interfere with the planned action. This is how Spencer et al. describe the architectonics of volitional actions: "Thinking about what we are going to do before we do it clearly requires some form of mental representation of intended actions.... The parietal lobe probably contains representations of intended actions.... DLPFC seems to be involved in keeping possible actions in mind before they are executed, and selecting which one will be performed" (Spence & Frith, 1999, p. 27). PPC contributes to the programming of movements in space, while the subcortical structures (SMA in particular) participate in the planning of behavioural acts in time. It is likely that these structures also participate in the execution of movements, perhaps after the selection is made by DLPFC, but before their 'delegation' to the motor cortex and spinal cord (Spence & Frith, 1999, p. 22). The experiments of Koechlin and colleagues (2003) demonstrated that the control that is executed by the frontal lobes is organized and functions in a nested top-down manner, supporting the above presented propositions that human volitions can be found in the systemic organization of the brain's regulatory systems.

Despite this relatively elaborated picture of the neurophysiological mechanisms of a free-chosen action, Spence and Frith (1999) rightly remarked that "even the most simple motor procedures require complex (and distributed) neuronal activity. This serves to emphasize the prematurity of pondering the 'localization of free will!'" (p. 23). When extended to the execution of self-determined actions within the course of one's autonomous life, this comment sends an even clearer message: that human autonomy is not a hard-wired neurologically function, rather it is an emergent property of a healthy brain and healthy social conditions that, in its fullest manifestation, could not be traced back to highly specialized regions of the brain. Another implication of this message is that neurophysiology alone cannot be the primary source of our understanding of the nature and basis of autonomy. As Martin et al. (2003) mentioned, the brain is *required* for autonomous agency to function, but this does not mean that the brain *determines* it. Thus, although human autonomy and self-determination are evolutionary evolved fundamental properties of each and every human being that are based on the functioning of the healthy human brain, these functions are not the ultimate sources for our understanding of human autonomy. In order to do this, we need to examine the role socio-cultural conditions play in the emergence and operation of human autonomy.

The Role of Culture and Society in Shaping Human Autonomy, Well-Being, and Their Relations

The application of the systems approach to the role of culture in the emergence of human autonomy requires dialectical thinking to understand the interactive dynamics among all the constituents (Kagan, 2004; McCrone, 1999). The thesis to defend here is: Culture[7] – a cultural community of people who, through sharing language and other symbolical features, negotiate the meanings and practices that govern their lives – is absolutely important for the emergence of symbolic representations as a necessary prerequisite for symbolic reflective actions. Any socio-cultural community and any language can serve this function of promoting the development of symbolic capabilities. As soon as the symbolic representations are in place, they start the realization of their four functions: (1) providing mental distance from and mediating interactions with one's immediate environment; (2) planning future actions and constructing various potential arrangements of these actions before executing them; (3) opening opportunities to reflect on the individual's own regulative activity: wants, desires, and thoughts; and (4) contributing to the understanding of the minds of people with whom an individual interacts. These four functions of the symbolic representations constitute the basis of people's autonomous agency. However, this agency can attain full capacity only if a person is trained in using these functions properly and efficiently.

This is the second point where the socio-cultural environment plays a decisive role in shaping human autonomy. This role is three-fold: to show young individuals that they have this symbolic reflective capacity, to stress its importance, and to train them in the appropriate use of it. This training could include learning the skills of postponing reactions to immediate environmental and internal (bodily and psychological) demands, gaining competence in reflecting on one's own reactions to these demands, developing the habits of contemplating and planning further actions, and taking into consideration the thoughts and feelings of other people in planning one's responses (Kagan, 2004; Martin, 2008). There is one more component that emerges during this process of socialization through the appropriate usage of the symbolic representations. In terms of systems theory, Murphy and Brown (2007) defined it

---

[7] By 'Culture' (capital 'C') I mean a fundamental capacity of human beings to construct a socio-symbolic reality that constitutes the essence of their living environments. By 'cultures' (small 'c'), I mean particular representations of these symbolic arrangements of living environments in the forms of ethnic and national cultures (Islamic cultures, the cultures of Aboriginal people, a culture of middle-class urban citizens, etc.).

a '*supervisory system*' which consists of 'meta-organizer' and 'meta-comparator' (pp. 129–131). The function of this system is to guide a goal-setting process for higher-order regulatory systems. In psychological terms this meta-supervisory system is represented by values, life-goals, and world-views that people internalize from their socio-cultural environments during their socialization and develop in later years as an autonomous system of their own moral laws and values. People use these life-values to inhibit their impulses and actions that do not correspond to the attainment of these values and to set goals for future actions.

When this system of symbolic representations at different levels is in place and all the relevant skills of using it are learned, a person has all the prerequisites to exercise his or her autonomy and enjoy all the benefits it provides: the feeling of freedom, the fullness of life, eudaimonic well-being, creativity, and many others. Moreover, as soon as people develop and endorse an autonomous way of living and acting, they become relatively free from the constraining demands of their socio-cultural contexts that provided the conditions for the emergence of their autonomy, as people now can reflect on these conditions, understand them, and act in accord or against their prescriptions. This is how sociologist Riesman, in his highly influential book "The Lonely Crowd" (2001/1961), described autonomous people and their relations with their society. "Autonomous person... possessed clear-cut, internalized goals..., was capable of choosing his goals and modulating his pace. The goals, and the drive toward them, were rational, nonauthoritarian and noncompulsive..." (p. 250). Autonomous individuals are "capable of transcending their culture" (p. 245); they "...are free to choose whether to conform or not" (p. 242); their "acceptance of social and political authority is always conditional" (p, 251); and they "can cooperate with others in actions while maintaining the right of private judgment" (p. 251). Thus, an autonomous person is a person who can understand his or her culture and overrule it. Martin et al. (2003) labeled this condition as the *under* determination of autonomous agents by culture, meaning that the determining power of the cultural context, which was crucial in the emergence and development of autonomous regulation, can now be overruled, resisted or even transformed. If an autonomous agency is *under* determined by both brain and culture (Martin, et al., 2003), then nothing is left to explain it except by referring to people's self-determination, the determination that is built on their own values, norms, and rules for acting. This self-determination is accompanied by people's reflections on external and internal demands and processes and provides a deeply gratifying experience of owing one's actions and a feeling of being the master of one's own behavior and destiny.

This is where the third aspect of cultural influence comes into play. After autonomous regulation has been developed in people, the socio-cultural community may play a twofold role in influencing the functioning of this regulation. It may facilitate the performance of autonomous agents by providing the means and conditions under which they can exercise this emergent capacity to the fullest extent, or the community may impede the realization of this ability and hinder its manifestation either partially or completely. A nearly complete obstruction of autonomy and freedom is observed in totalitarian regimes. As Riesman noted, "... while it is possible to be autonomous no matter how tight the supervision of behaviour as long as thoughts are free,... most men need the opportunity for some freedom of behaviour if they are to develop and confirm their autonomy of character " (p. 250). The majority of restrictive societies allow their members to exercise autonomy and freedom only in particular domains of their lives or at particular periods of their lives. For example, married women in South Asian families acquire their autonomy and a feeling of freedom when they have reached middle-age and have a fully-functioning household (Shweder, Much, Mahapatra, & Park, 2003), while Indians have a spiritual sphere to exercise their autonomy (Roland, 1988). But even in more restrictive periods of their lives people still have the capability for psychological autonomy, autonomy of thoughts, reflections and hopes (Ali & Haq, 2006; Devine, Camfield, & Gough, 2008; Ewing, 1991).

Why autonomy is considered the fundamental prerequisite for people's well-being and happiness? Following Kant's theorizing (Guyer, 2000, 2003), it is possible to state that our deepest pleasure in life is activity itself and the promotion of life through it. But the only human activity that can promote a full life is the activity that we execute freely. Thus, according to Kant, autonomy is essential to the promotion of life and the greatest pleasures that come with it (Guyer, 2000). Therefore, the well-being and happiness of an autonomous person depends mostly on the deepest feeling of vitality that comes with this, as Kant said, "free and regular play of all of the powers and faculties of the human being" (cited by Guyer, 2003, p. 84). As soon as people reach the state of autonomy and self-determination, their well-being becomes determined mostly by the life-force of their autonomy. In societies that thwart this capability, the manifestation of this state will be less behaviourally visible, but the autonomy of thoughts, reflections, and judgments may stay mostly intact. Thus, autonomy will never go away and never become detrimental to a person's well-being; in this state of autonomous agency, people acquire such great psychological strength and empowerment that no external circumstances can demolish. An autonomous person, as the Stoics said, can be happy in any dire situation and in any conditions (Irvine, 2009).

Cultures of Horizontality and Verticality in Promoting Autonomy and Self-Determination

No existing society is completely autonomy supportive or autonomy thwarting. Real communities have the elements of both tendencies, but in different proportions. In this section I want to ask the following questions: What types of societal, communal, and interpersonal relations are conducive toward the development and exercise of human autonomy? And which ones hinder it?

Two of the greatest philosophers of autonomy, Spinoza and Kant, highlighted the social conditions necessary for experiencing autonomy, freedom and the happiness that depends on them. These conditions are cooperation, friendship, sympathy to other human beings, and egalitarian associations (Guyer, 2003; Uyl, 2003). Based on these insights, and following the arguments of the modern scholars presented below, I want to argue that those communities that guide their citizens' social lives by the values of trust, respect toward people's privacy and individuality, tolerance to differences among people, feelings of equality between people, and willingness to share resources, ideas, feelings, and thoughts, are the communities that will be more successful in promoting autonomy and good lives for their members. The contrasting anti-egalitarian communities build their social relations around a hierarchical distribution of power by endorsing the values of obedience and loyalty to those in power and the practices of authoritarian control by powerful members of the community over less powerful members. I hypothesise that the nature of these hierarchical relationships works against supporting and facilitating human autonomy, self-determination and, correspondently, people's happiness. Such hierarchical communities will be much less conducive and, in the extreme forms of totalitarian regimes, strongly detrimental to the development and realization of autonomy and consequently to the promotion of people's good lives and happiness.

Chirkov, Lebedeva, Molodtsova, and Tatarko (in press) labelled the first type of societal arrangement as the *culture of horizontality* and the second one as the *culture of verticality*. Both cultures are multi-layered social arrangements that contain a proximal circle of corresponding relations that includes family, school, workplace, neighbourhood and similar communities/institutions wherein people usually interact with each other face to face. These cultures also encompass distal circles of social relationships, including governmental policies, systems of relations among different social institutions and the relations of these institutions with the members of a society. Important aspects of this distal circle are the political arrangements in a society, society's basic political values and the foundational principles of political governance.

On a political level, the culture of horizontality is represented by democratic, libertarian, and egalitarian systems of values and political arrangements. On a social level, it is well grasped by the notion of *social capital* in its different forms (Fukuyama, 2002; Grootaert & van Bastelaer, 2001; Portes, 1998), and on a socio-psychological level horizontality corresponds to 'authoritative/democratic parenting' (Baumrind, 1971), 'autonomy supportive relations' and 'relations that facilitate basic psychological needs satisfaction' (Grolnick, Ryan, & Deci, 1997; Ryan et al., 2006). The culture of verticality is comprised by autocratic political values and relations, by the vertical components of social capital (Grootaert & van Bastelaer, 2001), and by 'authoritarian parenting' (Baumrind, 1971) and 'controlling relationships' on a more proximal level of relations.

Following the conventional classification of cultures (Triandis, 1995), Chirkov et al. discussed the collectivistic and individualistic aspects of both horizontality and verticality. *Horizontal collectivism* is a set of norms and practices that are built around the values of cooperation, interdependence, and solidarity and that are practiced on the background of the norms of equality and respect for each member of a community regardless of his or her social status. People who endorse horizontal collectivism on a psychological level take into account and acknowledge other people's needs and goals and attribute to them the same level of respect as one gives to oneself. They mindfully listen to other people's opinions and perspectives and take them into account when making their decisions. This type of interpersonal relation has been labelled 'dialogical' (Bakhtin, 1984; Buber, 2002), 'democratic' (Lewin & Lippitt, 1938) and 'autonomy supportive' (Ryan et al., 2006).

Lawrence Kohlberg (Kohlberg, Boyd, and Levine, 1990), a moral developmental psychologist, is famous for his defence of the widely discussed Stage 6 of moral development. This stage, which could be labelled a stage of moral autonomy, represents the ability of a mature person to develop and act upon self-generated moral imperatives. When discussing the social conditions that facilitate the development of this type of autonomy, this scholar and his colleagues (Kohlberg et al., 1990) stressed such norms and practices as *respect for another person*, consisting of the feelings of *justice*, *benevolence*, and *active sympathy*. These conditions could also be accompanied by relations and attitudes of *reciprocity* and *equality*. According to Kohlberg, these social relations are crucially important in order to maintain an individual's personal and ego identity's integrity, which lies at the centre of the Stage 6 moral autonomy. Habermas (1990) complemented these conditions by emphasising *solidarity* as a necessary collectivistic component of horizontal relations. His point was that in addition to maintaining the identity integrity of an individual, it is crucially important to maintain one's group integrity, otherwise there will be no medium in which to exercise one's autonomy:

> Every autonomous morality has to serve two purposes at once: it brings to bear the inviolability of socialized individuals by requiring equal treatment and thereby equal respect for the dignity of each one [a horizontal component of the horizontal collectivistic dimension –VC]; and it protects intersubjective relationships of mutual recognition requiring solidarity of individual members of community, in which they have been socialized [the collectivistic component of the same dimension – VC]. Justice [another horizontal component– VC] concerns the equal freedoms of unique and self-determining individuals [an individualistic component of horizontal relations – VC], while solidarity concerns the welfare of consocates who are intimately linked in an intersubjectively shared form of life – thus also to the maintenance of the integrity of this form of life itself [underlined by me, VC] (p. 244).

If we interpret this statement not in terms of the purposes of autonomous morality, but as a description of the conditions in a community that promote this form of morality: respect, benevolence, justice, and solidarity, all of which facilitate and promote human personal autonomy, we will get a presentation of horizontal collectivism (and partially individualism) nearly in its purest form. Similar ideas have recently been expressed by Sen (2009).

Another component of the culture of horizontality is *horizontal individualism*. A full account of the ideology of horizontal individualism, as well as its antipode – the culture of verticality – was presented by Lukes (1973). He identified four fundamental ideas of this ideology: value for human dignity, autonomy, privacy, and self-development. Respect for human dignity is a paramount and fundamental moral value of individualism: every human being is an end in him or herself and cannot be a means for any other end. Value for human autonomy and privacy are two interconnected and pivotal concerns of the ideology of horizontal individualism. Lukes's understanding of autonomy is in full concordance with the above provided conceptualization of it.[8] But he also stressed that autonomy "has... been widely held as a moral value – a condition of the individual that should be increased or maximized. It is a value central to the morality of modern Western civilization, and it is absent or understressed in others (such as many tribal moralities or that of orthodox communism in Eastern Europe today [1973 – VC])" (p. 58). This statement is very important as it differentiates autonomy as a psychological phenomenon – a state of rational reflections – from autonomy as a value within the ideology of a society. Privacy is "an area within which the individual is or should be left alone by others and able to do and think whatever he chooses – to pursue his own good in his own way, as Mill put it" (p. 59). Respect for privacy is a respect for a person's right to have the space and time to be oneself in an unrestricted and self-determined way. The last value of individualism is the individual's right for self-development with regard to his or her uniqueness and individuality. To summarize the ideas of individualism, Lukes used the words of Mill that "the only freedom which deserves the name, is that of pursuing our own good in our own way, so long as we do not attempt to deprive others of theirs, or impede their efforts to obtain it" (p. 64). It is worth mentioning that Lukes warned against the dangers of overemphasizing people's embeddedness into sociality to the extent of washing out their right to be autonomous. He mentioned numerous past and current attempts to dissolve these four fundamental individualistic values in the embracing communalities of religion, political parties, or professional associations. If people's autonomy is shifted to the higher order 'social selves' and from there to the complete identification with one's collectivity, then, as Lukes warned, freedom can be turned into servitude.

The culture of verticality is also built around the ideologies of collectivism and individualism. *Vertical collectivism* is a dimension that emphasizes obedience and sacrifice to one's community (comparable to solidarity) and obedience and submission to authority figures (Lukes, 1973). *Vertical individualism* is represented by the competitiveness of an individual against other people within the existing hierarchy of power, wealth, and status (de Botton, 2004). People who endorse and exercise vertical relations do this at the expense of their own and other people's personal autonomy and freedom. Lukes (1973) connected the presence of verticality with a lack of horizontal individualism in all its four manifestations and with a lack of support for personal autonomy:

> We cease to respect someone when we fail to treat him as an agent and a chooser, as a self from which actions and choices emanate, when we see him and consequently treat him not as a person but as merely the bearer of a title or the player of a role, or as merely a means of securing a certain end, or worse of all, as merely an object. We deny his status as an autonomous person when we allowed our attitudes to him to be dictated solely by some contingent and socially defined attribute of him, such as his place in the social

---

[8] "... an individual is autonomous (at the social level) to the degree to which he subjects the pressures and norms with which he is confronted to conscious and critical evaluation, and forms intentions and reaches practical decisions as the result of independent and rational reflection" (Lukes, 1973, p. 52).

order or his occupational role.... There are other ways of denying someone's autonomy and thereby failing to respect him. One way is simply to control or dominate his will; another is unreasonably to restrict the range of alternatives between which he can choose; but perhaps the most insidious and decisive way is to diminish, or restrict the opportunity to increase, his consciousness of his situation and his activities. Secondly, one manifestly fails to respect someone if one invades his private space and interferes, without good reason, with the valued activities.... Finally, I claim that one also importantly fails to respect someone if one limits or restricts his opportunities to realize his capacities of self-development (pp. 133–134).

Thus, it is logical to conclude that the culture of horizontality, especially in its individualistic component, is a necessary condition for promoting people's autonomy and consequently for cultivating their happy lives, whereas the culture of verticality is detrimental to the development of these capacities. Current cross-cultural quality-of-life surveys convincingly support this conclusion (Veenhoven, 1999). Some of the empirical SDT-based evidence detailing the role the culture of horizontality plays in people's functioning is reported in the following section and also in other chapters.

To conclude this section, I want to state that human autonomy is a cross-culturally universal human capability even though it is dependent on Culture (capital 'C') for its emergence and complete functioning. Culture enables autonomy, but cultures may almost kill it. Culture leads human autonomy from potentiality to actuality, and people may exercise this capacity to different extents within their lives under the conditions of their particular cultures. In the societies where the culture of horizontality prevails over the culture of verticality and where horizontality is exercised in the most important areas of a society's functionings – parenting, education, work, and politics – autonomous individuals flourish. Because hierarchical relations are inevitable in any society, these horizontal societies exercise different measures to control the manifestations of the verticality, thus limiting its detrimental influences on human autonomy. But in the societies where the culture of verticality prevails over the culture of horizontality, especially if it is strong in parenting, education, work relations, and politics, the members of these societies have limited opportunities for developing their capacity for autonomy and self-determination and, as a result, to enjoy the benefits of it. As a result of the limits imposed on people's autonomy and freedom, these societies may suffer from poverty, corruption, low productivity and many other social and political diseases.

The Empirical Support of the Cross-National Universality of the Relations of Autonomy and Happiness

In this section I will provide some empirical evidence from various SDT-guided research that supports the above-presented arguments regarding the facilitating roles human autonomy and self-determination play in promoting people's happiness across cultures.

SDT is one of the few psychological theories that directly addresses the issue of the autonomous regulation of people's lives and behaviour and the consequences this type of regulation has for their health, well-being, and general functioning. This theory's operationalization of autonomy is based on above-presented definitions of motivational autonomy as a full endorsement of one's actions based on mindful reflections upon all internal and external forces of one's motivation. Following Heider's attributional theorizing (Heider, 1982/1958), SDT researchers have labelled the result of these reflections as the 'Perceived Locus of Causality' (PLOC) (Ryan et al., 2006). People may experience their motivations as coming either from within or from outside their selves. The former type of experience has been labelled 'internal locus of causality' and the corresponding motivational forces have been called 'autonomous or self-determined motivation'. If people experience these forces streaming from outside their selves, this 'external locus of causality' is believed to be accompanied by 'controlled motivation'. Consequently, people's experiences of these loci of causality and their reports about them are SDT's operational 'window' into the phenomenological dynamics of motivational autonomy. SDT researchers have standardized the experience of the autonomous and controlled forms of motivation along four types of motivational regulations (Ryan & Connell, 1989): *external* – the experience of being forced to do something through rewards, punishments or direct coercion; *introjected* – the experience of being driven by the internalized expectations of others; *identified* – value-based acting; and *integrated* – the decision to act in a certain way based on the reflections on one's needs, goals, values, and constraining circumstances. SDT researchers also distinguish *intrinsic motivation* as another type of self-determined motivation. Intrinsic motivation is not based on reasoning and reflections about being in a situation, but instead is generated by unconditional curiosity, interest, and the enjoyment of the process of behaviour regardless of the rewards and outcomes that may follow.

SDT is built upon the assumption that autonomous motivation can be experienced by people all over the world. In order to test this thesis, SDT researchers took great care to ensure that their operationalization of autonomous and controlled motivation was unanimously understandable and usable across different countries and societies. Several studies have directly addressed the statistical invariance of the SDT-based scales of autonomous motivation across time, genders and cultures (Chirkov & Ryan, 2001; Chirkov, Ryan, Kim, & Kaplan, 2003; Grouzet, Otis, & Pelletier, 2006; Legault, Green-Demers, & Pelletier, 2005; Roth, Assor, Kanat-Maymon, & Kaplan, 2006). When accompanied by the examination of the linguistic invariance of these scales across different languages, ethnicities, and nations (Hagger, Chatzisarantis, Barkoukis, Wang, & Baranowski, 2005; Hayamizu, 1997; Rudy, Sheldon, Awong, & Tan, 2007; Tanaka & Yamauchi, 2000; Vallerand, Blais, Brière, & Pelletier, 1989; Vansteenkiste, Zhou, Lens, & Soenens, 2005; Yamauchi & Tanaka, 1998), these studies demonstrate that these SDT-based operationalizations of autonomy are linguistically meaningful and applicable to participants from different nations, societies and ethno-linguistic groups.

According to SDT scholars, motivational autonomy is a fundamental factor in promoting people's optimal functioning, creativity, and physical and psychological well-being. Most of the chapters in this book deal with these topics, so I will not repeat them. Instead I will highlight only the most important aspects of the above thesis. As was mentioned above, the main argument of the psychologists who deny the universally beneficial role of autonomy in people's functioning is that the constructs of autonomy and self-determination, together with such cultural values as individualism, liberalism, independence, self-reliance and many others, are the socio-cultural constructions of the Western civilisation and are not (or are only partially) applicable to the rest of the world that is depicted as less individualistic and more collectivistic or group-oriented (Markus & Kitayama, 2003). According to this view, autonomy is a socially constructed value, and its meaning is differently negotiated in various socio-cultural contexts. Autonomy and self-determination are seen as culturally relative virtues, and the endorsement of the universalist view with regard to autonomy has been blamed as ethnocentric Western-based intellectual colonialism. According to SDT, personal and motivation autonomy are not cultural values but are fundamental conditions that must be in place for people's optimal functioning, and these conditions are universal across societies and cultures (see also the Chapter 1).

One study that directly addressed these debates applied the SDT construct of PLOC to various cultural practices that have been categorised in mainstream cross-cultural psychology as individualistic vs. collectivistic and horizontal vs. vertical (Chirkov et al., 2003; Chirkov, Ryan, & Willness, 2005). In these studies Chirkov and his colleagues suggested that the concepts of autonomous vs. controlled motivation could be applied to valued cultural practices the same way as to any other forms of social behaviour. They hypothesised that people could reflect on these practices and evaluate whether they fully endorse them or whether the motivation for these cultural practices is alien to their selves. Thus, the demarcation line between autonomy as an experiential feature of our personal causation and autonomy as a cultural value of individualism and independence could be drawn. The results supported the initial hypotheses. In particular, participants from six countries (Brazil, Canada, Russia, South Korea, Turkey and the USA) demonstrated that various cultural practices could be autonomously or control motivated, meaning that a person can be either autonomous or non-autonomous with regard to individualistic or collectivistic horizontal or vertical cultural practices. These data also demonstrated that higher levels of autonomous motivation were associated with better well-being outcomes in all countries. The most recent studies from a number of non-Western countries demonstrated the same pattern. Participants from South Korea and China, for example, countries where autonomy is not valued highly and is cultivated less than in Western nations, demonstrated the same understanding and endorsement of autonomous motivation and demonstrated the same beneficial effect on academic learning (Jang, Reeve, Ryan, & Kim, 2009; Vansteenkiste et al., 2005; Chapter 6 by Reeve & Assor, this volume; Chapter 11 by Helwig, this volume) work effectiveness (Chapter 8 by Gagné & Bhave, this volume), and physical health (Chapter 7 by Williams et al., this volume) as in their Western counterparts. Based on these and the numerous studies presented in other chapters of this volume, I may conclude that there is enough empirical evidence to support the statements that motivational autonomy constitutes a fundamental and universal condition for people's optimal functioning and well-being. This conclusion corresponds fully with the philosophical and psychological accounts of autonomy as a paramount state of human existence, a state in which people reach their highest point of understanding themselves in the world and which is accompanied by a full utilization of human beings' most prominent and distinguished capacities: reason, reflectivity, mindfulness, integrity, and concern for others. Without people who possess and exercise these capacities, none of the existing societies could survive.

Another set of empirical evidence is concerned with the role that socio-cultural environment – the culture of horizontality – plays in the development and functioning of motivational autonomy and, consequently, of people's well-being. Most SDT-guided studies have addressed the culture of horizontality at the most proximal levels of social psychological relations: relationships in families, schools, work settings, and health-care institutions. These researchers call them *autonomy-supportive social relationships*. The main argument of cultural determinists is that many cultures highly value obedience to authority, strict discipline, and a hierarchical, authoritarian style of parent–children, teacher–student or boss–employees relations. These scholars believe that in these societies supporting peoples' autonomy, providing them with choices, and acknowledging their feelings, thoughts, and opinions will not be appreciated and, even more, will work against their efficient functioning and optimal development (Miller, 1999). SDT researchers argue against this position, instead suggesting that autonomy support is a necessary condition to satisfy the need for autonomy to cultivate autonomous motivation, and it is universally beneficial, even within cultures in which parents or teachers do not endorse this mode of social interaction (Ryan & Deci, 2003).

The area of strongest debate around this issue regards teacher–students relations (see also Chapter 6 by Reeve & Assor, this volume). To measure perceived autonomy support, some SDT researchers have used modifications of the Teaching Climate Questionnaire, which has been translated into various languages and tested for cross-cultural validity and invariance (Chirkov & Ryan, 2001; Hagger et al., 2007). Studies of the positive role of autonomy-supportive academic and familial environments were conducted in some Western countries: Belgium (Soenens et al., 2007), Britain (Ntoumanis, 2005); Canada (Legault et al., 2005), France (Trouilloud, Sarrazin, Bressoux, & Bois, 2006), Germany (Levesque, Zuehlke, Stanek, & Ryan, 2004), Italy (Szadejko, 2003), Norway (Ommundsen & Kvalo, 2007), and the United States (Reeve & Jang, 2006; Ryan et al., 2006). Similar research was also done in many non-Western nations that strongly vary regarding collectivism, authoritarianism, patriarchy and other cultural dimensions. These countries include: Brazil (Chirkov et al., 2005), Israel (Assor, Kaplan, Kanat-Maymon, & Roth, 2005; Roth, Assor, Kanat-Maymon, & Kaplan, 2007), South Korea (Jang et al., 2009), Greece, Poland, and Singapore (Hagger et al., 2005), China (Vansteenkiste et al., 2005), Pakistan (Stewart et al., 2000), Russia (Chirkov & Ryan, 2001), Taiwan (Hardre et al., 2006); with multiethnic students in South Africa (Muller & Louw, 2004), and varied samples of immigrants and sojourners in Canada (Downie et al., 2007). In accord with the propositions of SDT, autonomy support from teachers and parents has been associated with or has predicted (in longitudinal studies) more autonomous motivation in students, higher academic outcomes, better psychological well-being, less problem behaviours, higher self-esteem, less dropping out, and stronger persistence in educational settings. These positive associations and predictions across a wide range of cultures that value autonomy support very differently provide substantial cross-cultural validation of the SDT hypotheses concerning the fundamentally important roles motivational autonomy and autonomy support play in students' functioning.

Some SDT researchers addressed the role the culture of horizontality plays in people's autonomous motivation and well-being at a more distal social level. Chirkov and his colleagues (Chirkov et al., in press) compared relations that indicators of the culture of horizontality have with people's motivation for health behaviour as well as their well-being, frequencies of health-maintaining (physical exercise and dieting) and health-risky (smoking and alcohol drinking) behaviours and health attitudes. This study was conducted in Canada and Russia, two countries that differ substantially with regard to the prevalence of the culture of horizontality (Canada has a much higher level of this culture). These researchers were interested in the role autonomous motivation plays in mediating the statistical predictions of various well-being indicators as well as health-related behaviours and attitudes by the indicators of horizontality and verticality. The measures of these cultures consisted of such indicators as national identity, the perception of trust in communal relations, the level of trust toward social institutions, and the perception of national cultural contexts along such dimensions as horizontal and vertical individualism and collectivism.

In summary, the perceived horizontal dimension of national cultures is positively related with the beneficial behavioural and cognitive aspects of health attitudes as well as with participants' psychological well-being in countries with both high (Canada) and low (Russia) levels of the culture of horizontality. These researchers discovered such correlations in the Canadian sample, and they were stronger than in the sample of Russian participants. Aspects of the culture of horizontality such as national identity, perceived trust in one's communities and perceived horizontal collectivism were related positively with autonomous motivation for health-promoting behaviours, whereas the vertical dimensions of the perceived national cultures were associated with the more controlled forms of health-promoting motivation. Path analysis revealed that in the Canadian sample both the culture of horizontality and autonomous motivation for health promotion positively predicted participants' psychological well-being, whereas the same indicator of horizontal social context predicted the frequencies of health-promoting behaviours only through the corresponding autonomous motivation. These data provided preliminary support for the prediction that the culture of horizontality, even at the distal social level, works positively toward people's healthy life-styles by promoting in them higher levels of motivational autonomy.

Conclusion

The goal of this chapter was to settle the dispute regarding the issue of the culturally universal versus culturally relative nature of psychological autonomy and the nature of its relations with people's well-being. The evidence from biological and system-theory sciences supports the idea that human autonomy is a natural and biologically based universal human capability. It encompasses the ability of people to consciously reflect on their own motivations, to set their own rules and norms for behaviour and to follow them in their actions and behaviours. There is no evidence to suggest that this capacity's existence depends on negotiations and agreements among the members of cultural communities. The psychological reality of a human autonomous capability is independent of its representation in the minds of people. Human autonomy is not a social construction but a natural capability of any human individual to be the master of one's own life, actions, and behaviours. Another powerful argument toward the same thesis stems from the philosophical, theoretical, and empirical evidence that being autonomous is one the most fundamental conditions for people to experience life in its fullest form and, because of this, to possess the highest levels of functioning, creativity, well-being and happiness. As numerous scholars argue, without autonomy and the feeling of freedom that accompanies it, it is not possible to be a healthy and fully functioning person. Without autonomous agency, the best qualities of humans cannot flourish. Autonomy and freedom are universally fundamental conditions required for people to thrive.

This universalist thesis does not deny the crucial and constitutive role that the cultural symbolic environments play in the emergence and development of human autonomy from potentiality to actuality. Culture is required for autonomy to evolve. Without a social, linguistic and cultural environment, the symbolic representations that lie at the basis of humans' reflective capacities cannot emerge, and human self-determination and freedom would not be possible. But the fact that human autonomy requires culture to emerge does not mean that culture determines autonomy. An autonomous person can reflect on his or her socio-cultural influences, endorse them or reject them, and act either along or against their prescriptions. Cultural communities negotiate the meaning and value of psychological autonomy in their members, who may be either in favour of or against its development and manifestation. At this stage, cultures play their important role in shaping the manifestation of autonomy, designating the appropriate areas and times for its exercise and providing conditions for it to flourish. Autonomy-restrictive cultural communities may strongly diminish and hinder the functioning of autonomous individuals, but as soon as autonomy emerges it will never go away and the beneficial role it plays in people's well-being and happiness will always be present, despite the suffering that striving for self-determination and freedom can bring in these restrictive societies. The provided empirical evidence based on SDT research supported the proposed propositions.

References

Ali, S. M., & Haq, R. U. (2006). Women's autonomy and happiness: The case of Pakistan. *Pakistan Development Review, 45*, 121–136.
Assor, A., Kaplan, H., Kanat-Maymon, Y., & Roth, G. (2005). Directly controlling teacher behaviors as predictors of poor motivation and engagement in girls and boys: The role of anger and anxiety. *Learning and Instruction, 15*(5), 397–413.
Baer, J., Kaufman, J. C., & Baumeister, R. F. (Eds.). (2008). *Are we free? Psychology and free will*. New York: Oxford University Press.

Bakhtin, M. (1984). *Problems of Dostoevsky's poetics*. Minneapolis, MN: University of Minnesota Press.
Bargh, J. A. (2008). Free will is un-natural. In J. Baer, J. C. Kaufman, & R. F. Baumeister (Eds.), *Are we free? Psychology and free will* (pp. 128–154). New York: Oxford University Press.
Bargh, J. A., & Ferguson, M. J. (2000). Beyond behaviorism: On the automaticity of higher mental processes. *Psychological Bulletin, 126*(6), 925–945.
Baumrind, D. (1971). Current patterns of parental authority. *Developmental Psychology Monograph, 4*, 1–103.
Buber, M. (2002). *Between man and man*. London: Routledge.
Chirkov, V. I., Lebedeva, N., Molodtsova, I., & Tatarko, A. (in press). Social capital, motivational autonomy, and health behavior: A comparative study of Canadian and Russian youth. In D. Chadee & A. Kostic (Eds.), *Research in social psychology*. Trinidad: University of West Indies Press.
Chirkov, V. I., & Ryan, R. M. (2001). Parent and teacher autonomy-support in Russian and US adolescents: Common effects on well-being and academic motivation. *Journal of Cross-Cultural Psychology, 32*(5), 618–635.
Chirkov, V. I., Ryan, R. M., Kim, Y., & Kaplan, U. (2003). Differentiating autonomy from individualism and independence: A self-determination theory perspective on internalization of cultural orientations and well-being. *Journal of Personality and Social Psychology, 84*(1), 97–110.
Chirkov, V. I., Ryan, R. M., & Willness, C. (2005). Cultural context and psychological needs in Canada and Brazil: Testing a self-determination approach to internalization of cultural practices, identity and well-being. *Journal of Cross-Cultural Psychology, 36*(4), 425–443.
Cooper, J. M. (2003). Stoic autonomy. In E. F. Paul, F. D. Miller, Jr., & J. Paul (Eds.), *Autonomy* (pp. 1–29). Cambridge: Cambridge University Press.
David, N., Newen, A., & Vogeley, K. (2008). The "sense of agency" and its underlying cognitive and neural mechanisms. *Consciousness and Cognition, 17*(2), 523–534.
de Botton, A. (2004). *Status anxiety*. Toronto, ON: Penguin.
Deacon, T. W. (1997). *The symbolic species: The co-evolution of language and brain*. New York: Norton.
Deci, E. L., & Ryan, R. M. (1985). *Intrinsic motivation and self-determination theory of human behavior*. New York: Plenum.
Deci, E. L., & Ryan, R. M. (Eds.). (2002). *Handbook of self-determination research*. Rochester, NY: The University of Rochester Press.
Dennett, D. C. (1986). *Elbow room: The varieties of free will worth wanting*. Cambridge, MA: The MIT Press.
Dennett, D. C. (2003). *Freedom evolves*. New York: Viking.
Devine, J., Camfield, L., & Gough, I. (2008). Autonomy or dependence-or both? Perspectives from Bangladesh. *Journal of Happiness Studies, 9*, 105–138.
Downie, M., Chua, S. N., Koestner, R., Barrios, M.-F., Rip, B., & M'Birkou, S. (2007). The relations of parental autonomy support to cultural internalization and well-being of immigrants and sojourners. *Cultural Diversity and Ethnic Minority Psychology, 13*(3), 241–249.
Ewing, K. P. (1991). Can psychoanalytic theories explain the Pakistani woman? Intrapsychic autonomy and interpersonal engagement in the extended family. *Ethos, 19*(2), 131–160.
Farrer, C., & Frith, C. D. (2002). Experiencing oneself vs another person as being the cause of an action: The neural correlates of the experience of agency. *NeuroImage, 15*(3), 596–603.
Frie, R. (2008). *Psychological agency: Theory, practice, and culture*. Cambridge, MA: The MIT Press.
Fukuyama, F. (2002). Social capital and development: The coming agenda. *SAIS Review, 22*(1), 23–37.
Fuster, J. M. (2002). Frontal lobe and cognitive development. *Journal of Neurocytology, 31*, 373–385.

Gallagher, S. (2000). Philosophical conceptions of the self: Implications for cognitive science. *Trends in Cognitive Sciences, 4*(1), 14–21.
Grolnick, W. S., Ryan, R. M., & Deci, E. L. (1997). Internalization within the family: The self-determination theory perspective. In J. E. Grusec & L. Kuczynski (Eds.), *Parenting and children's internalization of values* (pp. 135–161). New York: Wiley.
Grootaert, C., & van Bastelaer, T. (2001). *Understanding and measuring social capital: A synthesis of findings and recommendations from the Social Capital Initiative*. Washington, DC: The World Bank.
Grouzet, F. M. E., Otis, N., & Pelletier, L. G. (2006). Longitudinal cross-gender factorial invariance of the Academic Motivation Scale. *Structural Equation Modelling, 13*(1), 73–98.
Guyer, P. (2000). *Kant on freedom, law, and happiness*. Cambridge, UK: Cambridge University Press.
Guyer, P. (2003). Kant on theory and practice of autonomy. In E. F. Paul, F. D. Miller, & J. Paul (Eds.), *Autonomy* (pp. 70–98). Cambridge, UK: Cambridge University Press.
Habermas, J. (1990). Justice and solidarity: On the discussion concerning stage 6. In T. E. Wren, W. Edelstein, & G. Nunner-Winkler (Eds.), *The moral domain: Essays in the ongoing discussion between philosophy and the social sciences* (pp. 224–252). Cambridge, MA: The MIT Press.
Hagger, M. S., Chatzisarantis, N. L. D., Barkoukis, V., Wang, C. K. J., & Baranowski, J. (2005). Perceived autonomy support in physical education and leisure-time physical activity: A cross-cultural evaluation of the trans-contextual model. *Journal of Educational Psychology, 97*(3), 376–390.
Hagger, M. S., Chatzisarantis, N. L. D., Hein, V., Pihu, M., Soos, I., & Karsai, I. (2007). The perceived autonomy support scale for exercise settings (PASSES): Development, validity, and cross-cultural invariance in young people. *Psychology of Sport and Exercise, 8*, 632–653.
Hardre, P. L., Chen, C., Huang, S., Chiang, C., Jen, F., & Warden, L. (2006). Factors affecting high school students' academic motivation in Taiwan. *Asia Pacific Journal of Education, 26*, 198–207.
Hayamizu, T. (1997). Between intrinsic and extrinsic motivation: Examination of reasons for academic study based on the theory of internalization. *Japanese Psychological Research, 37*, 98–108.
Heider, F. (1982/1958). *The psychology of interpersonal relations*. Philadelphia: Psychology Press.
Irvine, W. B. (2009). *A guide to the good life: The ancient art of Stoic joy*. Oxford: Oxford University Press.
Jang, H., Reeve, J., Ryan, R. M., & Kim, A. (2009). Can self-determination theory explain what underlies the productive, satisfying learning experiences of collectivistically-oriented Korean students? *Journal of Educational Psychology, 101*(3), 644–661.
Juarrero, A. (1999). *Dynamics in action: Intentional behavior as a complex system*. Cambridge, MA: A Bradford Books.
Kagan, J. (2004). The uniquely human in human nature. *Daedalus, 133*(4), 77–88.
Koechlin, E., Ody, C., & Kouneiher, F. (2003). The architecture of cognitive control in human prefrontal cortex. *Science, 302*, 1181–1185.
Kohlberg, L., Boyd, D. R., & Levine, C. G. (1990). The return of stage 6: Its principle and moral point of view. In T. E. Wren (Ed.), *The moral domain: Essays in the ongoing discussion between philosophy and the social science* (pp. 151–181.). Cambridge, MA: The MIT Press.
Legault, L., Green-Demers, I., & Pelletier, L. (2005). Why do high school students lack motivation in the classroom? Toward an understanding of academic amotivation and the role of social support. *Journal of Educational Psychology, 98*(3), 567–582.
Levesque, C., Zuehlke, A. N., Stanek, L. R., & Ryan, R. M. (2004). Autonomy and competence in German and American university students: A comparative study based on Self-determination theory. *Journal of Educational Psychology, 96*(1), 68–84.
Lewin, K., & Lippitt, R. (1938). An experimental approach to the study of autocracy and democracy: A preliminary note. *Sociometry, 1*(3/4), 292–300.

Libet, B., Freeman, A., & Sutherland, K. (Eds.). (1999). *The volitional brain: Towards a neuroscience of free will*. Thorverton: Imprint Academic.
Lukes, S. (1973). *Individualism*. New York: Harper Row.
Markus, H. R., & Kitayama, S. (2003). Models of agency: Sociocultural diversity in the construction of action. *Nebraska Symposium on Motivation, 49*, 1–57.
Martin, J. (2008). Perspectival selves and agents: Agency within sociality. In R. Frie (Ed.), *Psychological agency: Theory, practice, and culture* (pp. 97–116). Cambridge, MA: The MIT Press.
Martin, J., Sugerman, J., & Thompson, J. (2003). *Psychology and the question of agency*. Albany, NY: State University of New York Press.
May, R. (1961). The emergence of existential psychology. In R. May (Ed.), *Existential psychology* (pp. 11–51). New York: Random House.
McCrone, J. (1999). A bifold model of free will. In B. Libet, A. Freeman, & K. Sutherland (Eds.), *The volitional brain: Towards a neuroscience of free will* (pp. 241–259). Thorverton: Imprint Academic.
McDonough, R. (1997). The concept of organism and the concept of mind. *Theory and Psychology, 7*(5), 579–604.
Mele, A. R. (2001). *Autonomous agents: From self-control to autonomy*. Oxford: Oxford University Press.
Mele, A. R. (2005). *Motivation and agency*. Oxford: Oxford University Press.
Miller, J. G. (1999). Cultural conceptions of duty: Implications for motivation and morality. In D. Munroe, J. F. Schumaker, & S. C. Carr (Eds.), *Motivation and culture* (pp. 178–192). New York: Routledge.
Muller, F. H., & Louw, J. (2004). Learning environment, motivation and interest: Perspectives on self-determination theory. *South African Journal of Psychology, 34*(2), 169–190.
Murphy, N. C., & Brown, W. S. (2007). *Did my neurons make me do it? Philosophical and neurobiological perspectives on moral responsibility and free will*. Oxford: Oxford University Press.
Murphy, N. C., & Stoeger, W. R. (2007). *Evolution and emergence: Systems, organisms, persons*. Oxford: Oxford University Press.
Ntoumanis, N. (2005). A prospective study of participation in optional school physical education using a self-determination theory framework. *Journal of Educational Psychology, 97*(3), 44–453.
Ommundsen, Y., & Kvalo, S. E. (2007). Autonomy-mastery supportive or performance focused? Different teacher behaviours and pupils' outcomes in physical education. *Scandinavian Journal of Educational Research, 51*(4), 385–413.
Oshana, M. (2003). How much should we values autonomy? In E. F. Paul, F. D. Miller, & J. Paul (Eds.), *Autonomy* (pp. 99–126). Cambridge: Cambridge University Press.
Paul, E. F., Miller, F. D., & Paul, J. (Eds.). (2003). *Autonomy*. Cambridge: Cambridge University Press.
Pink, T. (1996). *The psychology of freedom*. Cambridge: Cambridge University Press.
Portes, A. (1998). Social capital: Its origin and application in modern sociology. *Annual Review of Sociology, 24*, 1–24.
Reeve, J., & Jang, H. (2006). What teachers say and do to support students' autonomy during a learning activity. *Journal of Educational Psychology, 98*(1), 209–218.
Riesman, D., with, Clazer, N., & Denny, R. (2001/1961). *The lonely crowd: A study of the changing American character*. New Haven, CT: Yale University Press.
Roland, A. (1988). *In search of self in India and Japan: Toward a cross-cultural psychology*. Princeton, NJ: Princeton University Press.
Roth, G., Assor, A., Kanat-Maymon, Y., & Kaplan, H. (2006). Assessing the experience of autonomy in new cultures and contexts. *Motivation & Emotion, 30*(4), 361–372.
Roth, G., Assor, A., Kanat-Maymon, Y., & Kaplan, H. (2007). Autonomous motivation for teaching: How self-determined teaching may lead to self-determined learning. *Journal of Educational Psychology, 99*(4), 761–774.

Rudy, D., Sheldon, K. M., Awong, T., & Tan, H. H. (2007). Autonomy, culture, and well-being: The benefits of inclusive autonomy. *Journal of Research in Personality, 41*, 983–1007.

Ryan, R. M., & Connell, J. P. (1989). Perceived locus of causality and internalization: Examining reasons for acting in two domains. *Journal of Personality and Social Psychology, 57*, 749–761.

Ryan, R. M., & Deci, E. L. (2000a). The darker and brighter sides of human existence: Basic psychological needs as a unifying concept. *Psychological Inquiry, 11*(4), 319–338.

Ryan, R. M., & Deci, E. L. (2000b). Self-determination theory and the facilitation of intrinsic motivation, social development, and well-being. *American Psychologist, 55*(1), 68–78.

Ryan, R. M., & Deci, E. L. (2003). On assimilating identities to the self: A self-determination theory perspective on internalization and integrity within cultures. In M. R. Leary & J. P. Tangney (Eds.), *Handbook of self and identity* (pp. 253–272). New York: The Guilford Press.

Ryan, R. M., & Deci, E. L. (2004). Autonomy is no illusion: Self-determination theory and the empirical study of authenticity, awareness, and will. In J. Greenberg, S. L. Koole, & T. Pyszczynski (Eds.), *Handbook of experimental existential psychology*. New York: The Guilford Press.

Ryan, R. M., Deci, E. L., Grolnick, W. S., & La Guardia, J. G. (2006). The significance of autonomy and autonomy support in psychological development and psychopathology. In D. Cicchetti & D. J. Cohen (Eds.), *Developmental psychopathology* (2nd ed., Vol. 1, pp. 795–849). New York: Wiley.

Ryan, R. M., Kuhl, J., & Deci, E. L. (1997). Nature and autonomy: Organizational view of social and neurobiological aspects of self-regulation in behavior and development. *Development and Psychopathology, 9*, 701–728.

Schwabe, L., & Blanke, O. (2007). Cognitive neuroscience of ownership and agency. *Consciousness and Cognition, 16*(3), 661–666.

Sen, A. (2009). *The idea of justice*. Cambridge: Belknap Press of Harvard University Press.

Sheldon, K. M. (2004). *Optimal human being: An integrated multi-level perspective*. Mahwah, NJ: Psychology Press.

Shweder, R. A., Much, N. C., Mahapatra, M., & Park, L. (2003). The big three of morality (autonomy, community, and divinity) and the big three explanations of suffering. In R. A. Sweder (Ed.), *Why do men barbecue? Recipes for cultural psychology* (pp. 74–133). Cambridge, MA: Harvard University Press.

Soenens, B., Vansteenkiste, M., Lens, W., Luyckx, K., Goossens, L., Beyers, W., et al. (2007). Conceptualizing parental autonomy support: Adolescent perceptions of promotion of independence versus promotion of volitional functioning. *Developmental Psychology, 43*(3), 633–646.

Spence, S. A., & Frith, C. D. (1999). Toward a functional anatomy of volition. In B. Libet, A. Freeman, & K. Sutherland (Eds.), *The volitional brain: Towards a neuroscience of free will* (pp. 11–29). Thorverton: Imprint Academic.

Sperry, R. M. (1991). In defense of mentalism and emergent interaction. *The Journal of Mind & Behavior, 12*, 221–245.

Stewart, S. M., Bond, M. H., Ho, L. M., Zaman, R. M., Dar, R., & Anwar, M. (2000). Perceptions of parents and adolescent outcomes in Pakistan. *British Journal of Developmental Psychology, 18*, 335–352.

Szadejko, K. (2003). Percezione di autonomia, competenza e relazionalità. Adattamento italiano del questionario basic psychological needs scale. *Orientamenti Pedagogici, 5*, 853–872.

Tanaka, K., & Yamauchi, H. (2000). Influence of autonomy on perceived control beliefs and self-regulated learning in Japanese undergraduate students. *North American Journal of Psychology, 2*, 255–272.

Taylor, C. (1985). *Human agency and language. Philosophical papers* (Vol. 1). Cambridge: Cambridge University Press.

Taylor, J. S. (Ed.). (2005). *Personal autonomy: New essays on personal autonomy and its role in contemporary moral philosophy*. Cambridge: Cambridge University Press.

Triandis, H. C. (1995). *Individualism and collectivism*. Boulder, CO: Westview Press.
Trouilloud, D., Sarrazin, P., Bressoux, P., & Bois, J. (2006). Relation between teachers' early expectations and students' later perceived competence in physical education classes: Autonomy-supportive climate as a moderator. *Journal of Educational Psychology, 98*(1), 75–86.
Uyl, D. D. (2003). Autonomous autonomy: Spinoza on autonomy, perfectionism, and politics. In E. F. Paul, F. D. Miller, & J. Paul (Eds.), *Autonomy* (pp. 30–69). Cambridge, UK: Cambridge University Press.
Vallerand, R. J., Blais, M. R., Brière, N. M., & Pelletier, L. G. (1989). Construction et validation de l'échelle de motivation en éducation (ÉMÉ) [Construction and validation of the Échelle de Motivation en Éducation – ÉMÉ]. *Canadian Journal of Behavioural Science, 21*, 323–349.
Vansteenkiste, M., Zhou, M., Lens, W., & Soenens, B. (2005). Experiences of autonomy and control among Chinese learners: Vitalizing or immobilizing? *Journal of Educational Psychology, 97*(3), 468–483.
Varela, F. J. (1979). *Principles of biological autonomy*. New York: North Holland.
Varela, F. J., Thomson, E., & Rosch, E. (1991). *The embodied mind: Cognitive science and human experience*. Cambridge, MA: The MIT Press.
Veenhoven, R. (1999). Quality-of-life in individualistic society. *Social Indicators Research, 48*(2), 157–186.
Waller, B. N. (1998). *The natural selection of autonomy*. Albany, NY: State University of New York.
Wegner, D. M. (2002). *The illusion of conscious will*. Cambridge, MA: Bradford Books, The MIT Press.
Yamauchi, H., & Tanaka, K. (1998). Relations of autonomy, self-referenced beliefs and self-regulated learning among Japanese children. *Psychological Reports, 82*, 803–816.

Part II
Human Autonomy Across Cultures and Domains of Life: Health, Education, Interpersonal Relationships, and Work

Chapter 5
The Role of Autonomy in Promoting Healthy Dyadic, Familial, and Parenting Relationships Across Cultures

C. Raymond Knee and Ahmet Uysal

The quality of our close relationships has a major impact on our health and well-being. When asked "What is it that makes your life meaningful?" or "What is necessary for your happiness?" most people mention, before anything else, satisfying close relationships with friends, family, or romantic partners (Berscheid, 1985). Indeed, relationships are one of the most important sources of life satisfaction and emotional well-being (Berscheid & Reis, 1998). As noted by Reis and Gable (2003), the weight of evidence is so compelling that one commentator referred to the association between relationships and well-being as a "deep truth" (Myers, 1992), and virtually all reviews have drawn similar conclusions (e.g., Argyle, 1987; Berscheid & Reis, 1998; Diener, Suh, Lucas, & Smith, 1999). People are also better adjusted both physically and psychologically when they are in a close relationship than when they are not (Burman & Margolin, 1992). That said, when relationships are not going well, there can be substantial consequences. For example, relationship conflict and disruption has been shown to influence depression, the immune system, and mortality rate, among other things (Kiecolt-Glaser & Newton, 2001; Stroebe & Stroebe, 1987 In this way, close relationships can also be a major cause of emotional distress when difficulties and challenges arise.

But by what criteria do we define quality close relationships? Further, what factors promote versus thwart relational health and well-being? A motivational perspective on relational health emerges from self-determination theory (SDT; Deci & Ryan, 2000; La Guardia & Patrick, 2008) and specifies what optimal relationship development and functioning is likely to be. Whereas many close relationship theories posit satisfaction, intimacy, and perceived partner responsiveness as optimal outcomes, SDT argues that it is the motivational underpinnings of behavior and interactions that determine optimal development and outcomes. For example, one important relationship outcome is commitment, in which one feels determined to remain in the relationship. This criterion is typically considered so important in

---

C.R. Knee (✉)
University of Houston, Houston, TX 77024, USA
e-mail: knee@uh.edu

close relationships, that one of the more influential theoretical models in this literature focuses almost exclusively on what predicts commitment (Rusbult, 1983). But a motivational perspective derived from SDT would argue that not all forms of commitment are created equal. Specifically, if one feels committed to remain in a relationship because of perceived pressures from family and friends, the quality of this commitment will be significantly different than when commitment is motivated by personal endorsement and identification with the relationship oneself (Blais, Sabourin, Boucher, & Vallerand, 1990; Knee, Lonsbary, Canevello, & Patrick, 2005).

Self-determination theory posits that optimal psychological health and well-being emerge when basic psychological needs for autonomy, competence, and relatedness are supported rather than thwarted (Deci & Ryan, 2000). Need for autonomy reflects the need to feel that one's behavior is personally endorsed and self-initiated. Need for competence reflects the need to feel competent and effective at what one does. Need for relatedness reflects the need for strong, stable, healthy interpersonal bonds and attachments to others (e.g., Baumeister & Leary, 1995). For close relationships, this basic psychological needs perspective means that quality close relationships are thought to involve more than simply feeling satisfied with them. Relational well-being is thought to emerge as a function of the relationship context supporting the basic needs of both partners, promoting more autonomous motivation for being in the relationship, which in turn facilitates how the couple approaches and manages disagreements and conflicts (Patrick, Knee, Canevello, & Lonsbary, 2007). The SDT perspective on basic psychological needs is also important because these needs can account for the motivational underpinnings of relational well-being (La Guardia & Patrick, 2008). That is to say, a key reason why having secure attachments and relying emotionally on close others predict better relational outcomes is because these processes facilitate the fulfillment of basic psychological needs within one's relationships.

Autonomy and Openness Vs. Defensiveness

Autonomy benefits one's relationships in several ways. For example, when autonomously motivated, one is more open and receptive to events and information, regardless of whether autonomy is measured as a general motivation orientation, or whether it is experimentally induced (Hodgins & Knee, 2002; Hodgins, 2008; Hodgins et al., (in press). In contrast, when motivated by control, one feels pressured or guilty for one's decisions and actions, and thus one tends to behave from a defensive interpersonal stance, being less open and more reactive, displaying more avoidance, denial, and behavioral disengagement (Hodgins, Yacko, & Gottlieb, 2006; Knee & Zuckerman, 1998). Among couples, autonomous motivation, in terms of having more intrinsic reasons for being in the relationship, predicts less defensive responses to disagreements, and, in turn, more relative satisfaction following those disagreements (Knee et al., 2005, Study 3). Further, in another study of couples, those less defensive responses were observable in actual behaviors during a laboratory-induced conflict (Knee et al., 2005, Study 4). Why does autonomous motivation promote openness rather than defensiveness in social interactions? One reason is that autonomy reflects an integrated sense of self and authentic, or true, self-esteem whereby one's ego is not "on the line" and one is less concerned about proving oneself or feeling pressured to believe or think about oneself in a particular way (Deci & Ryan, 1995; Kernis, 2003; Ryan, 1995). As Hodgins et al. (in press) explained, "Integrated self-structures and stable, genuine self-esteem allow individuals to be relatively more aware of what is happening in the current moment and relatively less focused on proving themselves." According to recent empirical research, one consequence of this is a higher threat threshold and a shift in emotional regulation toward less avoidance, denial, and defensiveness (Hodgins et al., in press), all of which can facilitate open, honest communication in times of disagreement and conflict. This more recent research observes these effects from experimentally induced (primed) autonomous motivation, relative to experimentally induced (primed) controlled motivation. Thus, it appears that situationally induced autonomous motivation promotes more openness and less defensiveness as does more general autonomous motivation (measured as a trait or as reasons for engaging in behavior), although further research is needed.

This more open, authentic stance that is promoted by autonomy is not limited to romantic relationships. Autonomous motivation has also been found to predict more satisfying and honest, naturally occurring interactions with family and friends (Hodgins, Koestner, & Duncan, 1996), and fewer attempts to "save face," blame others, and aggravate the distress when awkward social events occur (Hodgins & Liebeskind, 2003; Hodgins, Liebeskind, & Schwartz, 1996). The more open and accepting orientation that autonomy promotes is not limited to only interpersonal events, but also minimizes the typical defensive attributions when one attempts to explain one's own behavior. For example, when higher on autonomy, and lower on controlled orientations (as measured by the General Causality Orientations scale, Deci & Ryan, 1985), one tends to make similar attributions after success and failure on a task, as opposed to the more typical acceptance of more responsibility for success, but less responsibility for failure (Knee & Zuckerman, 1998). When one's ego is less "on the line" and one feels less pressured to think, feel, or behave in a particular way, then as Rogers (1961) explained, "The facts are always friendly."

Another byproduct of autonomous motivation is less of a desire to present a particular self-image to others (Hodgins & Knee, 2002). Although everyone generally monitors and adjusts their behavior to fit the demands and expectations of specific environments and social settings, this tendency is likely to be weaker when autonomously motivated. While flexibility is also a hallmark of being autonomously motivated, the feeling that one must present a desirable (rather than authentic) image of oneself is likely to be less of a "prime directive." The ability to freely and mutually share oneself with close others, disclosing and responding with honest, emotionally relevant information, are major ingredients for the development of intimacy (Reis & Patrick, 1996). From an SDT perspective, genuine intimacy is less likely to emerge if partners are merely projecting the image they think the other person wants to see. The most profound connections are likely to emerge when two authentic selves are relating and responding to each others' needs openly and freely. That said, substantial research also indicates that people generally prefer to be viewed favorably, and viewing one's partner more favorably than the partner views him or herself predicts satisfaction in both dating relationships and marriages, and over time (e.g., Murray, Holmes, & Griffin, 1996). Still, "positive illusions" about one's romantic partner are probably not necessary for high relationship quality when one is autonomously motivated to be in one's relationship. This has already been shown for growth belief, a construct that is strongly associated with autonomous motivation (Knee, Patrick, Vietor, & Neighbors, 2004).

Having more autonomous reasons for being in one's relationship predicts more adaptive couple behaviors and greater satisfaction with one's relationship (Blais et al., 1990). We now know that a key part of why this is so concerns how feeling autonomous promotes more understanding and less defensive responses and behaviors during conflicts and disagreements (Knee, Patrick, Vietor, Nanayakkara, & Neighbors, 2002, 2005). Both those who are autonomous and, more specifically, those who are autonomously invested in a romantic relationship show less defensiveness and more understanding behavioral responses in the context of disagreements and in turn remain more satisfied with the relationship.

Thus far, most of this research has been conducted primarily on American and Canadian samples, so the generalization of these findings to more collectivist cultures is not yet proven. Still, when autonomy is defined in a manner similar to SDT, it appears to be associated positively, rather than negatively, with relatedness and predicts positive well-being in children and families in Turkish samples (Imamoglu, 2003; Kagitcibasi, 2005).

Need Fulfillment in Close Relationships

The concept of need fulfillment is central to why SDT is such a powerful theory of close relationships (La Guardia & Patrick, 2008). As stated earlier, SDT posits that optimal psychological health and well-being emerge from the satisfaction of basic psychological needs for autonomy, competence, and relatedness. Other relationship theories also tend to posit what produces high quality relationships and positive outcomes. For example, one of the most prominent and empirically validated theories on close relationships is attachment theory (Bowlby, 1969; see Simpson & Rholes, 2004 for review), which views felt security and appropriate responsiveness as important for maintaining secure attachments to close others. In this way, attachment theory spells out the processes whereby attachments to close others develop and change over time, as a function of the relational context in which they emerge. Attachment theory also allows for variation in how individuals become attached to different close others. Thus, one can have a relatively secure attachment to one's spouse, but a relatively less secure attachment to one's father, and so forth. Presumably, the different attachments people develop with close others are accounted for by different kinds of relational experiences across different contexts.

SDT is an especially powerful theory because its concept of basic psychological needs explicitly defines what kinds of experiences are needed for optimal development. While attachment theory primarily relies on felt security and feelings of relatedness in accounting for different attachments, SDT suggests that variations in the fulfillment of all three needs (autonomy, competence, and relatedness) in the relational context likely determine levels of felt security and qualities of attachment to close others.

Along these lines, an important series of studies by La Guardia and her colleagues (2000) examined the role of need fulfillment within attachment security. Across three studies, people tended to have different levels of attachment security in different relationships (e.g., friends, parents, romantic partners). More importantly, a significant degree of this within-person variation in attachments was predicted by the degree of need fulfillment within those specific relationships. People were more securely attached to those with whom they felt autonomous, competent, and related. In this way, need fulfillment may indeed reflect the motivational underpinnings of quality close relationships. Indeed, later work also found that emotional reliance can result in a similar way. Ryan, La Guardia, Solky-Butzel, Chirkov, and Kim (2005) found substantial within-person variation in emotional reliance across relationship partners. Importantly, the degree to which people's needs for autonomy, competence, and relatedness were met mediated the association between emotional reliance and well-being.

Another line of evidence that need fulfillment is beneficial for relationship well-being comes from studies that assessed the degree to which romantic partners felt that their needs for autonomy, competence, and relatedness were met, and tested whether this fulfillment predicted various relationship outcomes (Patrick et al., 2007). Just as research has shown that satisfaction of the three basic needs predicts positive health and well-being outcomes, it was hypothesized that satisfaction of the three basic needs in the context of one's close relationship would predict positive relational health and well-being outcomes. Study 1 found that fulfillment of autonomy uniquely predicted stronger relationship satisfaction and commitment, less perceived conflict, and more understanding and less defensive responses to conflict, even beyond the degree to which competence and relatedness were met. Study 2 found that the need fulfillment of each member within romantic couples uniquely predicts relationship outcomes such that one's partner's fulfillment of autonomy uniquely predicts one's own relationship outcomes. Thus, one's own feelings of autonomy in a relationship are not only important for how one feels about the relationship, but also uniquely extend to how the partner feels about it as well.

Overall, then, SDT is a powerful theory of close relationships because it explicitly defines three basic psychological needs that are at the core of developing optimal psychological well-being, and the satisfaction of these needs primarily occurs in interpersonal contexts such as one's close relationships with romantic partners, family, and friends. Our interactions with others either support or thwart the satisfaction of these basic needs. Whereas many relationship theories rely heavily on relatedness-type needs such as perceived responsiveness, intimacy, or felt security, SDT posits that more than the satisfaction of relatedness is at stake; without significant others supporting one's autonomy and competence, as well as relatedness, the quality of those relationships will be suboptimal. As La Guardia (2007) noted, "... even the best partners will not always be need supportive, understanding the regulation of needs—both their fulfillment and sacrifice in the service of the relationship—will be vital to predicting personal and relational health outcomes in the short and long term."

Autonomy and Interpersonal Conflict

Does being autonomously motivated pose a problem when one wants to do something that a friend or partner does not? While this has been an issue of some debate (see Ryan & Deci, 2000), the disagreement largely stems from confusion about what autonomy is, according to SDT, and what it is in other literature (e.g., Freud, 1958; Mahler, 1972; Murray, 1938). In SDT, autonomy is not akin to notions of independence, detachment, avoidance, or rebelliousness. To the contrary, Deci and Ryan's construct of autonomy reflects a deep personal endorsement of one's actions and involvements with others, and is associated with better personal and social adjustment (Hodgins et al., 1996; Koestner & Losier, 1996). Investigators have clarified these constructs by distinguishing between reactive and reflective autonomy, with the latter capturing the SDT notion (Koestner et al., 1999; Koestner & Losier, 1996). Reactive autonomy involves resisting influence, defying authority and striving for independence. On the other hand, reflective autonomy is about making informed choices based on an awareness of one's needs, interests, and values (Deci & Flaste, 1996). Similar theoretical approaches to autonomy have emerged elsewhere as well (Angyal, 1951; Imamoglu, 2003; Kagitcibasi, 2005). To the extent that one freely chooses to engage in behavior while considering one's needs, interests, and goals, one is fully autonomous. Autonomous behaviors result from a reflective evaluation of options and a consideration of one's interests and needs rather than from a reactive opposition to others (Koestner et al., 1999; Ryan, 1993).

As explained above, autonomy also comes with an openness to information that reduces defensiveness and promotes a full exploration and consideration of all the various features of one's situation, including the consideration of others' needs (Hodgins & Knee, 2002). It is perhaps this openness to information that most facilitates how conflicts are more successfully negotiated when autonomously motivated. Indeed, research has shown that autonomous motivation predicts more relative satisfaction after disagreements, and that this is accompanied by less defensive, more understanding perceptions and observable behaviors (Knee et al., 2005).

In sum, considerable theory and research suggests that when autonomy is defined as in SDT, it predicts a wealth of positive relationship processes and outcomes. This is partly due to individuals' basic need for autonomy (as well as competence and relatedness) and also because of the more open and less defensive interpersonal stance that feeling autonomous promotes. Results from studies employing a variety of designs, methods, and analytical approaches appear to converge on the notion that feeling autonomous, whether at the trait level, the relationship level, or the event-specific level, predicts more understanding and less defensive interpersonal responses toward peers and romantic partners, and, in turn, more positive interaction behaviors and relational outcomes.

Parental Autonomy Support

According to SDT, successful parenting hinges on the provision of autonomy support, structure, and involvement (for review, see Joussemet, Landry, & Koestner, 2008). These three qualities map onto the basic psychological needs of autonomy, competence, and relatedness rather nicely. A child's need for autonomy is fulfilled by the parents' provision of autonomy support. A child's need for competence is fulfilled by parents providing optimal structure, challenges, and setting reasonable and clear limits. A child's need for relatedness is fulfilled by parents being appropriately involved, caring for, and validating the child noncontingently. Parental autonomy support refers to the active support of the child's capacity to be self-initiating and autonomous (Ryan, Deci, Grolnick, & La Guardia, 2006). As with other forms of autonomy in the context of SDT, it is important to note that parental autonomy support is not akin to promoting permissiveness, neglect, or selfishness. Permissiveness would reflect a lack of structure rather than a lack of autonomy support. Neglect would reflect a lack of involvement rather than a lack of autonomy support. Supporting a child's autonomy has been shown to promote healthy internalization of behaviors and successful limit-setting (e.g., Joussemet, Koestner, Lekes, & Houlfort, 2004; Koestner, Ryan, Bernieri, & Holt, 1984). For example, in a classic experiment, Koestner and his colleagues operationalized autonomy support according to four key ingredients: (1) providing rationale and explanation for behavioral requests; (2) recognizing the feelings and perspectives of the child; (3) offering choices and encouraging initiative; and (4) minimizing controlling techniques. When limits were set with these principles in mind, children's intrinsic motivation was not affected whereas setting limits in a controlling manner undermined intrinsic motivation. More recently, research has distinguished clearly between autonomy support (the promotion of volition) and the promotion of independence (Soenens et al., 2007). The researchers assessed adolescents' perceptions of their parents' promotion of volition (e.g., "My parents let me make my own plans for things I want to do") versus independence (e.g., "My parents encourage me to be independent from them") their own perceived autonomy, and their own psychosocial functioning. Results showed that promotion of volition uniquely predicted psychosocial adjustment whereas promotion of independence did not.

The benefits of parental autonomy support have emerged from studies using a variety of methodologies. For example, observation studies have found that parental autonomy support predicts better motivation and persistence in infants and more complete internalization in toddlers (see Joussemet et al., 2008 for review). Further, parental autonomy support has also been coded in interviews and found to predict children's social and academic adjustment at school. Finally, adolescent children who can report their perceptions of their parents' autonomy support have found psychosocial and academic benefits as well. Researchers have examined the opposite of parental autonomy support as well, by focusing on consequences of controlling parental styles. This work has been careful to distinguish between psychological control and behavioral control. Psychological control involves pressuring a child to think, feel, or behave in certain ways through guilt induction, love withdrawal, and invalidation of feelings (Assor, Roth, & Deci, 2004; Ryan, 1982). Behavioral control refers to communicating clear expectations about appropriate behavior and monitoring the relevant behavior. The structure in behavioral control supports the child's competence and is consistent with providing structure, warmth, and democracy whereas the techniques employed in psychological control undermine the child's autonomy and competence, and predict detrimental outcomes (Grolnick, 2003).

Another feature of parenting that has been examined from an SDT perspective is parental conditional regard. Conditional regard involves providing love and affection when children execute specific behaviors and withholding love and affection when they do not. Despite being a common parenting practice that can, from an operant conditioning perspective teach kids what is expected fairly quickly, research also indicates that it comes with significant costs. For example, Assor and his colleagues (Assor et al., 2004) found that, although perceived parental conditional regard was related to behavioral enactment in several domains, it was also associated with negative affective consequences such as feelings of internal compulsion, short-lived satisfaction, shame after failure, fluctuations in self-esteem, poor coping skills, low self-worth, a sense of being disapproved of by parents, and resentment toward parents. Importantly, they also found evidence that the use of conditional regard may be passed down from one generation to the next as those parents who endorsed it tended to report that their own parents had done this as well.

More recent work has directly compared conditional positive regard (rewarding appropriate behaviors with love and affection) against conditional negative regard (punishing inappropriate behaviors by withholding love and affection), and parental autonomy support on a number of important developmental outcomes such as emotional health and academic consequences (Roth, Assor, Niemiec, Ryan, & Deci, 2009). Two sizeable samples of 9th-grade Israeli students provided data from multiple reporters. The researchers tested whether the three parenting styles (conditional negative regard, conditional positive regard, and autonomy support) would map roughly onto three forms of emotion regulation: emotion dysregulation, emotion suppression, and emotion integration, respectively. Their findings indeed supported models in which (a) conditional negative regard predicted resentment toward parents which in turn predicted emotion dysregulation and academic disengagement; (b) conditional positive regard predicted feelings of internal compulsion which then predicted emotion suppression and grade-focused academic engagement; and (c) autonomy support predicted a sense of choice which in turn predicted integrated emotion regulation and interest-focused academic engagement. Thus, it appears to be not only conditional negative regard that has emotion and academic consequences, but also positive conditional regard, and these different emotional and academic outcomes are easily distinguished and predicted by SDT.

Where do these controlling parenting styles originate? As mentioned above, some evidence suggests that parenting styles may be transferred from one generation to the next (Assor et al., 2004). But there are also contextual factors that can promote a controlling rather than supportive parental style. Grolnick (2003) suggested that when parents experience pressure, they are more likely to employ controlling behaviors because supporting autonomy may require more time and psychological availability. The child's behavior can also promote a controlling parental style such that oppositional behavior may be especially challenging to manage in an autonomy-supportive fashion, especially when the behavior is considered dangerous. Finally, parents can become ego-involved in their child's behaviors and performances, feeling as if the child's behavior reflects the parent's worth, and thus leading them to treat the child as they would treat their own controlled self. Grolnick, Price, Beiswenger, and Sauck (2007) studied 4th grade children and their mothers, some of whom were told that their children were to be evaluated by other children. These ego-involved mothers ended up being the most controlling toward their children. While this study demonstrated that evaluative pressure can lead to controlling parental behaviors, other research has already suggested that controlling contexts can promote intergenerational transmission of controlling behavior (e.g., Soenens, Duriez, Vansteenkiste, & Goossens, 2007; Soenens et al., 2005).

In sum, parental contexts that promote autonomy and provide structure and involvement are associated with more positive psychological, developmental, and educational outcomes in children. In contrast, parental contexts that promote contingent love, psychological control, permissiveness, and neglect are associated with more negative psychological, developmental, and educational outcomes. These findings have emerged from various research designs, in ages from young children to late adolescents, and across different methodologies such as parent observation, parent interviews, and children's reports of parents' behavior. Further, promoting autonomy (volition) in these contexts uniquely predicts positive outcomes whereas promoting independence does not. Moreover, behavioral control, which involves communicating clear expectations about appropriate behavior and monitoring the relevant behavior, has benefits whereas psychological control, which involves coercing the child to behave by means of guilt induction, love withdrawal, and invalidation of feelings, does not.

Autonomy and Relational Well-Being Across Cultures

We acknowledge that controversy exists regarding the importance of autonomy across cultures. While some of this controversy stems from misrepresentations of autonomy as independence, selfishness, avoidance, etc., more recent critiques have emerged from a cultural relativist perspective (e.g., Cross & Gore, 2003; Markus & Kitayama, 2003; Oishi & Diener, 2001). From this perspective, autonomy is viewed as a primarily Western cultural ideal rather than a universal psychological need. In this way, cultures that emphasize family, hierarchy, and group-based norms may have different ideals and may function just fine without feeling autonomous. In these more collectivist cultures, subordination of one's own will to the will of important and valued others may be preferred, and autonomy would presumably become less important for well-being (see Rudy, Sheldon, Awong, & Tan, 2007 for review). Indeed, there appears to be evidence for both the SDT and cultural relativist perspectives across cultures. Part of this puzzle may be in defining what exactly is meant by "subordinating one's will to others." It is conceivable that there are more autonomous and accepting ways to behave as important close others wish, and less autonomous, less accepting ways to behave as others wish.

Other cross-cultural perspectives on autonomy have emerged as well, and these offer creative synthesis of autonomy and relatedness dimensions, in a manner consistent with SDT. For example, Kagitcibasi (1996, 2005) defined the "autonomous-relational" self and reviewed cross-cultural evidence in support of this integration derived from the developmental and family systems literatures. This conceptualization recognizes that it is fully possible to parent in a manner that facilitates both autonomy and relatedness. Kagitcibasi believes that individualistic societies have recognized and nourished the need for autonomy at the cost of ignoring, even suppressing the equally important need for relatedness, whereas collectivistic societies have done the reverse.

With regard to whether fulfillment of relatedness predicts positive outcomes across cultures, Ryan et al. (2005) focused on emotional reliance, which was defined as people's self-reported willingness to turn to others during emotionally salient times. They found that while the degree of emotional reliance on others varied across cultures, reliance on others always predicted better well-being, and was always facilitated by autonomy support, as SDT would predict. In other cross-cultural research, culture moderated associations between perceived autonomy support and outcomes (Lynch, La Guardia, & Ryan, 2009). This study focused on discrepancies between one's ideal and actual self-concepts, and whether such discrepancies would be smaller in the context of autonomy-supportive relationships. Relationship partner was a within-participants variable such that participants rated their actual and ideal selves on several fundamental personality dimensions in each of several different relationships (i.e., mother, father, best friend, romantic partner, roommate, teacher). Culture was defined as participant location in terms of China, Russia, or the US. Results showed that culture moderated the degree to which partner autonomy support predicted smaller actual-ideal self discrepancies, and varied on certain personality dimensions as well. That said, the expected negative association between partner autonomy support and ideal-actual self discrepancies was significant and in the same direction in all three cultures.

What does all of this mean for the issue of whether the benefits of autonomous motivation in one's close relationships generalize across cultures? While research that specifically addresses this question is needed, we think that several points can be made. First, one reason that autonomous motivation facilitates more understanding and less defensive responses during interpersonal conflict is because of the increased openness to information and others' perspectives that it promotes. By openness, we mean a willingness to listen and hear another's perspective completely, without defending against it reactively; a reflective interest in another's viewpoint, rather than assuming that a viewpoint is wrong, reactively, and in order to defend one's own image or presentation.

Second, it is known that particular features of the social context can serve to thwart individuals' need for autonomy and thus be more likely to undermine intrinsic motivation and well-being (Deci & Ryan, 1987, 2000). To the extent that culture can be considered part of one's social context, and to also have more or fewer features that could undermine autonomy, it is possible that basic psychological needs could be more strongly thwarted in some places, in some people, at some times, relative to other places, people, and times. Further, long-term thwarting of basic psychological needs is thought to result in an "accommodative" process of devaluing of those needs which could manifest itself as an "I don't need it" type of reported devaluing (Deci & Ryan, 2000). Indeed, a recent series of experiments examined whether those low in satisfaction of the need for relatedness would experience less value from an experience that temporarily increased relatedness (Moller, Deci, & Elliot, in press). Results were consistent with a sensitization model in which those who were already higher in felt relatedness both anticipated and gained more value from an additional relatedness experience. Analogously, those who were lower in felt relatedness, both anticipated and gained less additional value from a relatedness experience. Thus, if there are cultural differences in reported need fulfillment, and its association with well-being, those who report lower fulfillment and seem fine with it, may have accommodated to the need-impoverished environment. In this way, experiencing autonomy may sensitize those who have gone without it to desire it and get more benefits from it.

Third, as stated earlier, the SDT definition of autonomy is not akin to independence or rugged individualism. That would be reactive autonomy as opposed to reflective autonomy (Koestner & Losier, 1996). It is relatively simple to think of cases in which reactive autonomy could undermine adaptive conflict resolution, and in many different cultures. It is much more difficult to think of convincing examples of how reflective awareness of and mindfulness of one's needs and actions in the context of all available information could actually exacerbate interpersonal conflict with close others. If anything, mindful reflection (as opposed to reaction) should make one more sensitive to and aware of others' needs as well. For instance, Koestner and colleagues (1999) found that highly reactive individuals rejected the recommendations of experts, whereas highly reflective individuals followed them. Thus even in some patriarchal cultures, where man is expected to make the final decisions for his family (even decisions like arranged marriages), a highly reflective husband would still make the final decisions but he would also take the suggestions of the family members into consideration, which would make the family members feel more valued. On the other hand, a highly reactive husband would disregard any advice from his family members, which would make the family members feel devalued. In both cases, the family members may feel controlled and less autonomous (as in the case of an arranged marriage); however this would especially be the case for the latter example.

Fourth, there may be times when satisfaction of one's need for autonomy and satisfaction of one's need for relatedness conflict, and this may seem more likely to happen in cultures that value "fitting in" and "getting along" over doing what one feels one wants to do. However, when this potential conflict occurs, it likely has more to do with the particular context rather than a general cultural norm, as in the research on contingent love and regard described above. Importantly, even if cultures vary on the importance of "going along to get along," the underlying dimension of more autonomously going along versus less autonomously going along, seems central in predicting what results in optimal outcomes (Chirkov, Ryan, Kim, & Kaplan, 2003; Rudy et al., 2007). In every case, more autonomously valuing one's in-group, family, or significant other should predict better individual and relational outcomes than less autonomously doing so.

Fifth, one can feel a range of autonomous motivation toward one's peer, family, and romantic relationships. For example, one can feel choicefully, reflectively, and authentically involved in a relationship; or one can feel coerced, pressured, and stuck in that relationship; or one can even not know why one is involved in a relationship. Cultures may vary in how socially acceptable and expected it is to feel coerced and pressured to remain in a relationship, even when it is not particularly satisfying. Further, the social and personal consequences of leaving that relationship, if it is even conceivable, could indeed vary considerably across cultures (Triandis, McCusker, & Hui, 1990).

We would expect those who feel more autonomously involved (relative to those who feel less autonomously involved) in their relationship to also generally experience better relationship quality, across cultures. Further, we would expect that on days in which one feels more autonomously involved (relative to days in which one feels less autonomously involved), one would tend to also experience better relationship quality, across cultures. However, these predictions seem to require an additional caveat. It is also important to consider the degree to which important others are included in one's self (Rudy et al., 2007), because the consequences of autonomously valuing one's relationship when one's family or an internalized cultural norm goes against it, could weaken that more general association.

Finally, maintaining relationships autonomously might appear hedonistic, akin to following one's interests, ephemeral and transitory as they might be. However, that is not what relationship autonomy means. According to SDT, not all forms of commitment are equal. Just as one's commitment to a task or job can be accepted and personally endorsed to varying degrees, one's commitment to a relationship can vary the same way. The kind of personally endorsed commitment that autonomy facilitates likely tends to be for the long haul, rather than ephemeral or transitory. When autonomously committed, one tends to be fully engaged, actively involved, and more likely to be invested with all of one's awareness. Autonomous commitment is akin to what health behavior therapists try to promote in patients and clients. Behavioral changes that are enacted out of guilt or pressure or someone else's expectations are more likely to fail in the long term whereas behavioral changes that are viewed as personally important and consistent with one's needs and desires, are likely to be adopted and internalized more fully, made one's own, and executed more completely, and over a longer time (Ryan, Patrick, Deci, & Williams, 2008). Thus, whereas controlled motivation and commitment likely promotes compliance, in that people can coercively comply with recommended behavioral changes, it is autonomous motivation that is needed for long-term adherence and self-regulated behavioral changes.

We think that a parallel can be drawn between autonomous motivation and the kind of personally endorsed commitment that emerges in the context of facilitating behavioral changes, and autonomous motivation and the kind of personally endorsed commitment that can emerge in the context of one's close relationships. When autonomously motivated within one's close relationships, one is more likely to naturally include close others within one's self-concept, and experience those relationships as deep, profound, personally endorsed and accepted commitments that are consistent and integrated with one's self and identity, rather than as merely obligations and promises to others.

In sum, whereas further research on cross-cultural generalization of the role and importance of autonomy, as defined within SDT, is needed, we feel that extant research and theory suggest that there is support for both universalist and cultural-relativist perspectives. In particular, continued research and conceptual clarification on the degree to which cultural norms and traditions are more autonomously versus less autonomously internalized and accepted seems especially promising. When one has autonomously included close others in one's self-concept, relationships with those close others probably benefit more than when one has less autonomously incorporated close others into one's self-concept.

References

Angyal, A. (1951). A theoretical model for personality studies. *Journal of Personality, 20,* 131–142.
Argyle, M. (1987). *The psychology of happiness.* London: Methuen.
Assor, A., Roth, G., & Deci, E. L. (2004). The emotional costs of perceived parental conditional regard: A self-determination theory analysis. *Journal of Personality, 72,* 47–87.
Baumeister, R. F., & Leary, M. R. (1995). The need to belong: Desire for interpersonal attachments as a fundamental human motivation. *Psychological Bulletin, 117,* 497–529.
Berscheid, E. (1985). Interpersonal attraction. In G. Lindzey & A. Aronson (Eds.), *Handbook of Social Psychology* (3rd ed., Vol. 2) pp. 413–484. New York: Random House.
Berscheid, E., & Reis, H. T. (1998). Attraction and close relationships. In D. T. Gilbert, S. T. Fiske, & G. Lindzey (Eds.), *The handbook of social psychology* (4th ed., Vol. 2, pp. 193–281). New York: McGraw-Hill.
Blais, M. R., Sabourin, S., Boucher, C., & Vallerand, R. J. (1990). Toward a motivational model of couple happiness. *Journal of Personality and Social Psychology, 59,* 1021–1031.
Bowlby, J. (1969). *Attachment and loss: Vol. 1: Attachment.* New York: Basic Books.
Burman, B., & Margolin, G. (1992). Analysis of the association between marital relationships and health problems: An interactional perspective. *Psychological Bulletin, 112,* 39–63.
Chirkov, V. I., Ryan, R. M., Kim, Y., & Kaplan, U. (2003). Differentiating autonomy from individualism and independence: A self-determination theory perspective on internalization of cultural orientations and well-being. *Journal of Personality and Social Psychology, 84,* 97–110.

Cross, S. E., & Gore, J. S. (2003). Cultural models of the self. In M. R. Leary & J. P. Tangney (Eds.), *Handbook of self and identity* (pp. 536–564). New York: Guilford Press.

Deci, E. L., & Flaste, R. (1996). *Why we do what we do: Understanding self-motivation.* New York: Penguin Books.

Deci, E. L., & Ryan, R. M. (1985). The general causality Orientations scale: self-determination in personality. *Journal of Research in Personality, 19*, 109–134.

Deci, E. L., & Ryan, R. M. (1987). The support of autonomy and the control of behavior. *Journal of Personality and Social Psychology, 53*, 1024–1037.

Deci, E. L., & Ryan, R. M. (1995). Human autonomy: The basis for true self-esteem. In M. Kernis (Ed.), *Efficacy, agency, and self-esteem* (pp. 31–49). New York: Plenum Publishing Co.

Deci, E. L., & Ryan, R. M. (2000). The 'what' and 'why' of goal pursuits: Human needs and the self-determination of behavior. *Psychological Inquiry, 11*, 227–268.

Diener, E., Suh, E. M., Lucas, R. E., & Smith, H. L. (1999). Subjective well-being: Three decades of progress. *Psychological Bulletin, 125*, 276–302.

Freud, A. (1958). Adolescence. *Psychoanalytic Study of the Child, 13*, 255–278.

Grolnick, W. S. (2003). *The psychology of parental control: How well-meant parenting backfires.* Mahwah, NJ: Erlbaum.

Grolnick, W. S., Price, C. E., Beiswenger, K. L., & Sauck, C. C. (2007). Evaluative pressure in mothers: Effects of situation, maternal, and child characteristics on autonomy supportive versus controlling behavior. *Developmental Psychology, 43*, 991–1002.

Hodgins, H. S. (2008). Motivation, threshold for threat, and quieting the ego. In H. A. Wayment & J. J. Bauer (Eds.), *Transcending self-interest* (pp. 117–124). Washington, DC: American Psychological Association.

Hodgins, H. S., & Knee, C. R. (2002). The integrating self and conscious experience. In E. L. Deci & R. M. Ryan (Eds.), *Handbook of self-determination research* (pp. 87–100). Rochester, NY: University of Rochester Press.

Hodgins, H. S., Koestner, R., & Duncan, N. (1996). On the compatibility of autonomy and relatedness. *Personality and Social Psychology Bulletin, 22*, 227–237.

Hodgins, H. S., & Liebeskind, E. (2003). Apology versus defense: Antecedents and consequences. *Journal of Experimental Social Psychology, 39*, 297–316.

Hodgins, H. S., Liebeskind, E., & Schwartz, W. (1996). Getting out of hot water: Facework in social predicaments. *Journal of Personality and Social Psychology, 71*, 300–314.

Hodgins, H. S., Yacko, H. A., & Gottlieb, E. (2006). Autonomy and nondefensiveness. *Motivation and Emotion, 30*, 283–293.

Imamoglu, E. O. (2003). Individuation and relatedness: Not opposing but distinct and complementary. *Genetic, Social, and General Psychology Monographs, 129*, 367–402.

Joussemet, M., Koestner, R., Lekes, N., & Houlfort, N. (2004). Introducing uninteresting tasks to children: A comparison of the effects of rewards and autonomy support. *Journal of Personality, 72*, 140–166.

Joussemet, M., Landry, R., & Koestner, R. (2008). A self-determination theory perspective on parenting. *Canadian Psychology, 49*, 194–200.

Kagitcibasi, C. (1996). The autonomous-relational self: A new synthesis. *European Psychologist, 1*, 180–186.

Kagitcibasi, C. (2005). Autonomy and relatedness in cultural context: Implications for self and family. *Journal of Cross-Cultural Psychology, 36*, 403–422.

Kernis, M. H. (2003). Toward a conceptualization of optimal self-esteem. *Psychological Inquiry, 14*, 1–26.

Kiecolt-Glaser, J. K., & Newton, T. L. (2001). Marriage and health: His and hers. *Psychological Bulletin, 127*, 472–503.

Knee, C. R., Lonsbary, C., Canevello, A., & Patrick, H. (2005). Self-determination and conflict in romantic relationships. *Journal of Personality and Social Psychology, 89*, 997–1009.

Knee, C. R., Patrick, H., Vietor, N. A., Nanayakkara, A., & Neighbors, C. (2002). Self-determination as growth motivation in romantic relationships. *Personality and Social Psychology Bulletin, 28*, 609–619.

Knee, C. R., Patrick, H., Vietor, N. A., & Neighbors, C. (2004). Implicit theories of relationships: Moderators of the link between conflict and commitment. *Personality and Social Psychology Bulletin, 30*(5), 617–628.

Knee, C. R., & Zuckerman, M. (1998). A nondefensive personality: Autonomy and control as moderators of defensive coping and self-handicapping. *Journal of Research in Personality, 32*, 115–130.

Koestner, R., Gingras, I., Abutaa, R., Losier, G. F., DiDio, L., & Gagné, M. (1999). To follow expert advice when making a decision: An examination of reactive vs. reflective autonomy. *Journal of Personality, 67*, 851–872.

Koestner, R., & Losier, G. F. (1996). Distinguishing reactive from reflective autonomy. *Journal of Personality, 64*, 465–494.

Koestner, R., Ryan, R. M., Bernieri, F., & Holt, K. (1984). Setting limits on children's behavior: The differential effects of controlling versus informational styles on children's intrinsic motivation and creativity. *Journal of Personality, 54*, 233–248.

La Guardia, J. G. (2007). On the role of psychological needs in healthy functioning: Integrating a self-determination theory perspective with traditional relationship theories. In J. V. Wood, A. Tesser, & J. Holmes (Eds.), *Self and relationships*. New York: Psychology Press.

La Guardia, J. G., & Patrick, H. (2008). Self-determination theory as a fundamental theory of close relationships. *Canadian Psychology, 49*, 201–209.

La Guardia, J. G., Ryan, R. M., Couchman, C. E., & Deci, E. L. (2000). Within-person variation in security of attachment: A self-determination theory perspective on attachment, need fulfillment, and well-being. *Journal of Personality and Social Psychology, 79*, 367–384.

Lynch, M. F., La Guardia, J. G., & Ryan, R. M. (2009). On being yourself in different cultures: Ideal and actual self-concept, autonomy support, and well-being in China, Russia, and the United States. *The Journal of Positive Psychology, 4*, 290–304.

Mahler, M. (1972). On the first three phases of the separation-individuation process. *International Journal of Psychoanalysis, 53*, 333–338.

Markus, H. R., & Kitayama, S. (2003). Models of agency: Sociocultural diversity in the construction of action. In V. Murphy-Berman & J. J. Berman (Eds.), *Nebraska symposium on motivation: Cross cultural differences in perspectives on the self* (pp. 18–74). Lincoln, NE: University of Nebraska Press.

Murray, H. A. (1938). *Explorations in personality*. New York: Oxford University Press.

Murray, S. L., Holmes, J. G., & Griffin, D. W. (1996). The benefits of positive illusions: Idealization and the construction of satisfaction in close relationships. *Journal of Personality and Social Psychology, 70*, 79–98.

Myers, D. G. (1992). *The pursuit of happiness: Who is happy – and why*. New York: William Morrow.

Oishi, S., & Diener, E. (2001). Goals, culture, and subjective well-being. *Personality and Social Psychology Bulletin, 27*, 1674–1682.

Patrick, H., Knee, C. R., Canevello, A., & Lonsbary, C. (2007). The role of need fulfillment in relationship functioning and well-being: A self-determination perspective. *Journal of Personality and Social Psychology, 92*, 434–457.

Reis, H. T., & Gable, S. L. (2003). Toward a positive psychology of relationships. In C. L. M. Keyes & J. Haidt (Eds.), *Flourishing: Positive psychology and the life well-lived*. Washington, DC: American Psychological Association.

Reis, H. T., & Patrick, B. P. (1996). Attachment and intimacy: Component processes. In E. T. Higgins & A. W. Kruglanski (Eds.), *Social psychology: Handbook of basic principles* (pp. 523–563). New York: Guilford.

Rogers, C. R. (1961). *On becoming a person: A therapist's view of psychotherapy*. London: Constable.

Roth, G., Assor, A., Niemiec, C. P., Ryan, R. M., & Deci, E. L. (2009). The emotional and academic consequences of parental conditional regard: Comparing conditional positive regard, conditional negative regard, and autonomy support as parenting practices. *Developmental Psychology, 45*, 1119–1142.

Rudy, D., Sheldon, K. M., Awong, T., & Tan, H. H. (2007). Autonomy, culture, and well-being: The benefits of inclusive autonomy. *Journal of Research in Personality, 41*, 983–1007.

Rusbult, C. E. (1983). A longitudinal test of the investment model: The development (and deterioration) of satisfaction and commitment in heterosexual involvements. *Journal of Personality and Social Psychology, 45*, 101–117.

Ryan, R. M. (1982). Control and information in the intrapersonal sphere: An extension of cognitive evaluation theory. *Journal of Personality and Social Psychology, 43*, 450–461.

Ryan, R. M. (1993). Agency and organization: Intrinsic motivation, autonomy and the self in psychological development. In J. Jacobs (Ed.), *Nebraska symposium on motivation: Developmental perspectives on motivation* (Vol. 40, pp. 1–56). Lincoln, NE: University Of Nebraska Press.

Ryan, R. M. (1995). Psychological needs and the facilitation of integrative processes. *Journal of Personality, 63*, 397–427.

Ryan, R. M., & Deci, E. L. (2000). The darker and brighter sides of human existence: Basic psychological needs as a unifying concept. *Psychological Inquiry, 11*, 319–338.

Ryan, R. M., Deci, E. L., Grolnick, W. S., & La Guardia, J. G. (2006). The significance of autonomy and autonomy support in psychological development and psychopathology. In D. Cicchetti & D. J. Cohen (Eds.), *Developmental psychopathology: Theory and method* (2nd ed., pp. 795–849). Hoboken, NJ: Wiley.

Ryan, R. M., La Guardia, J. G., Solky-Butzel, J., Chirkov, V., & Kim, Y. (2005). On the interpersonal regulation of emotions: Emotional reliance across gender, relationships, and cultures. *Personal Relationships, 12*, 145–163.

Ryan, R. M., Patrick, H., Deci, E. L., & Williams, G. C. (2008). Facilitating health behaviour change and its maintenance: Interventions based on self-determination theory. *The European Health Psychologist, 10*, 2–5.

Simpson, J. A., & Rholes, W. S. (Eds.). (2004). *Adult attachment: Theory, research, and clinical implications*. New York: Guilford Publications, Inc.

Soenens, B., Duriez, B., Vansteenkiste, M., & Goossens, L. (2007). The intergenerational transmission of empathy-related responding in adolescence: The role of maternal support. *Personality and Social Psychology Bulletin, 33*, 1–13.

Soenens, B., Elliot, A. J., Goossens, L., Vansteenkiste, M., Luyten, P., & Duriez, B. (2005). The intergenerational transmission of perfectionism: Parents' psychological control as intervening variable. *Journal of Family Psychology, 19*, 358–366.

Soenens, B., Vansteenkiste, M., Lens, W., Luyckx, K., Beyers, W., Goossens, L., et al. (2007). Conceptualizing parental autonomy support: Adolescent perceptions of promoting independence versus promoting volitional functioning. *Developmental Psychology, 43*, 633–646.

Stroebe, W., & Stroebe, M. S. (1987). *Bereavement and health: The psychological and physical consequences of partner loss*. New York: Cambridge University Press.

Triandis, H. C., McCusker, C., & Hui, C. H. (1990). Multimethod probes of individualism and collectivism. *Journal of Personality and Social Psychology, 59*, 1006–1020.

Hodgins, H. S., Weibust, K. S., Weinstein, N., Shiffman, S., Miller, A., Coombs, G., et al. (in press). The cost of self-protection: Threat response and performance as a function of autonomy and control motivation. *Personality and Social Psychology Bulletin*.

Moller, A. C., Deci, E. L., & Elliot, A. J. (2010). Person-level relatedness and the incremental value of relating. *Personality and Social Psychology Bulletin, 36*, 754–767.

Chapter 6
Do Social Institutions Necessarily Suppress Individuals' Need for Autonomy? The Possibility of Schools as Autonomy-Promoting Contexts Across the Globe

Johnmarshall Reeve and Avi Assor

Self-determination theory (SDT) emphasizes the important role that the experience of autonomy plays in a person's positive functioning and social adjustment (Ryan & Deci, 2000, 2002). Perceived autonomy is the subjective experience one feels during behavior that one's actions arise out of an internally locused, volitional sense of causality (Reeve, Nix, & Hamm, 2003). That is, the experience of autonomy is the inner endorsement of one's behavior as one's own. According to the theory, the experience of autonomy depends on the satisfaction of basic psychological needs (for autonomy, competence, and relatedness) and on the presence of environmental affordances that support these needs. While the needs for competence and relatedness have received considerable attention from other theories (Baumeister & Leary, 1995; Guisinger & Blatt, 1994; White, 1959), SDT is unique in its emphasis on and empirical exploration of the need for autonomy. As a psychological need, autonomy is the striving to feel that one is not compelled by external or by intra-personal forces to adopt goals and enact behaviors one does not fully identify with, as well as the striving to construct, maintain, and realize goals, values, and interests which can serve as an inner compass when choices are available (Assor, 2009a, 2010).

A core empirical finding is that people function positively in a variety of important ways when environments nurture and support their need for autonomy, while they function relatively poorly in terms of those same outcomes when their surroundings frustrate their need for autonomy (Assor, Kaplan, & Roth, 2002; Assor, Roth, & Deci, 2004; Black & Deci, 2000; Jang, Reeve, Ryan, & Kim, 2009; Roth, Assor, Niemiec, Ryan, & Deci, 2009; Vallerand, Fortier, & Guay, 1997; Vansteenkiste, Simons, Lens, Sheldon, & Deci, 2004). The practical implication of this research is that the more social institutions are sensitive to and supportive of individual's need for autonomy, the better individuals in those social institutions function.

A seemingly irreconcilable conflict with the aforementioned conclusion surfaces when considering societies that characterized themselves by hierarchical values

---

J. Reeve (✉)
World Class University Project Group, Department of Education, Korea University, Seoul 136-701, South Korea
e-mail: reeve@korea.ac.kr

and structures (Kohn, 1993; Ryan & Brown, 2005; Ryan & Weinstein, 2009). When societies and social institutions utilize a hierarchical structure to ensure the smooth transmission and enactment of dominant values and goals to children or employees and when that structure is paired with a carrot-and-stick approach to motivating them, then the idea of supporting or nurturing a person's need for autonomy seems out of place. For instance, in many schools, smooth functioning means (in part) that students are behaving well, acquiring valued skills, performing well on achievement tests, and graduating in a timely fashion. If schools perceive that such outcomes can best be attained by creating an authoritarian, evaluative, pressure-inducing, and high-stakes social context, then sacrificing students' need for autonomy is often viewed as a necessary side effect of such practices. Some school administrators even prioritize the use of shame-based motivators (publically and critically comparing one school to another) and threats of sanctions as the means to attain their desired outcomes (Nichols & Berliner, 2007). The theme that runs throughout this chapter is that this is a problem, and it is a problem because empirical research shows that neglecting or discounting the importance of students' need for autonomy is an administrative and curricular blunder—and this is true in the classroom (Assor, Kaplan, Kanat-Maymon, & Roth, 2005), at the level of the school (Kohn, 2000), and at the level of the culture more generally (Ryan & La Guardia, 1999).

This same conflict between sacrificing individuals' needs in favor of institutional goals plays itself out across a range of institutional settings, including the family, businesses, corporations, the military, religious institutions, sports teams, health care settings, governmental agencies, and so forth. While the present paper does examine social institutions in general, its specific focus will be on the social institution of the school—and on addressing the following five questions in particular:

- What makes a social institution controlling?
- Do social institutions necessarily need to be controlling?
- Can hierarchical social institutions be both smooth functioning and noncontrolling? Can they be both smooth functioning and autonomy-promoting?
- What would an autonomy-promoting school look like?
- Are autonomy-promoting schools cross-culturally feasible?

The present paper concerns the role that culturally embedded social institutions play in nurturing versus suppressing individuals' need for autonomy. Implied within the first half of the paper's title is the idea that social institutions often function in ways that suppress individuals' need for autonomy. The question of how and why social institutions pursue their goals in autonomy-suppressing ways occupies the first half of the chapter. Implied in the second half of the paper's title is the idea that social institutions—and schools in particular—can pursue societal goals in ways that support and even nurture the individual's need for autonomy. The question of how and why schools might function as autonomy-promoting cultural institutions occupies the second half of the chapter.

What Makes a Social Institution Controlling?

What makes any entity—an individual, a school, a government, an organization, a corporation, or a culture—controlling is that it intrudes into people's naturally occurring ways of thinking, feeling, and behaving to pressure them to change what they think, feel, or do, and it does so without respecting and considering their concerns or reasons for doing so. For instance, a teacher acts in a controlling way when she tells a student to quit procrastinating and complete her assignment immediately without asking why the student is having trouble finishing the project in the first place. Teachers vary in how controlling they are (Reeve, 2009), parents vary in how controlling they are (Grolnick, 2009), schools vary in how controlling they are (Moss, 2010), and it is also probably true that whole nations vary in how controlling they are (though we are not aware of such comparative data).

What are the attributes which make institutions or people controlling? First, a controlling entity adopts only its own perspective without considering or being sensitive to the perspective of others. This means that the controlling entity prioritizes its own needs and concerns over those of individuals, sometimes grossly so. Second, the controlling entity utilizes insensitive and disrespectful influence attempts to change the individual's thoughts, feelings, and behaviors into something prescribed by the social institution as more acceptable. This means that, rather than allowing individuals to have thoughts, feelings, and actions of their own, the controlling entity tells individuals what is right or what is desirable in terms of what to think, feel, or do. Further, a controlling entity applies pressure until individuals relent and change the way they think, feel, or behave (to be consistent with those of the institution's).

Research has explored why people adopt a controlling style toward others—that is, why any one person or any one representative of a social institution might adopt only his or her own perspective and why he or she might enact insensitive and disrespectful influence attempts (Grolnick, Price, Beiswenger, & Sauck, 2007; Pelletier & Sharp, 2009; Pelletier, Seguin-Levesque, & Legault, 2002; Reeve, 2009; Taylor, Ntoumanis, & Smith, 2009). Essentially, a controlling style becomes increasingly probable when people are subjected to pressures from above, pressures from below, and pressures from within (to borrow a framework first introduced by Pelletier and colleagues, 2002).

In the case of teachers, *pressures from above* include those from school administrators who impose demands such as time constraints (cover curricular material in a specific time), impose performance evaluations, pressure teachers to conform to certain teaching methods, and make teachers accountable and responsible for their students' level of performance (Pelletier & Sharp, 2009; Pelletier et al., 2002). Such pressures can originate from school administrators, but they can also originate from colleagues, departmental chairs, school boards, state legislators, and parents that demand results. *Pressures from below* include teachers' reactions to students' poor-quality motivation, lackluster performance, or irresponsible self-regulation (Pelletier et al., 2002). That is, teachers tend to adapt their motivating style according to their perceptions of the autonomous quality of students' motivation (i.e., they tend to become more controlling when they believe students have poor quality motivation; Pelletier & Vallerand, 1996). Finally, *pressures from within* include those that arise from within a teacher's own personality, values, and beliefs about motivation. When teachers themselves possess controlled motivations, are authoritarian and highly conservative, embrace a control causality orientation, and see utility in controlling motivational strategies (rewards, pressuring-inducing language), they tend to relate to students in controlling ways (Boggiano, Barrett, Weiher, McClelland, & Lusk, 1987; Nachtscheim & Hoy, 1976; Reeve, 1998; Roth, Assor, Kanat-Maymon, & Kaplan, 2007). This trichotomous framework explains why any one particular person adopts a controlling style toward others, but the question pursued in the present paper asks why an entire social institution (or even nation) tends to adopt a controlling style.

Do Social Institutions Necessarily Need to Be Controlling?

To understand the enactment of a controlling style at an institutional level, additional sources of influence need to be added to the trichotomous framework offered above, influences that explain how behavior arises from and reflects social norms as much as it might arise from and reflect personal attitudes. To provide such a framework, we apply the theory of planned behavior (TPB; Ajzen, 1988, 1991), as illustrated graphically in Fig. 6.1.

The TPB seeks to explain people's intentions to engage in a particular behavior and their actual engagement (or not) in that behavior—for instance, whether people intend to vote or exercise or quit smoking and then also whether they actually vote, engage in exercise, or quit smoking. In the TPB, behavior is mostly determined by the person's intentions to engage in the behavior, and intentions are determined by three sources. First, as shown in the three bold boxes in the center of Fig. 6.1, intentions are predicted by the ease of performing that course of action (perceived behavioral control), and that sense of ease is largely a function of how easy versus difficult the successful performance on the behavior is likely to be (e.g., one's intention to quit smoking will be low if quitting is perceived to be a very difficult thing to do). Second, intentions are predicted by the person's attitude toward the course of action (positive attitude), and attitudes in the TPB are essentially the person's beliefs about the value, importance, and enjoyment of the behavior (e.g., one's intention to quit smoking will be low if the person really likes smoking). Third, intentions are predicted by the person's perceptions of the social norms governing the behavior (subjective norm), and subjective norms involve the person's sense of the social pressure and the behavioral expectations of others that guide one in the direction of behaving in a particular way (e.g., one's intention to quit smoking will be high if the person perceives that smoking cessation is something important others expect him or her to do).

In trying to understand why a person (or people working within a social institution more specifically) might adopt an autonomy-supportive motivating style, we

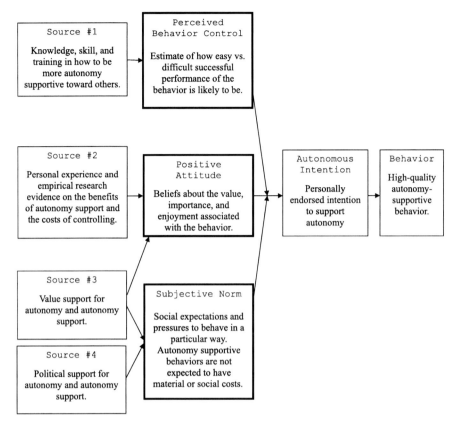

Fig. 6.1 (Modified) Theory of planned behavior to predict how likely it is that individuals will engage in autonomy-supportive behaviors

argue that the likelihood that a person will endorse the intention to act in highly autonomy-supportive ways toward others depends on (1) revising his or her expectation away from the idea that supporting autonomy is difficult and toward the idea that it is a relatively easy thing to do, (2) enhancing his or her positive attitude toward autonomy support (enhancing its perceived value, importance, and enjoyment), and (3) embedding the person's daily experience within a culture that makes autonomy support normative, expected, and unassociated with social costs (see Fig. 6.1).

Enhancing perceived behavioral control: Intervention training to learn how to support autonomy (source #1). In general, teachers rate an autonomy-supportive approach to instruction as a harder thing to do than they rate a controlling approach to instruction (Reeve et al., 2010). That is, teachers think that controlling others is relatively easy, while supporting autonomy is relatively hard. Put another way, teachers generally believe that taking students' perspectives, vitalizing their inner motivational resources, communicating with noncontrolling language, and acknowledging and accepting students' negative affect during instruction is more difficult than is simply telling students what to do and making sure they do it (i.e., a controlling style). While it is not clear if autonomy support is objectively a more difficult-to-apply approach to instruction, it does appear that teachers believe this to be true. Hence, if teachers could gain knowledge, skill, and training in how to be more autonomy-supportive toward students, then they might develop a greater intention to enact an autonomy-supportive style during instruction. Recognizing this, a meta-analysis of 20 independent, experimentally designed training intervention programs showed that teachers (and parents, coaches, workplace managers, physicians, and others) can learn how to be more autonomy-supportive (average effect size for the training intervention, $d = 0.63$; Su & Reeve, in press). That is, with training, autonomy support becomes easier to do (Reeve, Jang, Carrell, Barch, & Jeon, 2004). Thus, one path to help people in organizations adopt a more autonomy-supportive style would be to provide them with effective intervention training in how to do so (to enhance perceived behavioral control; Fig. 6.1).

Enhancing positive attitude: Learning the benefits of autonomy support (source #2). Empirical research affirms the validity of the conclusion that people benefit from autonomy support but suffer from behavioral control (Ryan & Deci, 2000). These benefits have been shown to be meaningful and wide spread, as support for autonomy has been shown to causally increase others' *motivation* (intrinsic motivation, perceived autonomy, perceived competence), *engagement* (effort, persistence, class participation, class attendance), *development* (self-worth, creativity), *learning* (deep processing of information, conceptual understanding, self-regulation strategies), *performance* (grades, standardized test scores), and *psychological well being* (vitality, positive affect, school satisfaction), as reviewed in Reeve (2009). As people learn of the benefits of autonomy support, they tend to adopt a significantly more positive attitude toward the practice (Reeve, 1998). Thus, a second path to help people in organizations adopt a more autonomy-supportive style would be to expose them to the wealth of evidence supporting the conclusion that people benefit from autonomy support but suffer from behavioral control (to enhance a favorable attitude; Fig. 6.1).

Enhancing subjective norm: Value support for autonomy (source #3). The values embraced by institutions and cultures influence individuals' capacity to satisfy their need for autonomy in their daily decisions and behaviors. In particular, when people rate the culture they live in as a relatively hierarchical one, they are less likely to feel that a subjective norm for autonomy-supportive social interactions exists within their culture and they are also less likely to feel autonomy in their daily lives (Chirkov, Ryan, Kim, & Kaplan, 2003; Downie, Koestner, ElGeledi, & Cree, 2004). Hence, social institutions that value hierarchy and social stratification pose a normative obstacle to its individual members' capacity to act in autonomy-supportive ways (Ryan & Sapp, 2007). On a more positive note, Downie, Koestner, and Chua (2007) showed that citizens in countries that embraced values supportive of autonomy relatively flourished and thrived (e.g., in terms of subjective and physical well-being), relative to citizens in countries that embraced values supportive of control. Thus, a third path to help people in organizations adopt a more autonomy-supportive style would be to move toward egalitarian values and therefore make autonomy support a socially valued thing to do (to enhance subjective norm; Fig. 6.1).

Enhancing subjective norm: Political support for autonomy (source #4). Political support for autonomy support has not been extensively studied in the SDT literature, but the research that has been done examined political support at the national level (Downie et al., 2007). National political support for autonomy is evidenced in societies rich in civil liberties and individual rights—that is, those that have governments that are accountable to the people, prioritize equality between individuals, apply the rule of law equally to all citizens, and enable citizens to exercise their right to vote in fair democratic elections. Downie and colleagues showed rather impressively that citizens in countries that provided high political support for daily autonomy relatively flourished and thrived (e.g., in terms of citizens' subjective and physical well-being) relative to citizens in countries that provide them with little or no political support for their autonomy. Thus, a fourth path to help people in organizations adopt a more autonomy-supportive style would be to surround them with a culture that highlighted the social importance of autonomy support and reduced fears that it might produce social or material costs (to enhance subjective norm; Fig. 6.1).

Hierarchical values and social structure. The common denominator underlying value- and politically-oriented influences on subjective norms for autonomy versus control is the concept of hierarchy (versus egalitarianism). Hierarchical organizations make salient and emphasize the legitimacy of authority, roles, social stratification, and unequal allocation of resources (Schwartz, 1994).

Nations can be scored and even rank ordered in terms of the hierarchical values its citizens embrace and depend upon for the culture's smooth functioning (Schwartz, 1994). It makes sense to extend this idea to propose that social institutions might similarly be scored and rank ordered on the extent to which they are hierarchical and dependent on such a structure for their smooth functioning. For instance, social institutions that would likely score as highly hierarchical (in most nations) would be prisons, the military, courts, and corporations, because organizational outcomes such as safety, the rule of law, and the bottom line (profit) are typically prioritized over the concerns and needs of the individuals in those organizations. Social institutions that would likely score as relatively more egalitarian (i.e., less hierarchical) might be hospitals, public services, and schools, as these social institutions generally value and serve the needs of both society and individuals in roughly equal weightings.

The basis for scoring a nation as hierarchical versus egalitarian is the value system that is internalized and endorsed by members of that nation, values that are rooted in the nation's historical, political, religious, and economic (e.g., seniority system) traditions. For a social institution, the basis for determining whether it is largely hierarchical or egalitarian is likely rooted in the purposes for which the social institution was created and continues to be maintained. Prisons are highly hierarchical because their chief function is to maintain order and protect public safety.

Individual rights of inmates are necessarily sacrificed to ensure that the valued institutional mission is accomplished. Of course, prisons could also serve the needs of inmates, as through the offering of educational and job-promotion programs, but the point here is that, generally speaking, hierarchical organizations prioritize institutional goals over individual goals and, in their day to day practice, view sacrificing the individual's concerns as acceptable if doing so helps them achieve their sought-after outcomes.

Can Hierarchical Social Institutions Be Both Smooth Functioning and Noncontrolling?

Social institutions have goals, priorities, and mission statements and they often use a hierarchical structure to make sure they realize their goals with minimum resistance and conflict. In that sense, then, hierarchical structures sometimes enhance smooth, conflict-free functioning that is consistent with the organization's goals. In many ways, the mere presence of a social hierarchy orients social interactants toward a controlling pattern of interaction that reflects influence, power, and control (Magee, Galinsky, & Gruenfeld, 2007). Hence, social hierarchies often achieve their smooth, conflict-free functioning through patterns of interaction that include controlling individuals' thoughts, feelings, and behaviors as a central element. Still, while a controlling hierarchical structure might yield smooth functioning, it nevertheless carries crucial risks to individuals' autonomy, development, and psychological well-being that simply cannot be ignored. So, a crucial question to ask is whether or not hierarchical social institutions can be smooth functioning and noncontrolling at the same time.

Hierarchical social institutions can certainly be smooth functioning. That is, by placing people into roles and by giving some roles the authority and legitimacy to tell others what to do, then social institutions can make progress toward realizing their goals and solving their problems. As an example, a school might want greater conformity from students and institute a dress code policy as a means toward that goal. The school would then give teachers the power to deliver rewards and sanctions to compliant and non-compliant students. The policy and its enforcement might very well yield smooth functioning and a lack of overt resistance to the extent that all students dress in a way that is desirable to the school authorities. But the crucial question is whether or not the social institution—the school, in this case—necessarily needs to be controlling to function in a harmonious way? That is, do hierarchical social institutions necessarily have to pursue their goals and solve their problems in ways that neglect or discount individuals' perspective and voice and do they necessarily have to pursue their goals and solve their problems in ways that are insensitive and disrespectful to individuals' needs and preferences? For a social institution (such as the school) to place individuals' perspective and ways of thinking, feeling, and behaving at the same level of importance as its own likely means it runs the risk of losing its capacity for smooth functioning, at least from the point of view of the social institution.

One contribution this chapter seeks to make is to show how schools can be structured to value and to meet the needs of both society and individuals. The provision of a structured learning environment is essential to meeting the needs, goals, and purposes of schools (e.g., preparing a skilled workforce, promoting the internalization of cultural values), and it is largely through the provision of structure that students become aware of what the social institution (the school) expects of them. The problem with structure, however, is that in many cases it is confused and used interchangeably with coercive control. Control involves demands, insistences, sanctions, and rigid rules; structure does not necessarily involve these components.

Classroom research shows that teacher-provided structure and teacher-provided autonomy support both contribute constructively to positive student outcomes, such as students' greater classroom engagement (Jang, Reeve, & Deci, 2010) and students' greater capacity for self-regulated learning (Sierens, Vansteenkiste, Goossens, Soenens, & Dochy, 2009). The conclusion is that the optimal learning environment for students is one that tends to be both structured and noncontrolling. This is so, because structure (formulating [with students' participation and input] clear goals, communicating reasonable expectations, providing guidance, offering feedback) is essential to meeting the needs, goals, and priorities of the school as well as for supporting students' sense of increased competence in mastering important skills and knowledge, while noncontrolling means that the structure is implemented in ways that value the students' perspectives and respect their concerns, needs, and preferences. So, potentially, hierarchical social institutions could be smooth functioning, harmonious, and noncontrolling. But, noncontrolling is not the same as autonomy supportive, a crucial distinction that leads us to ask whether hierarchical social institutions can be both smooth-functioning and autonomy supportive?

Can Hierarchical Schools Be Truly Autonomy Supportive?

Autonomy support means taking the perspective of the individual, welcoming and inviting individuals' thoughts, feelings, decisions, and actions, and supporting individuals' personal development and capacity for autonomous self-regulation (Reeve, 2009). In practice, autonomy support means creating (1) a structure and an atmosphere that affords choice and supports students as they formulate their inner compass—namely, direction-giving goals, values, and interests (Assor, 2009a, 2010), and (2) classroom conditions that allow students to experience autonomy (Reeve, 2006).

From this understanding of what it means to be autonomy supportive, it is apparent that hierarchical social institutions are structured in ways that work incompatibly against the offering of an environment that is deeply autonomy supportive. That is, by definition, hierarchical social institutions prioritize institutional (or societal) goals, needs, and perspective over individuals' goals, needs, and perspective. Also, by definition, autonomy-supportive environments take the individual's perspective, deeply value and honor that perspective, create opportunities to experience autonomy during action, and create opportunities for students to develop goals, values, and interests which they experience as authentic. This emphasis on the development of an authentic inner compass is a logical opposite to finding one's dutiful place within an imposed hierarchy.

The incompatibility between a hierarchical structure and full autonomy support increases when the hierarchical organization attempts to promote and transmit extrinsic values such as prestige, competitiveness, wealth, or risking your health in an attempt to abide by social conventions. According to SDT, such values do not really help to satisfy basic psychological needs and often make it more difficult to reach meaningful satisfaction of these needs. As a result, any institutional attempt to promote extrinsic values is likely to be experienced as controlling.

While the support of students' basic needs requires considerable material, emotional, and intellectual resources, schools can meet this demanding challenge. Autonomy-promoting schools would characterize themselves by two key features. First, they would be designed in ways that nurtured and satisfied students' need for autonomy. Second, they would offer frequently recurring opportunities for students to experience autonomy during learning activities.

What Would an Autonomy-Promoting School Look Like?

It Would Be Designed to Satisfy Students' Psychological Need for Autonomy

As discussed, the need for autonomy refers to a striving (a) to be able to choose and not be controlled, and (b) to formulate and realize values, goals, and interests which feel authentic and serve as an inner compass in one's life, thus providing inner criteria for making important decisions (when they are allowed to decide). It should be noted that direction-giving goals, values, and interests also provide people with internal criteria for evaluating others and themselves, provide a basis for feeling that one's actions are coherent and meaningful, and make one less dependent on others' evaluations (Assor, 2009a, 2010). SDT-based research has devoted considerable attention to school and classroom features which support students' striving for choice and lack of coercion (e.g., Assor et al., 2002; Reeve & Jang, 2006). However, the second propensity constituting the need for autonomy—the striving to form an inner compass—has received only little attention to date. Yet, there is some research on teacher and parent behaviors that do support the formation of authentic, direction-giving values, goals, and interests. After briefly surveying this research, we will describe the characteristics of schools supporting the formation of an authentic inner compass in students, based both on the surveyed research and on the larger educational literature.

Recent research by the Ben Gurion University motivation group (Assor, 2009b, 2010; Kanat-Maymon & Assor, 2010) suggests that there are two types of educators' behaviors which can support the formation of direction-giving values and goals. The first is educators' support of reflective value/goal exploration (SVE). SVE refers to discussions and activities that enable students to examine the extent to which they see various goals and values as worthy, desirable, and personally meaningful. The second is educators' support of the formation of integrated values, termed "Fostering inner directed valuing processes" (FIV), a construct with three components: helping students calm down before they have to make serious decisions, encouraging the examination of one's values and goals when faced with a difficult decision or external pressures, and encouraging the consideration of alternatives and relevant information before making a decision.

FIV differs from SVE in that it is a socializing practice that is used only when the child faces difficult decisions and social pressures and, unlike SVE, it provides a certain "training" in authentic and rational decision making under stress. In contrast, SVE refers to general encouragement of reflective discussion. FIV is hypothesized to contribute to the formation of integrated values and goals because it helps youth develop the capacity to withstand the difficulties involved in value exploration. Thus, youth who have often engaged in inner-directed valuing are assumed to develop skills and tendencies that would enable them to seriously examine their own thoughts, ideals, and inner feelings when they determine their important goals and form commitments.

Adolescents' perceptions of their parents as high on FIV predict identity-exploration and the formation of commitments that are experienced as autonomous (Assor, 2010; Assor, Eilot, & Roth, 2009). Moreover, FIV also predicts adolescents' capacity to experience anger and anxiety without losing control or immediately suppressing these feelings, as well as their tendency to try to understand the sources of these feelings and their implications for one's life and relationships.

Like parents, teachers too can support and guide youth's reflective value formation (Assor, 2010; Kanat-Maymon & Assor, 2010). For example, Kanat-Maymon and Assor (2010) showed, in three studies, that when teachers encourage students to openly discuss and explore values and goals, students engage in school activities with a strong sense of autonomy and volition, and they also report feeling well and vital. Importantly, these studies also suggest that teachers' SVE promotes not only students' sense of autonomy but students' engagement and grades as well. Thus, support for value and goal exploration might also have a salutary effect on positive academic functioning and in this way might be consistent with the goals of many hierarchical societies and schools.

The importance of SVE was demonstrated in research on modern-orthodox Jewish religious families who encourage open dialogue and reflection on religious principles. Thus, youth growing up in these families report feeling a higher level of integrated religious motivation, perceived autonomy, purpose, and well-being, relative to youth growing in families not supporting reflection and dialogue on religious principles (Assor, Cohen-Melayev, Kaplan, & Friedman, 2005).

The research surveyed makes it clear that schools aspiring to support the need for autonomy should do more than allow choice and avoid controlling teaching methods. Additionally, it appears important to foster students' capacity and inclination to engage in inner valuing (FIV), as well as create regular opportunities which support reflective discussion and exploration of goals and values (SVE). Therefore, these two inter-related supports for authentic value and goal formation constitute an essential element of the autonomy-promoting school. However, FIV and SVE might not be enough to support students' need for autonomy. To enable students to feel that they can truly have choice and influence on their life in school and to support the formation of authentic interests and values, additional school attributes are needed. Below is a brief description of six attributes of an autonomy-promoting school to supplement FIV and SVE.

(1) *Each teacher is responsible for a small number of students with whom he or she has regularly scheduled dialogues*. The first and perhaps most important feature of an autonomy-promoting school is the role-definition of teachers as *growth-promoting allies* who maintain regular dialogues with students. This role definition is not only one of the defining principles of the school, but more importantly, it is shared and internalized by the teachers, and the school further offers organizational supports, procedures, and regular in-service training to help teachers function and develop as growth-promoting allies. The growth-promoting teacher strives, and is expected, to create relationships with students which help them feel that the teacher is really interested in their growth and basic needs. This is facilitated by regularly scheduled and on-going teacher–student dialogues.

To become high-quality growth-promoting allies and to be able to conduct effective growth-promoting dialogues, most teachers have to go through training and consultation meetings to develop their skills and capacities in this domain. These meetings are most effective when they occur on a regular basis in small groups in which teachers can share their difficulties, clarify professional dilemmas, and plan ahead in a secure and accepting atmosphere that provides emotional and professional support (Assor, Kaplan, Feinberg, & Tal, 2009; Feinberg, Kaplan, Assor, & Kanat-Maymon, 2008; Kaplan & Assor, 2010). Such in-service support allows teachers the training they need to become growth-promoting allies in that they, first, decrease their own controlling behaviors, school violence decreases, and peer-to-peer caring increases (Feinberg et al., 2008); second, enhance their capacities to enact dialogue capable of enhancing students' positive affect and perceptions that their studies have relevance for students' lives and suppress violence in school (Kaplan & Assor, 2010), and; third, pave the wave for these teachers to find greater fulfillment and satisfaction in the profession and to understand students better and in ways that foster closer and less tense relationships (Assor, 2010; Feinberg et al., 2008).

While the above programs do not directly focus on teachers' ability to support the development of students' values, goals, and interests, it appears that the establishment of empathic, respectful, and trusting relations between teachers and students is a necessary foundation for teachers' ability to foster inner valuing processes and value and interest exploration in students. The next five attributes more directly support students' strivings for choice and for value and interest formation.

(2) *Students have considerable influence and responsibility (democratic participation)*. This feature refers to schools as democratic institutions in which students take part as citizens who have considerable influence as well as responsibility. Models of such schools and classrooms appear in Rogers and Freiberg (1994), Freiberg (1996) and also in Kohlberg's (1981) *Just Community* approach to moral development. This attribute refers to an organizational structure in which students are true partners in the determination of discipline laws, budget allocations, and even the selection of learning contents, knowledge objectives, and assessment procedures. It is assumed that adults' willingness to give students such influence and responsibility causes students to feel that their need for choice and their competence and inherent goodness are deeply respected. Moreover, the opportunity to participate in the determination of various objectives, in making highly consequential decisions, and the democratic deliberation procedures leading to various decisions enable students to reflect on various goals, values, and moral principles and then internalize them as integrated personal values and goals.

(3) *Foster the development of individual interests*. To allow the formation of individual interests, the autonomy-promoting school would allocate considerable time and resources to activities in which students' explore various domains of potential interest and then, with help and instruction from relevant people inside and outside of the school, they try to develop competence and skills which would enable them to develop enduring intrinsic interest in the domain they found to be satisfying and personally meaningful. Educational psychologists offer excellent insights into what relevant activities and structures help students develop individual interests (e.g., Hidi & Renninger, 2006). This feature of the autonomy-promoting school becomes increasingly important as students mature, so that in high school it can be expected to occupy a significant portion of the time students spend in school and after school.

(4) *Support exploration of and open reflection on important social and moral identity-defining values and issues (SVE)*. Post-modern societies and the information age are characterized by moral relativism, abundance of contradictory opinions, a huge volume of information, and the availability (or apparent availability) of many choice options in terms of life styles, world views, and careers. These circumstances, and particularly the absence of widely accepted authorities, make it especially difficult for youth to develop clear goals and values that are authentic and reflection based. To enable youth to develop such values and goals, it is important that schools institute regular activities and discussions in which youth are able to discuss their views on important social and moral issues. Such discussions should, of course, be carried out in an atmosphere that is accepting and tolerant to different views. Moreover, as part of such discussions, teachers should encourage skills and routines that foster inner directed valuing processes (FIV). Thus, before students arrive at a certain decision or make a commitment to some course of action (for example, volunteering), teachers should help students feel that it is okay to take the time to calm down, stay with the ambiguity for a while, avoid doing things as a result of social pressure, and examine why they really want to make the commitment. While

FIV can start in kindergarten, support for value exploration (SVE) likely becomes most important in adolescence.

(5) *Pro-social activities that are satisfying and choiceful.* In almost all societies children and youth are expected to internalize and enact pro-social and altruistic values, such as helping the needy, caring for others, and showing social involvement. Because such pro-social actions are not necessarily pleasant and often entail significant personal costs, authentic and deep internalization of such values is difficult to attain. Autonomy-promoting schools may therefore need to institute specific activities and structures that would allow students to discover the satisfactions that can be derived from meaningful pro-social action and social involvement. It is assumed that if students have satisfying experiences during these activities (e.g., while helping younger students in school, visiting the elderly, volunteering with a community organization), then they are likely to internalize the importance of pro-social activities and goals as an important aspect of their self and identity.

While youth identity includes interests, values, and goals other than pro-social goals and values, there is a good reason to believe that pro-social and moral values may be an especially important component of a healthy identity in post-modern societies, perhaps even form *the unshakeable core of one's inner compass.* These direction-giving goals and values may be a crucial source of a sense of autonomy and therefore vitality. They also are highly important across cultures, yield consistent psycho-social benefits, and appear to have at least a partly organismic (perhaps even evolutionary) foundation (Weinstein & Ryan, 2010). However, to increase the likelihood that pro-social activities will be satisfying and meaningful, it is important to create a school structure that allows pro-social activities to be experienced as need satisfying. That is, students need to feel that when they engage in helping or volunteering, their needs for choice and a lack of coercion, for competence, and for relatedness are being met. To insure such need satisfaction, it is important to allow students to choose the activities they engage in, and it is essential to provide guidance and support to help students cope with various difficulties in their pro-social activities. Thus, schools who would like to help students develop authentic pro-social goals and commitments cannot simply urge their students to get involved in pro-social activities. Rather, they can provide a structure that would insure that these involvements are need satisfying and therefore contribute constructively to the formation of authentic, direction-giving, pro-social goals and values.

(6) *Reduce the amount of information students are tested on and the frequency of comparative achievement tests.* Considerable research has shown that tests producing scores that allow students, teachers, and schools to be compared increase tension, create ego-involvement, and focus attention on ability demonstration rather than on ability improvement. Moreover, when schools and teachers have to demonstrate success in mastering great amounts of information they cannot devote sufficient time to participatory democratic procedures (including time-consuming discussions of conduct problems and rule violations), to regular teacher–student dialogues, to supervised pro-social activities, and to activities fostering the development of inner valuing, values, and interests.

Importantly, numerous educators have emphasized that in the information age, there is little sense in trying to transmit to children great amounts of information (including very specific mathematical or scientific procedures and detailed information in the social and biological sciences on which students are often tested). Rather, it is more important to develop basic language and math knowledge, skills allowing effective knowledge search and organization, and skills allowing logical and critical thinking. It therefore appears that schools can reduce the amount of information they test on and the frequency of comparative tests without harming their students' future ability to master difficult academic challenges or to obtain high-tech jobs.

When considering these attributes of autonomy-promoting schools, it is important *not* to view them simply as a list of separate components from which one can randomly pick. Rather, the first two components and the last one (regular teacher–student growth-promoting dialogues, students' influence on major aspects of school life, and reducing the amount of information to be tested on) appear to provide a necessary foundation which cannot be discarded. Components 3–5 then contribute to the construction of an authentic inner compass that includes goals, values, and interests.

What Would an Autonomy-Promoting School Look Like?

It Would Create Frequently Recurring Opportunities for Students to Experience Autonomy During Learning Activities

While the first key feature of autonomy-promoting schools is that they nurture and satisfy students' *need for autonomy*, the second is that they create ongoing opportunities for *autonomy experiences* during learning activities. Empirical, classroom-based research has identified four sets of teaching behaviors that reliably allow students to feel highly autonomous during learning activities: nurture inner motivational resources, rely on noncontrolling and informational language, display patience to allow for self-paced learning and personal development to occur, and acknowledge and accept expressions of negative feelings. Each of these four ways of relating to students will be discussed in the paragraphs below, but it is worth pointing out here that autonomy-supportive instructional behaviors (including those that extend beyond the four highlighted here) are simply those which effectively promote the subjective experience of autonomy—that is, feeling like an origin, engaging oneself in volitional action, experiencing a sense of choice, and learning to trust an inner voice.

(1) *Nurture inner motivational resources*. The first quality that makes a school autonomy-promoting is that it nurtures students' inner motivational resources during instruction. An autonomy-supportive approach to instruction rests on the assumption that students possess inner motivational resources that are fully capable of

energizing and directing their classroom activity in productive ways. Autonomy-promoting schools therefore strive to first gain awareness of what inner motivational resources students possess and then second find or create opportunities to nurture and develop those resources (Reeve & Halusic, 2009). What is meant by the term *inner motivational resources* are vitalizing sources of motivation such as intrinsic motivation, interests, self-set (intrinsic) goals, inner-directed valuing, among others (see Reeve, Deci, & Ryan, 2004). The fundamental importance of nurturing inner motivational resources during instruction becomes most obvious when teachers introduce a new learning activity and request that students engage themselves in it. To spark vitalized engagement, autonomy-promoting schools consistency involve and nurture students' inner resources that are too often latent (not activated) in students' classroom experiences, while controlling schools tend to just tell students what to do and then use extrinsic motivators and controlling language to make sure they do it. For instance, to vitalize an autonomy-rich learning experience, the teacher might begin the lesson by asking a curiosity-inducing question (e.g., "Where did the moon come from?"), pose an optimal challenge (e.g., "Here is a problem; see if you can figure it out."), or communicate that the learning activity represents an opportunity to make progress toward an intrinsic goal (e.g., to become a good writer), rather than artificially manufacture student initiative by telling them to obey a directive, fulfill a request, or earn extra credit points.

(2) *Rely on noncontrolling and informational language.* The second quality that makes a school autonomy-promoting is that it avoids controlling language and policies and, instead, relies on language and policies that are highly informational. Schools and classrooms invariably have rules, procedures, behavioral requests, and learning activities that are not inherently interesting and need-satisfying things for students to do. This creates a motivational problem for students who understandably have a difficult time generating the motivation they need to undertake such unappealing endeavors. To support students' volitional engagement in uninteresting (but important) activities, autonomy-promoting schools provide explanatory rationales that articulate clearly why the requested behavior is truly worth their effort, and they make a special effort to provide such rationales when choice is constrained or uninteresting endeavors are necessary. Such schools also frame unappealing requests and lessons (e.g., "You need to revise your paper again") within the context of pursuing and attaining intrinsic goals ("because it will help you become the writer you want to become"). What autonomy-promoting schools do not do (that controlling school do) is verbally push and pressure students toward predetermined answers, solutions, and desired behaviors through rigid, evaluative, and pressure-inducing communications, such as by uttering commands and directives (Assor et al., 2005), inducing feelings of shame, guilt, or anxiety (Ryan, 1982), cultivating perfectionistic standards and self-representations (Soenens, Vansteenkiste, Duriez, Luyten, & Goossens, 2005), or by offering "conditional regard" more generally (Assor et al., 2004).

(3) *Display patience to allow time for self-paced learning and personal development to occur.* The third quality that makes a school autonomy-promoting is that it allows students the time and space they need for self-paced learning and personal development to occur. Learning and personal development take time, as a

student who is trying to make sense of a learning activity or to understand and resolve a personal issue needs both time and opportunity to explore and manipulate materials and ideas, make plans, formulate and test hypotheses, evaluate evidence and feedback, adjust problem-solving strategies, monitor the progress they are making, revise their work, re-evaluate their goals, and so forth. In contrast, controlling schools short-cut this learning process (or even by-pass it altogether) and, instead, simply tell students answers and solutions before they have a chance to figure them out for themselves, as if the outcome was more important than the learning itself. So, instead of telling and showing students right answers and desired behaviors, a teacher in an autonomy-promoting school would take the time to listen, provide encouragement for initiative and effort, provide time and opportunities for students to work in their own way, offer helpful hints when students seem stuck, and postpone advice until they first understand the students' goals and perspective, though they also provide expectations, guidance, scaffolding, and feedback (i.e., structure) when it is needed and invited (Reeve & Jang, 2006).

(4) *Acknowledge and accept expressions of negative feelings*. The fourth quality that makes a school autonomy promoting is that it adopts the students' perspective to acknowledge and accept negative feelings and expressions of resistance. Students are bound to encounter motivational and behavioral problems in schools because schools necessarily have rules, requirements, and agendas that are sometimes at odds with their preferences and natural inclinations. The typical controlling reaction to student problems such as listlessness, complaining, whining, sloppy work, and irresponsible behavior is to counter students' negative affect and problematic behavior with power assertions designed to suppress these criticisms and complaints, or turn them into something more acceptable to the teacher (e.g., "quit your complaining and pay attention"; Assor et al., 2005). Such a reaction leaves students with the impression that the teacher is insensitive to their concerns. In contrast, autonomy-promoting schools acknowledge and accept such expressions of negative feelings in a way that students get the impression that the teacher understands that they are struggling and are in need of assistance and support. Acknowledging and accepting students' expressions of negative affect as a potentially valid reaction to an imposed rule or requirement is not about being permissive or relinquishing a teacher's authority. Rather, it is about giving students a voice and understanding their perspective. More proactively, it also means soliciting students' opinions, allowing (even encouraging) students to voice their preferences and opinions, and basically being more tolerant and appreciative of students' autonomy (Assor et al., 2005).

Are Autonomy-Promoting Schools Cross-Culturally Feasible?

So far, we have taken the position that schools can function as autonomy-promoting social institutions. We have further argued that we know what autonomy-promoting schools can look like in practice. We now turn to the question of whether autonomy-promoting schools are cross-culturally feasible. That is, autonomy-promoting schools might work in the United States and Canada, but will they work in Brazil

(Chirkov, Ryan, & Willness, 2005), Bulgaria (Deci et al., 2001), Korea (Jang et al., 2009), or China (Vansteenkiste, Zhou, Lens, & Soenens, 2005)?

To explain when people in social institutions (e.g., teachers in schools) enact autonomy-supportive or controlling behavior toward others, we offered Fig. 6.1, based loosely (but not directly) on the theory of planned behavior. In this theory, weights (weighted influence) are assigned to the three sources of influence—perceived behavioral control, personal attitude, and subjective norm. The magnitude of the weights is determined by the particulars of the behavior (e.g., how easy versus hard it is to do), the person's evaluation of that behavior (e.g., how valuable or enjoyable it has proven itself to be in the past), and the situational constraints and social forces operative when enacting the behavior (e.g., flexibility or inflexibility of school administrators).

In egalitarian countries where social norms expect and encourage autonomy and autonomy support, relatively little cultural press to enact a controlling motivating style is likely to exist. That is, in egalitarian countries, the subjective norm to engage in controlling behaviors is not likely to be a dominating behavioral influence. Hence, whether a school creates an autonomy-supportive climate for its students depends largely on how valuable teachers believe autonomy support to be (positive attitude) and how efficacious they perceive themselves to be when trying to teach in autonomy-supportive ways (perceived behavioral control). Such attitudes and perceptions of control can be (and have been) supported by professional developmental opportunities, as discussed earlier. This means that autonomy-promoting schools are quite feasible in egalitarian countries.

In hierarchical countries where social norms neither expect nor encourage autonomy and autonomy support, a relatively strong cultural press to enact a controlling motivating style is likely to be a dominating behavioral influence. Hence, in hierarchical countries, the offering of an autonomy-promoting school is not a likely cultural product, assuming the prevailing social norms expect and encourage control and discourage autonomy support. This means that autonomy-promoting schools will be less feasible in hierarchical countries.

Why go through all the trouble to create an autonomy-promoting school, especially when that school is situated within a hierarchical cultural context? We argue that an autonomy-promoting school is a social asset. This is so because the satisfaction of the need for autonomy and offering of recurring classroom opportunities to experience autonomy enable students to become more fully and more wholeheartedly immersed in the learning process. This, in turn, promotes optimal learning and personal growth, as well as the inclinations to internalize cultural values, care for others, and contribute to important social causes.

References

Ajzen, I. (1988). *Attitudes, personality, and behavior*. Chicago: Dorsey Press.
Ajzen, I. (1991). The theory of planned behavior. *Organizational Behavior and Human Decision Processes, 50*, 179–211.

Assor, A. (2009a). *Value/goal formation and inner valuing*. Paper presented in the convention of the American Educational Research Association, San Diego, CA.

Assor, A. (2009b). Enhancing teachers' motivation to apply humanist information technology innovations. *Policy Futures in Education, 66*, 662–669.

Assor, A. (2010). *Two under-emphasized components of autonomy support: Fostering value/goal exploration and inner valuing*. Paper presented in the 4th international conference on Self Determination Theory, Gent, Belgium.

Assor, A., Cohen-Melayev, M., Kaplan, A., & Friedman, D. (2005). Choosing to stay religious in a modern world: Socialization and exploration processes leading to an integrated internalization of religion among Israeli Jewish youth. *Advances in Motivation and Achievement, 14*, 105–150.

Assor, A., Eilot, K., & Roth, G. (2009). *In search of an optimal style of negative emotion regulation: Correlates and potential parental antecedents of integrated regulation*. Paper presented in the Society for Research in Child Development, Boston, MA.

Assor, A., Kaplan, H., Feinberg, O., & Tal, K. (2009). Combining vision with voice: A learning and implementation structure promoting teachers' internalization of practices based on self-determination theory. *Theory and Research in Education, 7*, 234–243.

Assor, A., Kaplan, H., Kanat-Maymon, Y., & Roth, G. (2005). Directly controlling teacher behaviors as predictors of poor motivation and engagement in girls and boys: The role of anger and anxiety. *Learning and Instruction, 15*, 397–413.

Assor, A., Kaplan, H., & Roth, G. (2002). Choice is good, but relevance is excellent: Autonomy-enhancing and suppressing teaching behaviors predicting students' engagement in schoolwork. *British Journal of Educational Psychology, 27*, 261–278.

Assor, A., Roth, G., & Deci, E. L. (2004). The emotional costs of parents' conditional regard: A self-determination theory analysis. *Journal of Personality, 72*, 47–88.

Assor, A. (in press). Autonomous moral motivation: Consequences, socializing antecedents and the unique role of integrated moral principles. In M. Mikulincer & P. R. Shaver (Eds.), *Social psychology of morality: Exploring the causes of good and evil*. Washington, DC: American Psychological Association.

Baumeister, R. F., & Leary, M. R. (1995). The need to belong: Desire for interpersonal attachments as a fundamental human motivation. *Psychological Bulletin, 117*, 497–529.

Black, A. E., & Deci, E. L. (2000). The effects of instructors' autonomy support and students' autonomous motivation on learning organic chemistry: A self-determination theory perspective. *Science Education, 84*, 740–756.

Boggiano, A. K., Barrett, M., Weiher, A. W., McClelland, G. H., & Lusk, C. M. (1987). Use of the maximal-operant principle to motivate children's intrinsic interest. *Journal of Personality and Social Psychology, 53*, 866–879.

Chirkov, V., Ryan, R. M., Kim, Y., & Kaplan, U. (2003). Differentiating autonomy from individualism and independence: A self-determination theory perspective on internalization of cultural orientation, gender, and well-being. *Journal of Personality and Social Psychology, 84*, 97–110.

Chirkov, V., Ryan, R. M., & Willness, C. (2005). Cultural context and psychological needs in Canada and Brazil: Testing a self-determination approach to the internalization of cultural practices, identity, and well-being. *Journal of Cross-Cultural Psychology, 36*, 423–443.

Deci, E. L., Ryan, R. M., Gagné, M., Leone, D. R., Usunov, J., & Kornazheva, B. P. (2001). Need satisfaction, motivation, and well-being in the work organizations of a former Eastern Bloc country: A cross-cultural study of self-determination. *Personality and Social Psychology Bulletin, 27*, 930–942.

Downie, M., Koestner, R., & Chua, S. N. (2007). Political support for self-determination, wealth, and national subjective well-being. *Motivation and Emotion, 31*, 174–181.

Downie, M., Koestner, R., ElGeledi, S., & Cree, K. (2004). The impact of cultural internalization and integration on well being among tricultural individuals. *Personality and Social Psychology Bulletin, 30*, 305–314.

Feinberg, O., Kaplan, H., Assor, A., & Kanat-Maymon, Y. (2008). *Self determination theory as a basis for a comprehensive school reform*. Poster presented at the convention of the American Educational Research Association, New York.

Freiberg, H. (1996). From tourists to citizens in the classroom. Creating a climate for learning. *Educational Leadership, 54*, 32–36.

Grolnick, W. S. (2009). The role of parents in facilitating autonomous self-regulation for education. *Theory and Research in Education, 7*, 164–173.

Grolnick, W. S., Price, C. E., Beiswenger, K. I., & Sauck, C. C. (2007). Evaluative pressure on mothers: Effects of situation, maternal, and child characteristics on autonomy-supportive versus controlling behavior. *Developmental Psychology, 38*, 143–155.

Guisinger, S., & Blatt, S. J. (1994). Individuality and relatedness: Evolution of a fundamental dialectic. *American Psychologist, 49*, 104–111.

Hidi, S., & Renninger, A. (2006). A four-phase model of interest development. *Educational Psychologist, 41*, 111–127.

Jang, H., Reeve, J., & Deci, E. L. (2010). Engaging students in learning activities: It's not autonomy support or structure, but autonomy support and structure. *Journal of Educational Psychology, 102*, 588–600.

Jang, H., Reeve, J., Ryan, R. M., & Kim, A. (2009). Can self-determination theory explain what underlies the productive, satisfying learning experiences of collectivistically-oriented Korean adolescents? *Journal of Educational Psychology, 101*, 644–661.

Kanat-Maymon, Y., & Assor, A. (2010). *Teachers' support for students' explorations of values and goals: Effects on perceived autonomy, engagement and grades*. Israel: Ben Gurion University.

Kaplan, H., & Assor, A. (2010). *Enhancing autonomy-supportive I-Thou dialogue in schools: Conceptualization and an interventions program*. Manuscript under review.

Kohlberg, L. (1981). *Essays on moral development*. New York: Harper & Row.

Kohn, A. (1993). *Punished by rewards: The trouble with gold stars, incentive plans, A's, praise, and other bribes*. Boston: Houghton Mifflin.

Kohn, A. (2000). *The case against standardized testing: Raising the scores, ruining the schools*. Portsmouth, NH: Heinemann.

Magee, J. C., Galinsky, A. D., & Gruenfeld, D. H. (2007). Power, propensity to negotiate, and moving first in competitive interactions. *Personality and Social Psychology Bulletin, 33*, 200–212.

Moss, J. D. (2010). *Autonomy support and engagement in prekindergarten: Training the teachers in traditional and Montessori environments*. Master's thesis, University of Wisconsin-Milwaukee, Milwaukee, WI.

Nachtscheim, N. M., & Hoy, W. K. (1976). Authoritarian personality and control ideologies of teachers. *Alberta Journal of Educational Research, 22*, 173–178.

Nichols, S. L., & Berliner, D. C. (2007). *Collateral damage: How high-stakes testing corrupts America's schools*. Cambridge, MA: Harvard Education Press.

Pelletier, L. G., Seguin-Levesque, C., & Legault, L. (2002). Pressure from above and pressure from below as determinants of teachers' motivation and teaching behaviors. *Journal of Educational Psychology, 94*, 186–196.

Pelletier, L. C., & Sharp, E. C. (2009). Administrative pressures and teachers' interpersonal behavior in the classroom. *Theory and Research in Education, 7*, 174–183.

Pelletier, L. G., & Vallerand, R. J. (1996). Supervisors' beliefs and subordinates' intrinsic motivation: A behavioral confirmation analysis. *Journal of Personality and Social Psychology, 71*, 331–340.

Reeve, J. (1998). Autonomy support as an interpersonal motivating style: Is it teachable? *Contemporary Educational Psychology, 23*, 312–330.

Reeve, J. (2006). Teachers as facilitators: What autonomy-supportive teachers do and why their students benefit. *Elementary School Journal, 106*, 225–236.

Reeve, J. (2009). Why teachers adopt a controlling motivation style toward students and how they can become more autonomy supportive. *Educational Psychologist, 44*, 159–175.

Reeve, J., Cheon, S. H., Assor, A., Kaplan, H., Moss, J. D., Vansteenkiste, M., Besbes, R., Jang, H., & Olaussen, B. S. (2010). *Testing cultural norms as the foundational basis for a teacher's motivating style toward students*. Unpublished manuscript, Korea University, Korea.

Reeve, J., Deci, E. L., & Ryan, R. M. (2004). Self-determination theory: A dialectical framework for understanding the sociocultural influences on student motivation. In D. McInerney & S. Van Etten (Eds.), *Research on sociocultural influences on motivation and learning: Big theories revisited* (Vol. 4, pp. 31–59). Greenwich, CT: Information Age Press.

Reeve, J., & Halusic, M. (2009). How K-12 teachers can put self-determination theory principles into practice. *Theory and Research in Education, 7*, 145–154.

Reeve, J., & Jang, H. (2006). What teachers say and do to support students' autonomy during a learning activity. *Journal of Educational Psychology, 98*, 209–218.

Reeve, J., Jang, H., Carrell, D., Barch, J., & Jeon, S. (2004). Enhancing high school students' engagement by increasing their teachers' autonomy support. *Motivation and Emotion, 28*, 147–169.

Reeve, J., Nix, G., & Hamm, D. (2003). Testing models of the experience of self-determination in intrinsic motivation and the conundrum of choice. *Journal of Educational Psychology, 95*, 375–392.

Rogers, C., & Freiberg, H. J. (1994). *Freedom to learn* (3rd ed.). New York: Macmillan/Merrill.

Roth, G., Assor, A., Kanat-Maymon, Y., & Kaplan, H. (2007). Perceived autonomy in teaching: How self determined teaching may lead to self-determined learning. *Journal of Educational Psychology, 99*, 761–774.

Roth, G., Assor, A., Niemiec, P. C., Ryan, R. M., & Deci, E. L. (2009). The negative consequences of parental conditional regard: A comparison of positive conditional regard, negative conditional regard, and autonomy support as parenting strategies. *Developmental Psychology, 4*, 1119–1142.

Ryan, R. M. (1982). Control and information in the intrapersonal sphere: An extension of cognitive evaluation theory. *Journal of Personality and Social Psychology, 43*, 450–461.

Ryan, R. M., & Brown, K. W. (2005). Legislating competence: The motivational impact of high-stakes testing as an educational reform. In C. Dweck & A. J. Elliot (Eds.), *Handbook of competence*. New York: Guilford Press.

Ryan, R. M., & Deci, E. L. (2000). Self-determination theory and the facilitation of intrinsic motivation, social development, and well-being. *American Psychologist, 55*, 68–78.

Ryan, R. M., & Deci, E. L. (2002). An overview of self-determination theory: An organismic-dialectical perspective. In E. L. Deci & R. M. Ryan(Eds.), *Handbook of self-determination research* (pp. 3–33). Rochester, NY: University of Rochester Press.

Ryan, R. M., & La Guardia, J. G. (1999). Achievement motivation within a pressured society: Intrinsic and extrinsic motivation to learn and the politics of school reform. In T. Urdan (Ed.), *Advances in motivation and achievement* (Vol. 11, pp. 45–85). Greenwich, CT: JAI Press.

Ryan, R. M., & Sapp, A. R. (2007). Basic psychological needs: A self-determination theory perspective on the promotion of wellness across development and cultures. In I. Gough &J. A. McGregor (Eds.), *Wellbeing in developing countries: From theory to research* (pp. 71–92). Cambridge: Cambridge University Press.

Ryan, R. M., & Weinstein, N. (2009). Undermining quality teaching and learning: A self-determination theory perspective on high-stakes testing. *Theory and Research in Education, 7*, 224–233.

Schwartz, S. H. (1994). Beyond individualism/collectivism: New cultural dimensions of values. In U. Kim, H. C. Triandis, C. Dagitcibasi, S. Choi, & G. Yoon (Eds.), *Individualism and collectivism: Theory, method, and applications* (pp. 85–119). Thousand Oaks, CA: Sage Publications.

Sierens, E., Vansteenkiste, M., Goossens, L., Soenens, B., & Dochy, F. (2009). The synergistic relationship of perceived autonomy support and structure in the prediction of self-regulated learning. *British Journal of Educational Psychology, 79*, 57–68.

Soenens, B., Vansteenkiste, M., Duriez, B., Luyten, P., & Goossens, L. (2005). Maladaptive perfectionistic self-representations: The mediational link between psychological control and adjustment. *Personality and Individual Differences, 38*, 487–498.

Su, Y.-L., & Reeve, J. (in press). A meta-analysis of the effectiveness of intervention programs designed to support autonomy. *Educational Psychology Review*.

Taylor, I., Ntoumanis, N., & Smith, B. (2009). The social context as a determinant of teacher motivational strategies in physical education. *Psychology of Sport and Exercise, 19*, 235–243.

Vallerand, R. J., Fortier, M. S., & Guay, F. (1997). Self-determination and persistence in a real-life setting: Toward a motivational model of high school dropout. *Journal of Personality and Social Psychology, 72*, 1161–1176.

Vansteenkiste, M., Simons, J., Lens, W., Sheldon, K. M., & Deci, E. L. (2004). Motivating learning, performance, and persistence: The synergistic role of intrinsic goals and autonomy support. *Journal of Personality and Social Psychology, 87*, 246–260.

Vansteenkiste, M., Zhou, M., Lens, W., & Soenens, B. (2005). Experiences of autonomy and control among Chinese learners: Vitalizing or immobilizing? *Journal of Educational Psychology, 97*, 468–483.

Weinstein, N., & Ryan, R. M. (2010). When helping helps: Autonomous motivation for prosocial behavior and its influence on well-being for the helper and recipient. *Journal of Personality and Social Psychology, 98*, 222–244.

White, R. W. (1959). Motivation reconsidered: The concept of competence. *Psychological Review, 66*, 297–333.

Chapter 7
Physical Wellness, Health Care, and Personal Autonomy

Geoffrey C. Williams, Pedro J. Teixeira, Eliana V. Carraça, and Ken Resnicow

In this chapter, we will review the self-determination theory (SDT; Deci & Ryan, 2000) perspective and the current empirical evidence linking personal autonomy with physical wellness within and across cultures. We define physical wellness as indicators of physical health, including health behaviors of tobacco use, nutrition, physical activity, medication adherence, disease risk, and disease status. We will also examine studies that have tested the relations between change in personal autonomy and physical wellness and interventions intended to change personal autonomy and a health outcome. In addition, it is our thesis that a clear understanding of the relation between autonomy and physical well-being is relevant for all cultures. Moreover, respect for patient autonomy is now considered to be an explicit, highest level goal of health care along with patient well-being and social justice (ABIM, 2002; Beauchamp & Childress, 2009). Personal autonomy and values are now recognized as important elements of informed decision making (Braddock, Edwards, Hasenberg, Laidley, & Levinson, 1999; Woolf et al., 2005). Together these changes foretell a potentially rapidly expanding role of personal autonomy in the delivery of health care. Self-determination theory uniquely identifies autonomy as a psychological need and provides for several measures of autonomy that are appropriate for workplace health and medical settings.

SDT posits that all humans are intrinsically oriented toward growth, psychological well-being, and physical well-being. As described in Chapter 2, human's need for autonomy is considered to be universal, although its expression may differ across cultures. The core component of this type of motivation relates to the quality of the psychological energy that energizes the behavior and the direction (or target) of the behavior. The fact that these tenets have been criticized as being Western or American ideals and thus are not generalizable to other cultures has been addressed in other chapters (see Chapter 3 and 4). In this chapter, and we will examine the relation of perceived personal autonomy and physical health within individual and across cultures, as the data allow. Multi-cultural studies (e.g., a study that included

---

G.C. Williams (✉)
Department of Medicine, Center for Community Health, University of Rochester, Rochester, NY 14607, USA
e-mail: Geoffrey_Williams@URMC.Rochester.Edu

more than one culture) are expected to be few in number as SDT has only recently been applied into heath care outside of the United States and Canada, and only within these countries since around 1990.

Self-determination theory is a general theory of human motivation and behavior which has guided a growing number of studies in health care and health promotion settings. Many health care studies have now tested the link between personal autonomy and health-related behaviors. Specifically, physical health and well-being are predicted to be enhanced by SDT when people's basic psychological needs of autonomy, perceived competence, and relatedness are satisfied. Further, satisfaction of these needs, and pursing intrinsically satisfying aspirations, facilitate the internalization autonomous self-regulations for health behaviors and perceived competence for desired healthy behaviors (e.g., not using drugs or tobacco, regular physical activity, healthy nutrition, maintained energy balance, and appropriate use of medications). Figure 7.1 illustrates the self-determination theory Model for Health Behavior. This model of need supportive-based health care delivery, although initially developed in the US (Williams et al., 2006), has been replicated in three other Western countries (Canada, Fortier, Sweet, O'Sullivan, & Williams, 2007, Norway, Munster Halvari & Halvari, 2006, and Portugal Silva et al., 2008). To the extent to which it is generalizable to other cultures, including non-Western societies is discussed below.

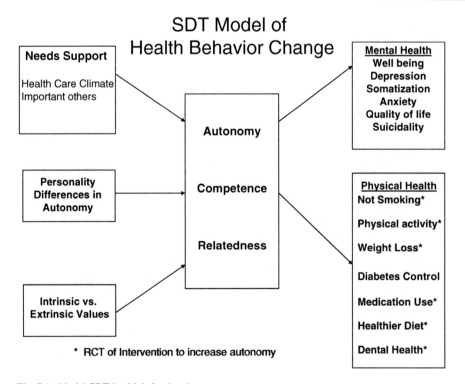

Fig. 7.1 Model SDT health behavior change

Autonomy-related measures, as depicted in SDT, have been assessed with several types of measures. These include: treatment self-regulation questionnaire (TSRQ); general causality orientation scale (GCOS); locus of causality (LOC); intrinsic motivation (IM); and the aspirations index (AI). Some measures are behavior specific, such as the exercise self-regulation questionnaire (SRQ-E), the TSRQ, and the Behavioral Regulation in Exercise Questionnaire (BREQ). Others refer to the perception of need support by participants, or treatment climate measured, for instance by the Health Care Climate Questionnaire (HCCQ). Vitality is a positive form of life energy within the SDT framework.

As we review each study, we will refer to all the various measures of autonomy as "personal autonomy," and also indicate the specific measure that was used in that study. Treatment self-regulation is the measure of personal autonomy that is most frequently used. It yields up to five subscale scores. Two autonomous levels of self-regulation (1) identified (ID-TSRQ), (2) integrated (IN-TSRQ) and two controlled forms of self-regulation, (3) introject (IJ-TSRQ), and (4) external control (EX-TSRQ). Amotivation is the final category and it will be designated as AM-TSRQ. Amotivation is the lowest form of self-regulation in that it is not volitional and is not directed at achieving an outcome. Internalization is the proactive process of change in personal autonomy and perceived competence within SDT. In the remainder of the chapter, we will outline what is known about how personal autonomy relates to health behaviors and physical well-being, and how interventions to promote personal autonomy may enhance physical well-being.

Systematic Search of the Literature

Inclusion Criteria

We searched Medline and PsychInfo through October of 2009 for manuscripts that include self-determination theory and autonomy, and health (including physical health, and health behaviors) that allow for cross-cultural comparisons in title, abstract, or key words. We accepted studies that provided quantitative measures of these relations within one culture, or in multiple cultures. We divided the manuscripts according to the health topics that were studied (e.g., tobacco abstinence, nutrition, physical activity, medication taking, physical diseases, or physical wellbeing) and then again within those outcomes by whether they provided data from multiple cultures, single non-US cultures, and single US cultures.

Exclusion Criteria

We excluded manuscripts that reported only personal autonomy and well being (well being, vitality, or quality of life) that were assessed in non-health care settings (education, home, business) unless a specific health outcome (physical health, functional incapacity, or health behavior) was also reported. We also excluded non-quantitative papers and those studies with measures of autonomy that were not defined as volition and were inconsistent with self-determination theory. A total of 54 manuscripts were identified, and selected for review in this chapter.

We hypothesized that various forms of personal autonomy would be positively predictive of physical well-being and healthier behaviors and health behavior change and that personal autonomy would be predictive of an increase in perceived competence. Controlled and amotivated self-regulation would be neutral or negatively predictive of physical well-being, healthier behaviors, and health behavior change. We will first turn to the studies that linked autonomous self-regulation to tobacco outcomes, and then other medical outcomes, before reviewing the physical activity, weight loss, and nutrition studies. Most of the tobacco and medical studies were conducted in the US. We now turn to the selected studies of personal autonomy and tobacco dependence treatment, chronic disease management (e.g., diabetes regulation, and medication adherence), dental outcomes, substance abuse, and surgical outcomes.

Personal Autonomy and Tobacco Outcomes

Abstinence from tobacco (e.g., smoking cessation without use of other tobacco products) has been associated with personal autonomy in 7 studies that span 20 years. The initial association using a measure of intrinsic (IM—concerns about health and desire for self-control) relative to extrinsic (EX—immediate reinforcement and social influence) motivation for smoking cessation was tested in two samples (ns = 1217 and 151) of smokers requesting smoking cessation materials in the Seattle, Washington area (Curry, Wagner, & Grothaus, 1991). They found that higher relative intrinsic motivation was associated with greater likelihood of abstinence. Further, a randomized trial with the larger sample found that smokers receiving personalized feedback (intrinsic motivation intervention) versus those receiving a monetary reward for completing a smoking cessation workbook (extrinsic motivation intervention), and those receiving both interventions, and those receiving neither intervention had significantly higher abstinence rates at 3 and 12 months (Curry et al., 1991). This was the first study indicating that higher levels of personal autonomy were associated with health behavior change, and it replicated Deci's (1971) findings and a subsequent meta-analysis (Deci, Koestner, & Ryan, 1999) that rewards undermine autonomously motivated behaviors.

In Williams, Cox, Kouides, and Deci (1999) reported that the 2- and 4-month change in personal autonomy (TSRQ) for not smoking was predictive of reduction in smoking for over 150 9–12th graders in upstate New York (Beta = 0.22, $p < 0.01$, and Beta = 0.26, $p < 0.001$). These adolescents had been randomized to receive an SDT intervention called "It's your Choice" versus a "Fear and Demand" (terror inducing intervention). Those in the choice intervention perceived greater autonomy support, but were not found to have greater levels of personal autonomy. In this same sample, a second measure of personal autonomy was assessed called relative intrinsic aspirations (IA) along with perceived parental autonomy support (PAS). Both personal autonomy (AI—beta = 0.21, $p < 0.001$) and parental autonomy support (PAS—beta, $p < 0.001$) predicted lower levels of a composite of health risk behaviors as well as each of the individual risk behaviors making up the composite. The composite included smoking, alcohol use, marijuana use, and early onset intercourse. These adolescents were predominantly white and of mid-level socioeconomic status in a suburban high school. Thus, no racial or ethnic subgroups were analyzed.

In a trial of adult smokers receiving a brief cessation intervention in two styles (Williams, Gagné, Ryan, & Deci, 2002), personal autonomy (ID IN-TSRQ) measured within the week following the intervention predicted 6, 12, and 30 month abstinence and continuous abstinence at all three times (parameter estimates = 0.12–0.14, p's < 0.001). No racial or ethnic subgroups were analyzed in this study. This study was the first to report that long-term maintenance of abstinence is predicted by personal autonomy following an intervention.

In Williams et al. (2006) reported on a randomized trial of 1,006 adult smokers that demonstrated that an intensive self-determination theory based intervention for tobacco dependence increased 6 and 18 month prolonged abstinence by more than 2.5 times compared to community care. This finding held independent of baseline willingness to quit in the next 30 days. The effect of this intervention was partially mediated by the change (internalization) in personal autonomy (ID IN-TSRQ) and perceived competence during the intervention period. Internalization of autonomy and perceived competence also explained abstinence in the community care group, thus supporting the concept that internalization is an innate potential, independent of intervention. These findings are consistent with a hypothesized causal relationship that changes in personal autonomy (ID IN-TSRQ) and perceived competence play in abstinence from tobacco. There were no differences found between the relation between personal autonomy and abstinence between whites and African Americans in this trial. Thirty-two-month data from this study still showed a between group effect on abstinence from tobacco, and found evidence that the 6-month change in autonomy that occurred within the 6 months of the intervention predicted 7 day point prevalence abstinence measured a full 24 months after the intervention ended. This latter finding suggests that change in personal autonomy may motivate future abstinence attempts (Williams, Niemiec, Patrick, Ryan, & Deci, 2009).

This study also provided initial evidence that the self-determination intervention can enhance personal aspirations for health and that increases in the health intrinsic aspiration (AI) is associated with long-term abstinence from tobacco (Niemiec, Ryan, Deci, & Williams, 2009). Vitality (psychological energy that is not directed at a specific outcome) was also found to increase significantly with personal autonomy (TSRQ—beta = 0.11, $p < 0.001$), and with decreased cigarette use over the time of the intervention (Williams et al., 2009), and the change in personal autonomy (ID IN-TSRQ) during the intervention increased vitality over the next 12 months (Beta = 0.07, $p < 0.05$). While these results represent small effects that need replication, they suggest that as smokers experience higher levels of personal autonomy they are more likely to abstain from tobacco and they experience a greater level of vitality, or well being. Also, this study found no differences for African Americans compared with whites in the relation of autonomous self-regulation and prolonged abstinence, thus suggesting no cross-cultural differences exist between these two groups.

Finally, a small randomized trial measuring autonomy support (HCCQ) and hypnosis ($n = 48$) conducted in England found that the autonomy support group had significantly higher levels of personal autonomy (ID IN-TSRQ), but no between group difference was found in abstinence from tobacco (Solloway, Joseph, 2006). Autonomous self-regulation accounted for 16% of the variance in smoking abstinence ($p < 0.01$). There were no cross-cultural comparisons made in this study.

Overall, the results of these studies in the US and England consistently reported weak to moderate effects of personal autonomy (ID IN-TSRQ) on tobacco abstinence or reduction in tobacco use, and improved well-being. Randomized controlled trials indicate that internalization of autonomous self-regulation can be facilitated by need supportive interventions, suggesting a causal relationship between autonomous self-regulation and abstinence from tobacco. While not mentioned in this review, the controlled forms of self-regulations (IJ, EX-TSRQ) were not significantly related to tobacco outcomes in several of the tobacco studies (Williams et al., 1999, 2006, 2002, 2009), thus these relations were not reported in the papers or discussed here. Only one study explicitly tested whites versus African Americans and found no difference. Cross-culture tests of SDT-based interventions intended to increase personal autonomy (ID IN-TSRQ or AI) and tobacco abstinence have not been conducted.

Diabetes Self-Management

Diabetes is a common disease that lowers quality and length of life. Almost one-third of Americans will be diagnosed with diabetes that are born after the year 2000 (Narayan, Boyle, Thompson, Sorenson, & Williamson, 2003). Further, it is a disease that can be prevented (DPP, 2002) and if patients manage their glucose control tightly, measured on hemoglobin A1c (HbA1c), they will experience fewer complications (DCCT). Chronic conditions such as diabetes mellitus offer a unique opportunity to examine the process of internalization of personal autonomy (ID IN-TSRQ) and perceptions of competence. Motivation is particularly relevant for people with chronic diseases because humans need energy for the day-to-day effective management of their diseases. Internalization is expected to begin with diagnosis and is expected to differ as a function of the need supportiveness of the health care climate and important others in the diabetics life, as well as personality differences in causality orientation. Autonomous self-regulation is expected to be important in long-term adherence to lifestyle and persistent use of medications. Personal autonomy and perceived competence were predicted to energize diabetes self-management behaviors and reducing disease complications such as blindness, kidney failure, and numbness that affect quality of life. This is somewhat different than motivation to prevent onset of a disease in that symptoms of a disease that has set in are frequently experienced, and the complications can be monitored with feedback for the patient. Several studies of motivation regarding diabetes mellitus have been conducted.

In a 12-month longitudinal study of 128 patients with diabetes (Williams, Freedman, & Deci, 1998), personal autonomy (ID IN-TSRQ) was significantly correlated with HbA1c at baseline ($r = -0.40$), 4 months ($r = -0.28$) and 12 months ($r = -0.30$, all p's < 0.001). In a second study of 159 patients with diabetes (Williams, McGregor, Zeldman, Freedman, & Deci, 2004), increase in personal autonomy (TSRQ) over the initial 6 months in the study predicted improvement in glycemic control ($r = -0.24$, $p < 0.01$). Life satisfaction was significantly correlated with personal autonomy (ID IN-TSRQ—beta = 0.34) even after controlling for dietary self-efficacy in a study of 638 French Canadian patients with diabetes (Senecal, Nouwen, & White, 2000). Personal autonomy (ID IN-TSRQ) for using medication to control diabetes and cholesterol was positively correlated with quality of life ($r = 0.19$, $p < 0.01$) measured on the Short-Form 12 Health Survey (SF-12v2; Ware, Kosinski, & Keller, 1996) in a study of approximately 2,000 patients with diabetes. In addition, personal autonomy (ID IN-TSRQ) predicted adherence to diabetes and cholesterol medications and diabetes control ($r = -0.12$, $p < 0.01$) and healthier cholesterol ($r = -0.09$, $p < 0.01$). Nearly 40% of this sample was non-white (36.5% African American, and 3.8% other), but when race was controlled for it didn't significantly effect the findings.

In summary, personal autonomy, in the form of autonomous self-regulation (ID IN-TSRQ) for diabetes self-management behaviors, has been consistently associated with improved diabetes control, quality of life, and life satisfaction in Western cultures. Non-white subgroups have participated in these studies and autonomous self-regulation appears to have similar associations with disease outcomes in both groups.

Medication Adherence and Use

Adherence is defined as the percentage of patient behavior/the "recommended" amount of behavior. The "recommended" amount is usually from treatment guidelines or from health care practitioners, but it could also be based on what patients agree to take. Adherence particularly to long-term regimens is an important outcome because it is a motivated behavior that requires psychological energy to maintain and it has a major effect on health outcomes (Osterberg & Blaschke, 2005). In the clinical world (as opposed to within controlled research studies) as much as a third of prescriptions are never filled and, only about 50% of prescriptions are taken as prescribed once started.

In a US study (Williams, Rodin, Ryan, Grolnick, & Deci, 1998) of 30 different long-term medications (mean time taken = 6.5 years) over a 14-day window of time, personal autonomy (ID IN-TSRQ) accounted for nearly half the variation in medication adherence (parameter estimate = 0.78, $p < 0.001$). A second study examined the relations between personal autonomy (ID IN-TSRQ) for adherence to more complex medication regimens prescribed for 205 HIV positive patients. These patients had been HIV positive for over 7 years on average and needed to take these HIV medications multiple times a day at specific intervals in order to suppress the virus. Personal autonomy (ID IN-TSRQ) was weakly but significantly correlated with adherence over the 3-day assessment period ($r = 0.15, p < 0.05$).

In summary, both studies of medication adherence were in US samples and no racial or cultural variables were reported. Both studies report moderate to strong positive relations between personal autonomy and adherence.

Substance Use and Abuse

Several studies of substance abuse and its treatment have been conducted. Ryan, Plant, and O'Malley (1995) found that personal autonomy (IJ ID-TSRQ; note that in this study here internalized motivation was the sum of introjected + identified self-regulation), and external motivation (EX-TSRQ; external control and pressure) interacted to predict a composite treatment outcome (completing treatment and number of the 8 planned therapy sessions attended) for alcohol-dependent clients seeking treatment. Racial and cultural demographics were unrelated to personal autonomy and the outcome variables, in this US sample of 100 clients (80% were Caucasian). In another US study, drinking alcohol was predicted by extrinsic reasons (EX IJ-TSRQ; introject + external control) in 78 undergraduates ($r = 0.42, p < 0.01$), and 53 members of college fraternities ($r = 0.40, p < 0.01$; Knee & Neighbors, 2002). While these studies included multiple ethnicities, the sample sizes didn't allow for subgroup analyses. Personal autonomy related to drinking or not drinking was not assessed in this study. Personal autonomy (IJ ID-TSRQ) for treatment in a methadone maintenance program for opioid dependence was reported for 74 clients, 52% of whom were white (Zeldman, Ryan, & Fiscella, 2004). Autonomous self-regulation was significantly correlated with all three treatment outcomes; percent of sessions missed ($r = -0.28, p < 0.01$), percent of positive urine tests ($r = -0.27, p < 0.05$), and number of days between entering treatment and being allowed to receive take-home doses of methadone ($r = -0.25, p < 0.05$). Racial differences were not reported.

Wild, Cunningham, and Ryan (2006) assessed personal autonomy (ID-TSRQ) for 300 addicts in Toronto Canada and found identified regulations predicted reduction in alcohol use (beta = 0.26, $p < 0.001$), alcohol use (beta = $-0.28, p < 0.05$), therapist ratings of client interest in treatment (beta = 0.18, $p < 0.05$), and client perceived benefits of reducing drug use (beta = 0.31, $p < 0.01$). No racial or ethnicity data are reported in this study. Finally, personal autonomy (GCOS autonomy and controlled subscales) predicted average daily alcohol consumption (r autonomy = -0.14 and r controlled = -0.10, p's < 0.05) in 818 first year college students who reported a heavy drinking episode in the previous month (Chawla, Neighbors, Logan, Lewis, & Fossos, 2009). This sample was collected online a large public US in the northwestern United States, and 65% were white, 24% Asian, and 11% other. Relations between personal autonomy (TSRQ) and drinking behaviors for the different races and ethnicities were not reported in this study.

In summary, studies of substance abuse and its treatment showed weak to moderate strength relations between various measure of autonomy, and control from self-determination theory. Controlled self-regulations (EX IJ-TSRQ; introject is typically unrelated and TSRQ external control is usually somewhat negatively predictive of physical health outcomes) have typically been found to be unrelated to physical health outcomes, or they have been unreported in physical health studies. All these studies were conducted in the US or Canada, and while some samples had diverse racial and ethnic make up, few of these relations were reported.

Autonomy and Other Medical, Surgical, and Dental Outcomes

One 5 country study of nurses offering information to 1,500 surgical patients found that desire for input into decision making regarding their care predicted independence level in daily activities ($r = 0.24$, $p < 0.001$) and subjective health status ($r = 0.12$, $p < 0.01$). SDT informed the measurement model that was assessed, but the construct representing autonomy (desire for input into decision making) was based on biomedical ethics definition of autonomous decision making (Beauchamp & Childress, 2009) and was not consistent with the SDT construct of autonomy. The mean levels of the desire for input into decision making were reported for the patients in Finland, Spain, Greece, Germany, and Scotland, and they were significantly different and ranged from 2.2 in Greece to 3.8 in Scotland ($F = 75.8\ df = 4.1$, $p < 0.005$). However, differences in parameter estimates by country are not reported. Further, the IRB did not allow the assessment of race and ethnicity in this study.

Personal autonomy (ID IN-TSRQ) was assessed in 50 residents of a nursing home in upstate New York and found to be predictive of patient vitality ($r = 0.36$, $p < 0.05$), mortality ($r = -0.36$, $p < 0.05$) and days lived ($r = 0.31$, $p < 0.05$) over a 13-month period (Kasser, & Ryan, 1999). No assessment of ethnicity or race was reported for the study participants. This study is notable for many reasons, but in particular, the association found between personal autonomy and mortality (length of life) is striking and calls for replication.

Personal autonomy (IM) related to the intrinsic motivational factors of job creativity, job autonomy, and job complexity were found to be similarly predictive of functional incapacity in a 5 country study (Canada, China, Finland, France, and Sweden) of 13,795 employees of a single global forest industry corporation (Vaananen et al., 2005). Interestingly, the strength of associations between personal autonomy (IM) and functional incapacity were the strongest among the Chinese employees then in the "Western" countries. The authors suggest that "the Chinese, as employees of an economy in transition, may particularly value intrinsic motivational factors of work in their cultural context." They also note the studies limitation of being cross-sectional, and call for longitudinal cross-national research. This study supports the SDT assumption that autonomous and intrinsic motivations are present in all humans, even those in Eastern cultures. These findings directly contradict the criticism that autonomy is a westernized concept, and suggests that the link between personal autonomy and functional status and possibly physical health is stronger in Eastern versus Western cultures.

Personal Autonomy and Testing for Coronary Artery Disease. Change in personal autonomy (ID IN-TSRQ) for 252 patients being evaluated for coronary disease predicted healthier diet ($r = 0.19$, $p < 0.01$) and physical activity ($r = 0.15$, $p < 0.05$) over a 3-year period of time (Williams, Gagne, Mushlin, & Deci, 2005). Three quarters of this cohort were white and the study was conducted in upstate New York. No racial or ethnicity data were analyzed in this study.

Personal Autonomy and Dental Health Behaviors. A randomized trial in Norway with 86 social science and school of medicine students demonstrated a large between group effect of an SDT intervention increasing autonomous self-regulation for flossing and brushing which mediated the effect of the intervention on the reduction in gingivitis and dental plaque over 7 months (Munster Halvari & Halvari, 2006). The change in personal autonomy (ID IN-TSRQ) on improving self-reported dental behaviors after controlling for change in perceived competence was significant (parameter estimate = 0.20, $p < 0.05$), and personal autonomy (ID IN-TSRQ) at 7-month follow-up was strongly correlated with lower levels of plaque ($r = -0.38$, $p < 0.001$). No racial or ethnicity data were analyzed in this trial. This trial provides strong evidence that change in autonomous self-regulation is associated with positive dental outcomes in a westernized culture.

In summary, medical studies outside of tobacco and diabetes, a surgical and a dental study have demonstrated consistent positive relationships between personal autonomy and physical health. However, only one study related to job autonomy assessed the strength of this relation in multiple cultures. This one study found that job autonomy and intrinsic motivations were stronger negative predictors of functional incapacity in Chinese workers than in four Western countries. We now turn to studies of within and cross-cultural associations between personal autonomy, physical activity, and physical well-being.

Personal Autonomy and Physical Activity/Exercise[1]

The relationship between perceptions of personal autonomy and exercise behaviors (e.g., intentions to exercise, exercise stages of change, minutes of moderate and vigorous physical activity, etc.) has been reported in several studies (e.g., Ryan, Williams, Patrick, & Deci, 2009). To empirically test SDT's tenets when applied to exercise promotion several questions have been addressed by previous studies, which can typically be included into one (or several) of the following categories:

---

[1] Although not strictly the same ("exercise" is typically considered a *structured* form of voluntary "physical activity"), we will use the terms "exercise" and "physical activity" indiscriminately in this text. In most studies we reviewed, subjects were measured as to their level of leisure time activity, often to improve health or fitness, or to control body weight (thus predominantly "exercise").

(i) testing whether different behavioral regulations (or *regulatory motives*) distinctly predict exercise behaviors; for instance, if autonomous regulations are stronger predictors than controlled motivations; (ii) evaluating whether reasons for exercising (or *participatory motives*), namely more "intrinsic" (e.g. challenge, health) vs. more "extrinsic" reasons/goals (e.g. social recognition), make a difference in the perceived locus of causality of exercise behaviors; (iii) testing the extent to which basic psychological needs are satisfied in exercise contexts and how that relates to the development of exercise motivation; and (iv) testing if interventions are successful in promoting personal autonomy by providing need-supportive contexts.

We identified 39 studies published since 1993 that address autonomy and exercise behaviors, varying substantially in design (largely observational but also including some experimental research), sample characteristics (healthy or presenting a clinical condition), and measures used to assess exercise/PA. Because there are many more studies in this area, it allows for more fine grained examination of the relations between the various types of personal autonomy and exercise behaviors outlined above. We will now briefly review those findings, drawing also on previous reviews on this topic (Chatzisarantis, Hagger, Biddle, Smith, & Wang, 2003; Hagger & Chatzisarantis, 2007; Wilson, Mack, & Grattan, 2008).

Overwhelmingly, evidence confirms that more self-determined regulations, namely identified, integrated, and intrinsic forms of motivation are significantly associated with increased physical activity adherence and related measures, such as intentions or stages of change (Brickell, Chatzisarantis, & Pretty, 2006; Chatzisarantis & Biddle, 1998; Daley & Duda, 2006; Edmunds, Ntoumanis, & Duda, 2006a; Edmunds, Ntoumanis, & Duda, 2008; Edmunds, Ntoumanis, & Duda, 2006b; Hagger, Chatzisarantis, Culverhouse, & Biddle, 2003; Hagger, Chatzisarantis, & Harris, 2006; Ingledew, Markland, & Ferguson, 2009; Landry & Solmon, 2004; Markland, 2009; Matsumoto & Takenaka, 2004; McNeill, Wyrwick, Brownson, Clarck, & Kreuter, 2006; Milne, Wallman, Guilfoyle, Gordon, & Corneya, 2008; Mullan & Markland, 1997; Peddle, Plotnikoff, Wild, Au, & Courneya, 2008; Rose, Parfitt, & Williams, 2005; Sebire, Standage, & Vansteenkiste, 2009; Thogersen-Ntoumani & Ntoumanis, 2006; Wilson, Blanchard, Nehl, & Baker, 2006; Wilson & Rodgers, 2004; Wilson, Rodgers, Blanchard, & Gessell, 2003; Wilson, Rodgers, & Fraser, 2002; Wilson, Rodgers, Fraser, & Murray, 2004; Wilson, Rodgers, Loitz, & Scime, 2006; Wininger, 2007). It is presently unclear precisely which specific type(s) of self-determined regulations is/are more closely associated with behavior outcomes. While many studies have not included a measure of integrated motivation, most have shown slightly higher association scores for identified motivation (for exercise) compared to intrinsic motivation (e.g., Edmunds et al., 2006a; Ingledew et al., 2009; Standage, Sebire, & Loney, 2008; Wilson & Rodgers, 2004). Although theoretically they are clearly separable, in the exercise context identified and intrinsic measures have tended to be collinear when tested in multivariate models (e.g., Standage et al., 2008). The same point has been made about integrated and intrinsic regulations (Ingledew et al., 2009). For this reason, some studies have chosen to use an autonomous scale instead of separate scales for identified and intrinsic regulations (Ingledew & Markland,

2007; Silva et al., 2010; Standage et al., 2008). In fact, some instruments do not assess integrated regulations (e.g., BREQ-2, D. Markland & Tobin, 2004). In real life, it is likely that people who have successfully integrated the regulation of exercise behaviors (e.g., who have come to see physical activities as contributing to highly valued outcomes or perceive a physically active lifestyle as an integral part of their sense of self) also find the experience of exercise interesting and enjoyable for its own sake. Likewise, individuals who have always enjoyed sports and exercise (e.g., based on positive experiences as a physically active teenager) are very likely to also identify with activity behaviors and/or value it highly during adulthood.

Regarding controlled motivations, while measures of external regulation are clearly not associated, or are negatively associated with initial or continued exercise participation (e.g., Ingledew & Markland, 2007), introjected regulations are sometimes positively related to exercise/PA outcomes (e.g., Edmunds et al., 2006a; Thogersen-Ntoumani & Ntoumanis, 2006; Wilson et al., 2003), although to a lesser extent than autonomous regulations. One recent study using objective measures of physical activity (accelerometry) showed no association between introjected motivation and behavior (Standage et al., 2008) supporting other studies with self-report measures (e.g., Ingledew & Markland, 2007; Ingledew et al., 2009). Since many reports have been cross-sectional and short-term, and have generally used simple self-reported measures to assess behavior, future studies, especially longitudinal, should clarify the role of introjected motivation in short-term and especially sustained exercise adherence. For instance, in a sport setting, introjected regulation predicted short-term but not long-term behavioral persistence (Pelletier, Fortier, Vallerand, & Brière, 2001). It should be noted that different regulations (more and less autonomous) can and most likely do co-exist for any given behavior, especially those involving complex tasks such as engaging in a regular exercise routine, which can include multiple behaviors and be subject to various influences (e.g. time- and job-related, access to facilities and other aspects of the built environment, weather, social influences, etc.). Indeed, it is the relative preponderance of each form of regulation that should, in the end, determine behavioral outcomes such as persistence vs. dropout. For instance, it is possible that some degree of introjection (e.g., feeling internal pressure every time several days without exercise go by) may not be detrimental to long-term adherence when in the presence of strong and concurrent regulations of a more autonomous nature, whether extrinsic (e.g., valuing the opportunity for meaningful social interaction) or intrinsic.

Other variables which have been used in exercise studies include participatory motives (or goal contents) in exercise (Ingledew & Markland, 2007; Ingledew et al., 2009; Markland & Tobin, 2010; Sebire et al., 2009; Segar, Eccles, & Richardson, 2008; Vansteenkiste, Simons, Soenens, & Lens, 2004). Collectively, results appear to concur with the tenets of self-determination, showing that more "intrinsic" goals (e.g., health, affiliation, challenge, and social engagement) are associated with more autonomous exercise self-regulation and/or with higher exercise adoption, when compared with "extrinsic" goals (e.g. appearance/attractiveness, social recognition). Two recent studies by Ingledew and Markland (2007, 2009) used mediation analysis to show that nominally intrinsic goals predicted exercise participation indirectly through autonomous forms of self-regulation; health/fitness and stress management goals predicted identified regulation whereas affiliation and challenge goals predicted intrinsic motivation. Contrarily, as expected from theory, controlled participatory motives (social recognition, appearance/weight) predicted external and/or introjected regulations.

According to SDT, there is a link between endorsing more intrinsic goals and the development of autonomous motivation through basic psychologic needs (Kasser & Ryan, 1996). Studies have also investigated perceived need satisfaction in exercise settings and the extent to which it contributed to motivation and behavioral outcomes (Edmunds et al., 2006a; Hagger et al., 2006; Markland, 1999; Markland & Hardy, 1997; Markland & Tobin, 2010; Wilson et al., 2003). For example, Markland and Tobin showed different pathways linking perceived need support (including autonomy, structure, and involvement), need satisfaction (autonomy, competence and relatedness) and behavioral regulations, in exercise-referral participants. Confirming previous studies (See Edmunds, Ntoumanis, & Duda, 2007b for a review), results supported SDT propositions for the mediating role of need satisfaction, in particular of autonomy, for the development of self-determined motivation.

Recently, in Portuguese women, perceived need support during an SDT-based intervention was associated not only with more autonomous exercise self-regulation but also with the development of introjected regulations (Silva, et al., 2010; See Fig. 7.2 below). The authors commented on this unexpected finding by suggesting that a cultural background where external approval is learned to be contingent on

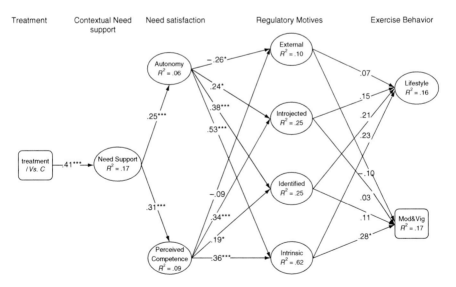

Values in the Paths represent the standardized bootstrap estimate, *p<.05, **p<.01, ***p<.001.

Fig. 7.2 Causal pathways linking an autonomy-promoting intervention with exercise behaviors in 239 overweight and obesity women (from Silva et al., 2009)

compliance and conformity (e.g. to God or expert opinion) could partially explain how an autonomy-promoting treatment climate also led to increased introjected regulations. Willing compliance could in fact be a common form of behavioral regulation in the Portuguese culture, strongly influenced by Catholic ethics and ideal. Interestingly, there were significant associations between introjected and both identified and intrinsic motivations (IM), but no association between introjected and external regulations. Additionally, in a subsequent analysis, we found no association between controlled exercise regulations (external and introjected scales together) and reduced psychological well-being in the same sample (Vieira, et al., in press), suggesting that the intervention effects on introjected regulation were perhaps not perceived as externally controlling and also not detrimental to well-being. This notwithstanding, the positive association between need satisfaction and introjection was not interpreted as supportive of using guilt or promoting contingent self-worth to motivate Portuguese weight loss program participants. In fact, the same study showed that introjected regulations failed to predict physical activity behaviors across multiple time points (Silva et al., 2010; Silva, et al., in press).

To date, only a few interventions have been designed to specifically increase personal autonomy in the form of autonomous self-regulation for exercise in adults (Edmunds et al., 2008; Fortier et al., 2007; Jolly et al., 2009; Silva et al., 2008). Some of these studies are still ongoing and all have been conducted in Western cultures. Fortier et al. (2007) tested an autonomy-promoting counseling protocol for promoting physical activity in sedentary primary care patients, for 13 weeks. Results showed that the intervention was successful in changing autonomous self-regulation to reach activity goals (vs. a brief counseling protocol) and that higher autonomous regulation for exercise mid-intervention predicted higher levels of physical activity at the end of the intervention, in the intervention group. In an exercise on prescription program, Edmunds et al. (2007a) showed increases in introjected and decreases in autonomous motivation during the course of the 3 month study. In spite of this fact, which authors attributed to the relative lack of contact with exercise specialists and low provision of structure during the program, relatedness need satisfaction predict higher levels of exercise autonomous self-regulation and higher attendance, while autonomous self-regulation predicted improved psychological well-being and positive affect; conversely, introjected exercise regulations predicted less subject vitality. At each time point, identified exercise regulation was associated with higher adherence whereas introjected regulations predicted less participation.

The longest RCT to date that evaluated autonomy support and physical activity behaviors was implemented in 239 overweight women, through 30 weekly group sessions for about 1 year (Silva et al., 2008). Strategies used to promote personal autonomy and the development of intrinsic motivation for exercise in this intervention are described in detail elsewhere (Silva et al., 2008, 2009). Results showed that the intervention was successful in changing exercise participatory motives, exercise autonomous self-regulation and exercise behavior (Silva et al., 2009). Additionally, it also indicated that the motivational sequence proposed by SDT (i.e., need-supportive health care climate need satisfaction for autonomy and competence autonomous exercise regulation exercise behaviors) was empirically supported using structural equation modeling (Silva et al., 2009). Figure 7.2 shows a Partial Least Squares model (and standardized coefficients) for predicting two different forms of exercise at intervention's end. The role of the intervention through perceived autonomy and competence support was particularly effective in increasing intrinsic motivation (IM), which in turn significantly predicted minutes of moderate and vigorous physical activity.

Collectively, available evidence supports the positive role of personal autonomy in adopting and maintaining physical activity and exercise behaviors. Furthermore, it appears that perceptions of autonomy need-support on the part of study participants significantly predict more autonomous self-regulation and improved behavioral outcomes. However, because most studies have been cross-sectional, more experimental data is needed to assess how manipulating social conditions (e.g., health care environments) can induce increases in personal autonomy and how, in turn, this leads to short- and long-term behavior change. Virtually all studies in this domain have been conducted in Western societies (mostly USA, UK, and Canada, but also Greece (Mildestvedt, Meland, & Eide, 2008), Australia (Vlachopoulos, Karageorghis, & Terry, 2000), Norway (Milne et al., 2008), and Portugal (e.g. (Silva et al., 2008)) with one exception from Japan (Matsumoto & Takenaka, 2004), a cross-sectional study of 486 men and women, where more advances stages of changes were predicted by intrinsic (IM), identified (ID-TSRQ) and introjected exercise regulation (IJ-TSRQ). Although no indication in the exercise domain exists that would suggest that the relations between personal autonomy and behavioral outcomes differs across cultures, the available evidence is clearly lacking in cultural diversity for firmer conclusions to be drawn.

Autonomy and Weight Regulation

Only a few studies have tested personal autonomy or related constructs as predictors of outcomes in obesity studies. Williams, Grow, Freedman, Ryan, and Deci (1996) studied severely obese patients in the context of a 6-month medically supervised very-low-calorie diet, where participants also received weekly group counseling, of a general nature, intended to provide peer support, facilitate discussion, promote self-monitoring, etc. Perceived autonomy support and treatment self-regulation were assessed immediately after the intervention. Perceived need support predicted autonomous reasons to continue to participate in treatment, which in turn predicted higher attendance and improved weight loss. Path analysis supported these same mediation paths for outcomes at treatment's end. Autonomous regulations at 6 months also correlated with self-reported exercise and weight loss at a 20-month follow-up (Williams et al., 1996). No cross-cultural analyses were reported in this study.

Between 2005 and 2007, a randomized controlled trial based on self-determination theory was implemented to identify mediating factors for long-term weight control, in premenopausal overweight and mildly obese women (Silva et al., 2008). Results thus far (Silva et al., 2009; Silva et al., 2010; Silva et al., (in press)) support a mediation effect of need support and need satisfaction (of autonomy and competence needs) for developing identified regulations and intrinsic motivation for exercise, which in turn were found to predict 3-year weight control.

Within the same trial—the PESO study—an empirical test of a more diverse set of psychological and behavioral variables showed that change in exercise motivation variables during the 12-month program (self-efficacy, perceived barriers, and intrinsic motivation) were significant predictors of 2-year weight change. Self-efficacy and flexible dietary restraint were found to partially mediate treatment effects on 2-year weight outcomes (Teixeira et al., 2009). A similar study had been conducted in US women who participated in a 4-month behavior weight control trial (Teixeira et al., 2006). In this analysis, changes in intrinsic motivation were found to be the best predictor of 16-month weight changes (no mediation analyses were conducted due to the absence of a control group).

Mata et al. (2009) analyzed whether, in overweight and obese women, treatment and exercise self-regulations predicted successful eating behavior and mediated the association between actual physical activity and eating behavior measures. Results were consistent with the hierarchical model of motivation (Vallerand, 1997), suggesting that the *quality* of motivation may be one mechanism through which successful self-regulation in one area may affect ("spill-over") into other behavioral domains. If confirmed, this could help explain how autonomously-motivated exercise behavior contributes to improved weight control; not only via the effects of physical activity itself (e.g., Silva et al., 2009) but also positively influencing the regulation of other relevant behaviors such as eating. In fact, the same eating variables studied in the Mata et al. report (flexible restraint, disinhibition, emotional eating, eating self-efficacy) were, in a subsequent analysis from the same trial, shown to predict weight change and partially mediate the effects of some forms of physical activity on weight control (Andrade, et al., in press).

Recently, Gorin and colleagues (2008) explored whether baseline levels of autonomous and controlled self-regulation, and changes in self-regulation over 6 months, were associated with 6-month weight outcomes in overweight women. Higher controlled self-regulation at baseline was associated with worse weight loss results. Conversely, increases in autonomous self-regulation and decreases in controlled self-regulation over the 6-month period predicted improved weight loss (Gorin, et al., 2008). Ongoing work from the same team appears supportive of autonomy support provided by other adults (Important Other Climate Questionnaire) in the home environment leading to more autonomous self-regulation for weight control, in turn predicting weight loss (Patrick, Gorin, & Williams, 2010).

In summary, although based on a somewhat limited set of studies, results to date suggest a positive association between experiences of personal autonomy and improved weight management in the short and long-term. In some studies, analyses have highlighted potential causal mechanisms linking personal autonomy with behavior change for exercise (e.g., Ingledew et al., 2009; (Silva, et al., in press) and eating behavior (e.g., Pelletier & Dion, 2007; Pelletier, Dion, Slovinec-D'Angelo, & Reid, 2004), in some cases leading to improved weight control. At the present time, and notwithstanding the previous point about the impact of an autonomy-promoting intervention on introjected regulations (in Portuguese women), there is no evidence upon which to discuss culture-specific issues regarding the impact of personal autonomy on obesity-related health behaviors.

Personal Autonomy and Dietary Behavior

The TSRQ has been used in several studies to measure autonomous (ID IN-TSRQ) and controlled self-regulation (EX IJ-TSRQ) of dietary behavior, each of which was conducted with African Americans. In the Healthy Body Healthy Spirit trial (Resnicow et al., 2005, 2002) our team (KR) recruited over 1,000 African American participants from 16 black churches in Atlanta Georgia. Participants completed the TSRQ at baseline and 1-year follow-up. Fruit and vegetable intake was assessed with food frequency questionnaires and serum carotenoids (sum of lutein, cryptoxanthin, carotene, and carotene) were obtained from most participants to supplement self report. Self-efficacy to eat more F & V was assessed at baseline and 1-year follow-up.

As shown in Table 7.1, autonomous regulation was moderately correlated with F & V intake at baseline and posttest, $r = 0.35$ and $r = 0.14$, respectively. Interestingly, controlled regulations (EX IJ TSRQ) was also significantly correlated with F & V intake at baseline and posttest though the magnitude of the association was weaker, $r = 0.15$ and $r = 0.11$ respectively. This pattern is consistent with other studies in health care settings using the TSRQ, where some of the controlled regulations (namely IJ-TSRQ) have been found to relate positively to health outcomes. In other domains (e.g. education, parenting) external and introjected self-regulations (EX IJ-TSRQ) typically relate negatively to outcomes in those domains. It is not yet known how to intervene to change controlled levels of personal autonomy. Amotivation (AM-TSRQ) was uncorrelated with intake.

Autonomous regulation (ID IN-TSRQ) was also related to serum carotenoids, an unbiased measure of dietary intake, at baseline, $r = 0.17$, but not posttest. Neither controlled regulation (EX IJ-TSRQ) nor amotivation (AM-TSRQ) were related to carotenoid levels at either time point.

Table 7.1 Correlations of TSRQ scores with fruit and vegetable intake, serum carotenoids, and self-efficacy in the healthy body trial

	Baseline ($n = 1,021$)			Post ($n = 942$)		
	FV	Carot	SE	FV	Carot	SE
Autonomous intrinsic motivation	0.35*	0.17*	0.29*	0.14*	0.06	0.29*
Controlled extrinsic motivation	15*	0.01	0.02	0.11*	0.01	−0.07
Amotivation	−0.06	−0.03	−0.12*	−0.06	−0.04	−0.15*

SE = Self Efficacy; Carot = Sum of total serum carotenoids.
*$p < 0.01$.

SDT posits that autonomous regulation will be more strongly associated with self-efficacy than controlled regulation (Markland, Ryan, Tobin, & Rollnick, 2005; Ryan & Deci, 2000; Williams et al., 1998). Individuals who have greater personal autonomy (ID IN-TSRQ, IM) are predicted to, SDT suggests, express greater persistence in their behavioral effort. Our findings strongly supported this assumption. Autonomous regulation was correlated $r = 0.29$ with self-efficacy at baseline and also at 1-year follow-up, whereas controlled regulation was uncorrelated with efficacy. Interestingly, amotivation (AM-TSRQ) was significantly inversely associated with efficacy, which also appears consistent with SDT assumptions, as amotivated regulation represents the person feeling dissociated from the outcome, and self-efficacy and perceived competence represent the extent to which the person feels the outcome is achievable.

Another diet-related study that used the TSRQ to measure personal autonomy was Body and Soul (B & S; Campbell, Resnicow, Carr, Wang, & Williams, 2007; Fuemmeler et al., 2006; Resnicow et al., 2004). B & S was a randomized effectiveness trial, testing the impact of a multi-component dietary intervention in 14 black churches recruited through local American Cancer Society (ACS) offices in California and in the Southeast (Georgia, North Carolina, and South Carolina) and Mid-Atlantic (Delaware and Virginia) regions of the US (Fuemmeler et al., 2006). Baseline and 6-month follow-up data were obtained from self-report. Measures of motivation (TSRQ), diet, efficacy, and social support were similar to those used in Healthy Body Health Spirit and prior studies.

As shown above in Table 7.2, autonomous regulation (ID IN-TSRQ) was significantly correlated with both the 2-item and 19-item F & V measure at baseline and 6-month follow-up. Controlled regulation (EX IJ-TSRQ) was more weakly correlated with intake at baseline and follow-up. Again, as in Healthy Body, autonomous regulation but not controlled regulation was significantly correlated with efficacy at both time points. In addition to cross sectional correlations of TSRQ with efficacy and diet, mediating effects of SDT and other variables were also reported for B & S.

Table 7.2 Correlations among study variables, reprinted with the permission from American Psychological Association (Fuemmeler et al., 2006)

Variables	1	2	3	4	5	6
1. 2-items measures	–	0.50**	0.23**	0.07*	0.31**	0.21**
2. FV FFQ	0.53**	–	0.20**	0.06	0.28**	0.19**
3. Autonomous motivation	0.25**	0.19**	–	0.25**	0.31**	0.23**
4. Controlled motivation	0.12**	0.09*	0.28**	–	−0.04	0.26**
5. Self-efficiency	0.28**	0.22**	0.33**	0.04	–	0.015**
6. Social support	0.19**	0.09*	0.20**	0.26**	0.16**	–

Note: Correlations displayed below the diagonal represent correlations at baseline and correlation above the diagonal represent correlation at follow-up. FV FFQ – 19-items food frequency questionnaire, excluding fried potatoes.
*$p < 0.05$.
**$p < 0.01$.

7 Physical Wellness, Health Care

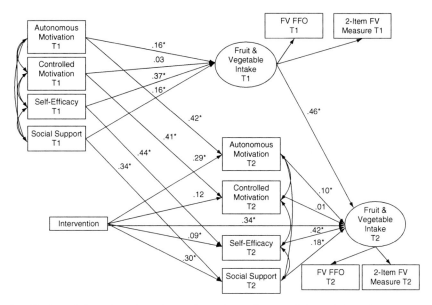

Fig. 7.3 Association of psychosocial mediators in the Body and Soul trial, reprinted with the permission from American Psychological Association (Fuemmeler et al., 2006)

As shown in the Fig. 7.3 the intervention had an impact on post test psychosocial outcomes (autonomous regulation, efficacy, and social support) as well as F & V intake, both prerequisites for mediation analyses. Moreover, change in autonomous regulation, efficacy and social support were significantly related to change in F & V intake. Not surprising, the intervention pathway was attenuated by the inclusion of these mediating variables in the model (0.47; $p = 0.01$ without mediators vs. 0.34; $p < 0.01$, with mediators). However, since the effect of the intervention on changes in FV intake remained significant, the intervention effect was only partially mediated by these variables.

One final diet study that included the TSRQ was the recently published Eat for Life trial (Resnicow et al., 2008). This study was designed to test whether tailoring a print-based fruit and vegetable (F & V) intervention on constructs from self-determination theory (SDT) and motivational interviewing (MI) increased intervention impact. Another aim was to examine possible user characteristics that may moderate intervention response. The primary user characteristic assessed was preference for an expert recommendation.

For this study, African American adults were recruited from two integrated health care delivery systems, one based in the Detroit Metro area and the other in the Atlanta Metro area, and then randomized to receive three tailored newsletters over 3 months. One set of newsletters was tailored only on demographic and social cognitive variables (control condition) whereas the other (experimental condition) was tailored on SDT and MI principals and strategies. The primary focus of the newsletters and the primary outcome for the study was fruit and vegetable intake, assessed with two brief self-report food frequency measures (FFQ) measures. Preference for an expert recommendation was assessed at baseline with a single item: "In general, when it comes to my health I would rather an expert just tell me what I should do." A total of 512 (31%) eligible participants, of 1,650 invited, were enrolled, of which 423 provided complete 3-month follow-up data. Considering the entire sample, there were no significant between-group differences in daily F & V intake at 3-month follow-up. Both groups showed similar increases of around 1 serving per day of F & V on the short form FFQ and half a serving per day on the long form FFQ. There were however, significant interactions of intervention group with preference for a recommendation. Specifically, individuals in the experimental intervention who at baseline preferred an expert recommendation increased their F & V intake by 1.07 servings compared to 0.43 servings among controls. See Fig. 7.4 below.

In this study, the TSRQ was also administered, which allowed us to examine the association between preference for a recommendation and TSRQ values. We split the expert recommendation preference variable above and below 6 (below 6 indicating lower desire for a recommendation, or structure, from the practitioner), and then looked at means of the three TSRQ variables. In this study, we split the controlled regulation scale into its two subscales, i.e., introjected and external control. As shown below, at baseline, individuals who expressed high preference for a recommendation (i.e., they agreed with the "tell me what to do" item), had significantly higher introject and external control scores on the TSRQ than those indicating low preference for an expert recommendation. As would be predicted by SDT, those who suffer with higher levels of guilt and perceptions of being externally controlled around these behaviors may feel uncomfortable in making their own decision. Thus,

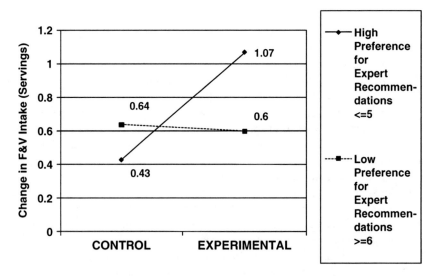

Fig. 7.4 Interaction of F & V change* with preference for expert recommendation

Table 7.3 Association of baseline TSRQ values and "preference for an expert recommendation (ER)": Eat for Life ($n = 528$)

	Autonomous	Introjected	External others
Expert ≤ 5 (high preference for ER)	6.2	3.7	2.5
Expert > 5 (low preference for ER)	6.3	4.5*	3.0*

Adjusted for age and gender.
*$p < 0.01$.

high levels of introject and perceived external controls are associated with greater dependence on external advice and direction. Variation in level of identified and integrated regulation (autonomy-TSRQ) was unrelated to whether the patient preferred a recommendation to be made. See Table 7.3. This pattern is possible because controlled regulations (EX IJ-TSRQ) are typically orthogonal (largely uncorrelated) with autonomous regulations (ID IN-TSRQ) in the health care domain. The same pattern of findings for the three subscales and preference for a recommendation was evident using posttest TSRQ values as well.

Are There Subgroups Who Express Greater Preference for Expert Recommendations?

In the EFL sample, there were several demographic characteristics associated with differences in preferences for expert recommendations. Males as well as individuals with income above $40 k, those under age 40, and those with higher educational attainment all showed a lower preference for expert recommendation in their health decisions. See Table 7.4. This suggests a potential benefit in tailoring the degree of direct recommendations made according to individual or group differences. Perhaps not all individuals want to be fully independent in their health care decision making. Some may in fact respond better when practitioners use a more directive style of communication. This raises some interesting questions about the difference between the two main definitions of autonomy as independence (the non SDT definition of personal autonomy—actions that are done without relation to others) and volition (the SDT definition of personal autonomy—willingness to engage in the behavior for oneself). Thus, the practitioner who provides an expert recommendation would likely be perceived as autonomy supportive if a recommendation is desired by the patient. Conversely, the practitioner would be more likely to be perceived as controlling if he forces the patient to make the choice without him (e.g., independently), if the patient desires practitioners input. When forced to make a decision that the patient may not feel competent to make would be expected to resulting lower energy for maintaining the behavior would be expected to lessen, may raise the patient's anxiety level and possibly to amotivation. If there is no evidence available on which the practitioner can base make a clear recommendation for treatment, it is the responsibility of the practitioner to inform the patient of that, and then to

Table 7.4 Preference for recommendation by demographic characteristics in the Eat for Life trial

	Prevalence of high preference for expert recommendation ($n = 562$)
Gender	
Male	50%
Female	40%
Income	
<40 k	36%
>40 k	49%
Age	
<40	53%
>40	40%
Education	
<HS	38%
Some college	42%
Complete college	46%

Response 5 or lower on the 7-point item: "In general, when it comes to my health I would rather an expert just tell me what I should do."

work with the patient to decide on the best direction for the patient to go given the lack of evidence (Woolf, 2005), and to provide ongoing care.

Autonomy (e.g., volitionally) supportive practitioners offer a menu of known effective options for treatment, and then provide their recommendation after exploring the patients' wishes about which option to pursue. If the practitioner reflects the patient's perspective back to the patient, and offers a rationale about why to pursue a treatment, if the practitioner wants to check back with her patient to elicit patients' perspective on the advice, it is expected that personal autonomy is increased (e.g., internalized). Thus, providing a menu of effective options for treatment along with an option for not changing is part of the definition of autonomy support.

Summary Personal Autonomy and Dietary Behavior

Across several studies, most of which were conducted among African Americans, there was considerable consistency in the relationship between dietary behavior and motivation. First, personal autonomy, most commonly measured with the TSRQ (ID IN-TSRQ, and IM), was more strongly related to diet behavior than was controlled regulations and amotivation (AM EX IJ-TSRQ). Second, only autonomous regulation was related to self efficacy. Both of these findings are consistent with suppositions of SDT.

However, although controlled regulation (EX IJ) was more weakly correlated with diet behavior than was autonomous regulation, in several instances the association was nonetheless significant. Given that these studies comprised exclusively African American participants, it is unclear if the moderately strong association between controlled regulations and diet is unique to this population. This pattern was also found in Portuguese women in the PESO trial (Silva et al., 2009) who are highly Catholic. Previous research has identified associations of religious self-regulations and mental health (Ryan, Rigby, & King, 1993), and perhaps there are common underlying regulations based on religious upbringing that account for these relations. Future cross-cultural studies are needed to explore this issue.

A key issue from an SDT perspective is whether behavior change driven by controlled regulation is less stable than that driven by more autonomous regulation. SDT might, for at least two reasons, posit that changes driven by more controlled regulation would be less enduring than those rooted in more autonomous regulation. First, given that lack of association between controlled regulation and self-efficacy, it is likely that the individual who is externally motivated by exhibit less behavioral persistence in their efforts. Second, because behavior energized by controlled regulations result in poorer well being as shown in many SDT studies described in other chapters in this text, or may be motivated by a form of internal control used by the patient to force himself to behave, or if the individual can learn to manage their negative introjects, through for example a cognitive shift, or an affective shift, or become less susceptible to social pressure, than the behavior from controlled forms of regulation to behave would be attenuated. On the other hand, more autonomously regulated behavior change, particularly when connected to one's deeper values and goals through internalization, would be more enduring. These are important theoretical questions that merit future research.

Overall Summary

Our aim was to review the literature on the relation between personal autonomy and physical well being and the extent to which the association of these constructs generalizes across cultures. The within culture results demonstrate a clear and consistent positive relation between personal autonomy and physical well being in westernized cultures. Four of these studies are randomized clinical trials and provide causal level evidence that interventions intending to facilitate internalization of personal autonomy and did so, and that change in personal autonomy mediated (at least partially) the effect of the intervention on the outcomes of physical activity, abstinence from tobacco, weight loss, dental outcomes and medication use. This pattern is consistent with a causal relation between personal autonomy and health behavior change. Other chapters in this book establish that personal autonomy is associated with psychological well-being. Both improved physical and psychological well-being are important individual outcomes in health care and become combined in important outcomes such as quality adjusted life years used in comparative effectiveness studies that will determine which interventions will be adopted into health care. Thus, not only are interventions intending to increase personal autonomy consistent with biomedical ethics and medical professionalism, evidence reviewed in this book suggests that enhancing personal autonomy will also extend expect life years, and that those life years will be of better quality.

Limitation of our review includes that most of the research reviewed here involved only a single nationality or ethnic group, typically, northern European, and North American whites. A few studies, mostly involving dietary behavior, and one in tobacco dependence treatment, demonstrated this same positive relation in African Americans. Only one true cross cultural study was found linking personal autonomy in the work place with lower levels of functional incapacitation, and this provided evidence that this relation was stronger in China then in the Western countries. Clearly, much more research is needed to confirm that personal autonomy has a stronger relation (or even the same) to physical health in Eastern cultures. This finding is intriguing as it is in the opposite direction then most critics of self-determination theory who consider "autonomy to be a western concept not relevant in collectivist societies." Perhaps, this stems from SDT's critics' confusion over the distinction between volition and independence. In addition, cost-effectiveness of interventions to increase personal autonomy has not been published.

In addition, we noted that introjected self-regulation, which is a less internalized form of personal autonomy, has been found to positively predictive of greater levels of physical activity and dietary intake, and lower levels of relapse in substance abuse. Why this type of motivation may function differently across health behaviors or cultures merits comments. In Portugal, a culture which is highly shaped by the Catholic Church, introjects may be strong enough to energize some modest amount of long-term health behavior. This pattern was also found in some North American African American church-based samples as well, suggesting that physical health related behaviors maybe weakly motivated by this less internalized form or personal autonomy. We note that in these studies the simplex pattern is still intact, and that only perceived external control is negatively associated with the health outcomes. We do not know how long lasting introjected motivated behavior would be sustained. This is important because SDT predicts that an introject is an impoverished form of energy and isn't expected to be sustained as long as more autonomous based change. It is likely that some level of introject is internalized while higher levels of self-regulation were internalized in these studies and that it was the autonomous levels of self-regulation (identified, integrated and intrinsic) that sustained the behavior change over time. Further, we would not recommend that clinicians of any type try to motivate others by inducing guilt or shame in their patients as we would expect that it would be associated with poorer emotional well-being as well as less positive long term outcomes. Instead, clinicians are encouraged to facilitate greater levels of autonomous levels self-regulations (identified, integrated, and intrinsic) for their patients. We would also recommend that practitioners elicit patient preferences for treatment, but be willing to provide expert advice in the form of a menu of effective options, when the patient is open to the recommendations.

In conclusion, the evidence in this chapter indicates strong, perhaps causal, evidence that increasing personal autonomy improves physical health. Other chapters indicate that increase in personal autonomy increases psychological well-being. Biomedical ethics has already established that personal autonomy and well-being are the highest level outcomes for health related interventions. Thus, studies that focus on increasing personal autonomy (at the identified, integrated and intrinsic levels) as the primary outcome are called for and are needed to guide clinical care, medical decision making, and biomedical ethics in all cultures around the world.

References

ABIM Foundation. European Federation of Internal Medicine. (2002). Medical professionalism in the new millennium: A physician charter. *Annals of Internal Medicine, 136*, 243–246.

Andrade, A. M., Coutinho, S. R., Silva, M. N., Mata, J., Vieira, P. N., Minderico, C. S., Melanson, K. J., Baptista, F., Sardinha, L. B., & Teixeira, P. J. (2010). The effect of physical activity on weight loss is mediated by eating self-regulation. *Patient Education and Counseling, 79*, 320–326.

Beauchamp, T. L., & Childress, J. F. (2009). *Principles of biomedical ethics* (6th ed.). New York: Oxford University Press.

Braddock, C. H., Edwards, K. A., Hasenberg, N. M., Laidley, T. L., & Levinson, W. (1999). Informed decision making in outpatient practice: Time to get back to basics. *Journal of the American Medical Association, 282*(24), 2313–2320.

Brickell, T., Chatzisarantis, N. L., & Pretty, G. M. (2006). *Autonomy and control: Augmenting the validity of the theory of planned behaviour in predicting exercise. Journal of Health Psychology, 11*, 51–63.

Campbell, M. K., Resnicow, K., Carr, C., Wang, T., & Williams, A. (2007). Process evaluation of an effective church-based diet intervention: Body & Soul. *Health Education and Behavior, 34*(6), 864–880.

Chatzisarantis, N. L., & Biddle, S. J. (1998). Functional significance of psychological variables that are included in the Theory of Planned Behaviour: A self-determination theory approach to the study of attitudes, subjective norms, perceptions of control, and intentions. *European Journal of Social Psychology, 28*, 303–322.

Chatzisarantis, N. L. D., Hagger, M. S., Biddle, S. J. H., Smith, B., & Wang, J. C. K. (2003). A meta-analysis of perceived locus on causality in exercise, sport, and physical education contexts. *Journal of Sport and Exercise Psychology, 25*, 284–306.

Chawla, N., Neighbors, C., Logan, D., Lewis, M. A., & Fossos, N. (2009). Perceived approval of friends and parents as mediators of the relationship between self-determination and drinking. *Journal of Studies on Alcohol and Drugs, 70*(1), 92–100.

Curry, S., Wagner, E. H., & Grothaus, L. C. (1991). Evaluation of intrinsic and extrinsic motivation interventions with a self-help cessation program. *Journal of Consulting and Clinical Psychology, 59*(2), 318–324.

Daley, A. J., & Duda, J. (2006). Self-determination, stage of readiness to change for exercise, and frequency of physical activity in young people. *European Journal of Sport Sciences, 6*, 231–243.

Deci, E. L. (1971). Effects of externally mediated rewards on intrinsic motivation. *Journal of Personality and Social Psychology, 18*, 105–115.

Deci, E. L., Koestner, R., & Ryan, R. M. (1999). A meta-analytic review of experiments examining the effects of extrinsic rewards on intrinsic motivation. *Psychological Bulletin, 125*, 627–668.

Deci, E. L., & Ryan, R. M. (2000). The "what" and "why" of goal pursuits: Human needs and the self-determination of behavior. *Psychological Inquiry, 11*, 227–268.

Diabetes Prevention Program Research Group. (2002). Reduction in the incidence of type 2 diabetes with lifestyle intervention. *The New England Journal of Medicine, 346*(6), 393–403.

Edmunds, J., Ntoumanis, N., & Duda, J. (2006a). A test of self-determination theory in exercise domain. *Journal of Applied Social Psychology, 36*, 2240–2265.

Edmunds, J., Ntoumanis, N., & Duda, J. L. (2006b). Examining exercise dependence symptomatology from a self-determination perspective. *Journal of Health Psychology, 11*(6), 887–903.

Edmunds, J., Ntoumanis, N., & Duda, J. (2007a). Adherence and well-being in overweight and obese patients referred to an exercise on prescription scheme: A self-determination theory perspective. *Psychology of Sport and Exercise, 8*, 722–740.

Edmunds, J., Ntoumanis, N., & Duda, J. (2007b). Perceived autonomy support and psychological need satisfaction in exercise. In M. S. Hagger & N. L. Chatzisarantis (Eds.), *Intrinsic motivation and self-determination in exercise and sport*. Champaighn, IL: Human Kinetics.

Edmunds, J., Ntoumanis, N., & Duda, J. (2008a). Testing a self-determination theory-based teaching style intervention in the exercise domain. *European Journal of Social Psychology, 38*, 375–388.

Fortier, M. S., Sweet, S., O'Sullivan, T. L., & Williams, G. C. (2007). A self-determination process model of physical activity adoption in the context of a randomized controlled trial. *Psychology of Sport and Exercise, 8*(5), 741–757.

Fuemmeler, B. F., Masse, L. C., Yaroch, A. L., Resnicow, K., Campbell, M. K., Carr, C., et al. (2006). Psychosocial mediation of fruit and vegetable consumption in the Body and Soul effectiveness trial. *Health Psychology, 25*(4), 474–483.

Gorin, A. A., Pinto, A., West, D., Niemeier, H., Fava, J., & Wing, R. R. (2008, October). Losing weight because you want to rather than because you feel you have to: Motivational predictors of weight loss outcomes. Poster presented at the annual meeting of the Obesity Society, Phoenix, AZ. *Obesity, 16*(Supplement), S214.

Hagger, M. S., & Chatzisarantis, N. L. D. (2007). Advances in self-determination theory research in sport and exercise (Editorial). *Psychology of Sport and Exercise, 8*, 597–599.

Hagger, M. S., Chatzisarantis, N. L., Culverhouse, T., & Biddle, S. J. (2003). The processes by which perceived autonomy support in physical education promotes leisure-time physical activity intentions and behavior: A trans-contextual model. *Journal of Educational Psychology, 95*, 784–795.

Hagger, M. S., Chatzisarantis, N. L., & Harris, J. (2006). From psychological need satisfaction to intentional behavior: Testing a motivational sequence in two behavioral contexts. *Personality and Social Psychology Bulletin, 32*, 131–148.

Ingledew, D. K., & Markland, D. (2007). The role of motives in exercise participation. *Psychology and Health, 23*, 807–828.

Ingledew, D. K., Markland, D., & Ferguson, E. (2009). Three levels of exercise motivation. *Applied Psychology: Health and Well-Being, 1*, 336–355.

Jolly, K., Duda, J., Daley, A. J., Eves, F. F., Mutrie, N., Ntoumanis, N., et al. (2009). Evaluation of a standard provision versus an autonomy promotive exercise referral programme: Rationaly and study design. *BMC Public Health, 9*, 176.

Kasser, G. V., & Ryan, R. M. (1999). The Relation of Psychological Needs for Autonomy and Relatedness to Vitality, Well-Being, and Mortality in a Nursing Home. *Journal of Applied Social Psycology. 29*(5), 935–954.

Kasser, T., & Ryan, R. M. (1996). Further examining the American dream: Differential correlates of intrinsic and extrinsic goals. *Personality and Social Psychology Bulletin, 22*, 80–87.

Knee, C. R., & Neighbors, C. (2002). Self-determination, perception of peer pressure, and drinking among college students. *Journal of Applied Social Psychology, 32*, 522–543.

Landry, J. B., & Solmon, M. (2004). African American women's Self-determination across the stages of change for exercise. *Journal of Sport and exercise Psychology, 26*, 457–469.

Markland, D. (1999). Self-determination moderates the effects of perceived competence on intrinsic motivation in an exercise setting. *Journal of Sport and Exercise Psychology, 21*, 351–361.

Markland, D. A. (2009). The mediating role of behavioural regulations in the relationship between perceived body size discrepanices and physical activity among adult women. *Hellenic Journal of Psychology. 6*, 169–182.

Markland, D., & Hardy, L. (1997). On the factorial and construct validity of the Intrinsic Motivation Inventory: Conceptual and operational concerns. *Research Quarterly Exercise and Sport, 68*(1), 20–32.

Markland, D., Ryan, R. M., Tobin, V. J., & Rollnick, S. (2005). Motivational interviewing and self-determination theory. *Journal of Social and Clinical Psychology, 24*(6), 811–831.

Markland, D., & Tobin, V. (2004). A modification of the behavioural regulation in exercise questionnaire to include an assessment of amotivation. *Journal of Sport and Exercise Psychology, 26*, 191–196.

Markland, D., & Tobin, V. (2010). Need support and behavioural regulation for exercise among exercise referral scheme clients: The mediating role of psychological need satisfaction. *Psychology of Sport and Exercise, 11*, 91–99.

Mata, J., Silva, M. N., Vieira, P. N., Carraca, E. V., Andrade, A. M., Coutinho, S. R., et al. (2009). Motivational "spill-over" during weight control: Increased self-determination and exercise intrinsic motivation predict eating self-regulation. *Health Psychology, 28*(6), 709–716.

Matsumoto, H., & Takenaka, K. (2004). Motivational profiles and stages of exercise behavior change. *International Journal of Sport and Health Science, 2*, 89–96.

McNeill, L. H., Wyrwick, K. W., Brownson, R. C., Clarck, E. M., & Kreuter, M. W. (2006). Individual, social environmental, and physical environmental influences in physical activity among black and white adults: A structural equation analysis. *Annals of Behavioral Medicine, 31*, 36–44.

Mildestvedt, T., Meland, E., & Eide, G. E. (2008). How important are individual counseling, expectancy beliefs and autonomy for the maintenance of exercise after cardiac rehabilitation? *Scandinavian Journal of Public Health, 36*, 832–840.

Milne, H. M., Wallman, K. E., Guilfoyle, A., Gordon, S., & Corneya, K. S. (2008). Self-determination theory and physical activity among breast cancer survivors. *Journal of Sport and exercise Psychology, 30*, 23–38.

Mullan, E., & Markland, D. (1997). Variations in self-determination across the stages of change for exercise in adults. *Motivation and Emotion, 21*, 349–362.

Munster Halvari, A. E., & Halvari, H. (2006). Motivational predictors of change in oral health: An experimental test of self-determination theory. *Motivation and Emotion, 30*, 294–305.

Narayan, K. M. V., Boyle, J. P., Thompson, T. J., Sorenson, S. W., & Williamson, D. F. (2003). Lifetime risk for diabetes mellitus in the United States. *JAMA, 290*, 1884–1890.

Niemiec, C. P., Ryan, R. M., Deci, E. L., & Williams, G. C. (2009). Aspiring to physical health: The role of aspirations for physical health in facilitating long-term tobacco abstinence. *Patient Education and Counseling, 74*(2), 250–257.

Osterberg, L., & Blaschke, T. (2005). Adherence to medications. *New England Journal of Medicine, 353*, 487–497.

Patrick, H., Gorin, A. A., & Williams, G. C. (2010). Lifestyle change and maintenance in obesity treatment and prevention: A self-determination theory perspective. In L. Dube, A. Bechara, A. Dagher, A. Drewnowski, J. LeBel, P. James, and R. Y. Yada (Eds.), Obesity prevention: The role of the brain and society on individual behavior, (pp. 365–374). New York: Academic Press.

Peddle, C. J., Plotnikoff, R. C., Wild, T. C., Au, J., & Courneya, K. S. (2008). Medical, demographic, and psychosocial correlates of exercise in colorectal cancer survivors: An application of self-determination theory. *Supportive Care in Cancer, 16*, 9–17.

Pelletier, L. G., & Dion, S. C. (2007). An examination of general and specific motivational mechanisms for the relations between body dissatisfaction and eating behaviors. *Journal of Social and Clinical Psychology, 26*, 303–333.

Pelletier, L. S., Dion, S., Slovinec-D'Angelo, M., & Reid, R. D. (2004). Why do you regulate what you eat? Relationships between forms of regulation, eating behaviors, sustained dietary behavior change, and psychological adjustment. *Motivation Emotion, 28*(3), 245–277.

Pelletier, L. G., Fortier, M. S., Vallerand, R. J., & Brière, N. M. (2001). Associations among perceived autonomy support, forms of self-regulation, and persistence: A prospective study. *Motivation and Emotion, 25*, 279–306.

Resnicow, K., Campbell, M. K., Carr, C., McCarty, F., Wang, T., Periasamy, S., et al. (2004). Body and soul. A dietary intervention conducted through African-American churches. *American Journal Preventive Medicine, 27*(2), 97–105.

Resnicow, K., Davis, R. E., Zhang, G., Konkel, J., Strecher, V. J., Shaikh, A. R., et al. (2008). Tailoring a fruit and vegetable intervention on novel motivational constructs: Results of a randomized study. *Annals of Behavioral Medicine, 35*(2), 159–169.

Resnicow, K., Jackson, A., Blissett, D., Wang, T., McCarty, F., Rahotep, S., et al. (2005). Results of the healthy body healthy spirit trial. *Health Psychology, 24*(4), 339–348.

Resnicow, K., Jackson, A., Braithwaite, R., DiIorio, C., Blisset, D., Rahotep, S., et al. (2002). Healthy body/healthy spirit: A church-based nutrition and physical activity intervention. *Health Education Research, 17*(5), 562–573.

Rose, E., Parfitt, G., & Williams, G. (2005). Exercise causality orientations, behavioral regulation for exercise and stage of change for exercise: Exploring their relationships. *Psychology Sport Exercise, 6*, 399–414.

Ryan, R. M., & Deci, E. L. (2000). Self-determination theory and the facilitation of intrinsic motivation, social development, and well-being. *The American Psychology, 55*(1), 68–78.

Ryan, R. M., Plant, R. W., & O'Malley, S. (1995). Initial motivations for alcohol treatment: Relations with patient characteristics, treatment involvement and dropout. *Addictive Behaviors, 20*, 279–297.

Ryan, R. M., Rigby, S., & King, K. (1993). Two types of religious internalization and their relations to religious orientation and mental health. *Journal of Personality and Social Psychology, 65*, 586–596.

Ryan, R. M., Williams, G. C., Patrick, H., & Deci, E. L. (2009). Self-determination theory and physical activity: The dynamics of motivation in development and wellness. *Hellenic Journal of Psychology, 6*(2), 107–124.

Sebire, S., Standage, M., & Vansteenkiste, M. (2009). Examining goal content in the exercise domain: Intrinsic versus extrinsic goals and cognitive, affective, and behavioural outcomes, and psychological need satisfaction. *Journal of Sport and exercise Psychology, 31*, 189–210.

Segar, M. L., Eccles, J. S., & Richardson, C. R. (2008). Type of physical activity goal influences participation in healthy midlife women. *Women's Health Issues, 18*, 281–291.

Senecal, C., Nouwen, A., & White, D. (2000). Motivation and dietary self-care in adults with diabetes: Are self-efficacy and autonomous self-regulation complementary or competing constructs? *Health Psychology, 19*, 452–457.

Silva M. N., Markland D., Carraça, E. V., Vieira P. N., Coutinho S. R., Minderico, C. S., et al. Exercise autonomous motivation predicts 3-year weight loss in women. Medicine and Science in Sports and Exercise (in press).

Silva, M. N., Markland, D., Minderico, C. S., Vieira, P. N., Castro, M. M., Coutinho, S. R., et al. (2008). A randomized controlled trial to evaluate self-determination theory for exercise adherence and weight control: Rationale and intervention description. *BMC Public Health, 8*, 234.

Silva M. N., Markland D., Vieira P. N., Coutinho S. R., Palmeira A. L., et al. (2010). Helping overweight women become more active: need support and motivational regulations for different forms of physical activity. *Psychology of Sport and Exercise 11*, 591–601.

Silva, M. N., Vieira, P. N., Coutinho, S. R., Matos, M. G., Sardinha, L. B., and Teixeira, P. J. (2010). Using self-determination theory to promote physical activity and weight control: a randomized control trial in women. *Journal of Behavioral Medicine. 33*, 110–22.

Solloway, V., Solloway, K., & Joseph, A. (2006). A hypnotherapy for smoking intervention investigates the effects of autonomy support on motivation, perceived competence and smoking abstinence. *European Journal of Clinical Hypnosis. 7*(2), 26–40.

Standage, M., Sebire, S., & Loney, T. (2008). Does exercise motivation predict engagement in objectively assessed bouts of moderate-intensity exercise? A self-determination theory perspective. *Journal of Sport and exercise Psychology, 30*, 337–352.

Teixeira, P. J., Going, S. B., Houtkooper, L. B., Cussler, E. C., Metcalfe, L. L., Blew, R. M., et al. (2006). Exercise motivation, eating, and body image variables as predictors of weight control. *Medicine and Science in Sports and Exercise, 38*(1), 179–188.

Teixeira, P. J., Silva, M. N., Kiernan, M., Coutinho, S. R., Palmeira, A. L., Mata, J., Vieira, P. N., Carraça, E. V., Santos, T. C., Sardinha, L. B. (2010). Mediators of weight loss and weight loss maintenance in middle-aged women. *Obesity (Silver Spring) 18*(4), 725–735.

Thogersen-Ntoumani, C., & Ntoumanis, N. (2006). The role of self-determined motivation in the understanding of exercise-related behaviours, cognitions and physical self-evaluations. *Journal Sports Science, 24*(4), 393–404.

Vaananen, A., Pahkin, K., Huuhtanen, P., Kivimaki, M., Vahtera, J., Theorell, T., et al. (2005). Are intrinsic motivational factors of work associated with functional incapacity similarly regardless of the country? *Journal of Epidemiology and community Health, 59*, 858–863.

Vallerand, R. J. (1997). Toward a hierarchical model of intrinsic and extrinsic motivation. In M. P. Zanna (Ed.), *Advances in experimental social psychology* (Vol. 29, pp. 271–360). London: Academic Press.

Vansteenkiste, M., Simons, J., Soenens, B., & Lens, W. (2004). How to become a persevering exerciser: The importance of providing clear, future goals in an autonomy-supportive way. *Journal of Sport and exercise Psychology, 26*, 232–249.

Vieira, P. N., Mata, J., Silva, M. N., Coutinho, S. R., Santos, T. F., Minderico, C. S., Sardinha, L., & Teixeira, P. J. Predictors of psychological well-being during behavioral obesity treatment in women. *Journal of Obesity* (in press).

Vlachopoulos, S. P., Karageorghis, C. I., & Terry, P. C. (2000). Motivational profiles in sport: A self-determination perspective. *Research Quarterly for Exercise and Sport, 71*, 387–397.

Ware, J., Jr., Kosinski, M., & Keller, S. D. (1996). A 12-item short form health survey: Construction of scales and preliminary tests of reliability and validity. *Medical Care, 34*, 220–233.

Wild, T. C., Cunningham, J. A., & Ryan, R. M. (2006). Social pressure, coercion, and client engagement at treatment entry: A self-determination theory perspective. *Addictive Behaviors, 31*, 1858–1872.

Williams, G. C., Cox, E. M., Kouides, R., & Deci, E. L. (1999). Presenting the facts about smoking to adolescents: The effects of an autonomy supportive style. *Archives of Pediatrics and Adolescent Medicine, 153*(9), 959–964.

Williams, G. C., Freedman, Z. R., & Deci, E. L. (1998). Supporting autonomy to motivate patients with diabetes for glucose control. *Diabetes Care, 21*(10), 1644–1651.

Williams, G. C., Gagne, M., Mushlin, A. I., & Deci, E. L. (2005). Motivation for behavior change in patients with chest pain. *Health Education, 105*(4), 304–321.

Williams, G. C., Gagné, M., Ryan, R. M., & Deci, E. L. (2002). Facilitating autonomous motivation for smoking cessation. *Health Psychology, 21*, 40–50.

Williams, G. C., Grow, V. M., Freedman, Z. R., Ryan, R. M., & Deci, E. L. (1996). Motivational predictors of weight loss and weight-loss maintenance. *Journal of Personality and Social Psychology, 70*, 115–126.

Williams, G. C., McGregor, H. A., Sharp, D., Levesque, C., Kouides, R. W., Ryan, R. M., et al. (2006). Testing a self-determination theory intervention for motivating tobacco cessation: Supporting autonomy and competence in a clinical trial. *Health Psychology, 25*(1), 91–101.

Williams, G. C., McGregor, H. A., Zeldman, A., Freedman, Z. R., & Deci, E. L. (2004). Testing a self-determination theory process model for promoting glycemic control through diabetes self-management. *Health Psychology, 23*(1), 58–66.

Williams, G. C., Niemiec, C. P., Patrick, H., Ryan, R. M., & Deci, E. L. (2009). The importance of supporting autonomy and perceived competence in facilitating long-term tobacco abstinence. *Annals of Behavioral Medicine, 37*(3), 315.

Williams, G. C., Rodin, G. C., Ryan, R. M., Grolnick, W. S., & Deci, E. L. (1998). Autonomous regulation and long-term medication adherence in adult outpatients. *Health Psychology, 17*(3), 269–276.

Wilson, P. M., Blanchard, C. M., Nehl, E., & Baker, F. (2006). Predicting physical activity and outcome expectations in cancer survivors: An application of self-determination theory. *Psycho-Oncology, 15*, 567–578.

Wilson, P., Mack, D., & Grattan, K. (2008). Understanding motivation for exercise: A self-determination theory perspective. *Canadian Psychology, 49,* 3.

Wilson, P. M., & Rodgers, W. M. (2004). The relationship between perceived autonomy support, exercise regulations and behavioral intentions in women. *Psychology of Sport and Exercise, 5,* 229–242.

Wilson, P. M., Rodgers, W. M., Blanchard, C. M., & Gessell, J. (2003). The relationship between psychological needs, self-determined motivation, exercise attitudes, and physical fitness. *Journal of Applied Social Psychology, 33,* 2373–2392.

Wilson, P. M., Rodgers, W. M., & Fraser, S. N. (2002). Examining the psychometric properties of the behavioral regulation for exercise questionnaire. *Measurement in Physical Education and Exercise Science, 6,* 1–21.

Wilson, P. M., Rodgers, W. M., Fraser, S. N., & Murray, T. C. (2004). The relationship between exercise regulations and motivational consequences. *Research Quarterly for Exercise and Sport, 75,* 81–91.

Wilson, P. M., Rodgers, W. M., Loitz, C. C., & Scime, G. (2006). "It's who I am...really!": The importance of integrated regulation in exercise contexts. *Journal of Applied Biobehavioral Research, 11,* 79–104.

Wininger, S. R. (2007). Self-determination theory and exercise behavior: An examination of the psychometric properties of the exercise motivation scale. *Journal of Applied Sport Psychology, 19,* 471–486.

Woolf, S. H., Chan, E. C. Y., Harris, R., Sheridan, S. L., Braddock, C. H., Kaplan, R. M., et al. (2005). Promoting informed choice: Transforming health care to dispense knowledge for decision making. *Annals of Internal Medicine, 143*(4), 293–300.

Zeldman, A., Ryan, R. M., & Fiscella, K. (2004). Motivation, autonomy support and entity beliefs: Their role in methadone maintenance treatment. *Journal of Social and Clinical Psychology, 23,* 675–696.

Chapter 8
Autonomy in the Workplace: An Essential Ingredient to Employee Engagement and Well-Being in Every Culture

Marylène Gagné and Devasheesh Bhave

Notions of autonomy underlie many old and new organizational practices. Japanese quality practices, empowerment, autonomous work teams, and many more organizational practices are grounded in giving employees more discretion over their work. Autonomy also captures the popular imagination: from the bumbling attempts of Michael Scott to empower his employees in television series "The Office" to the Dilbert comic strip's sense of helplessness related to the workplace. *Modern Times*, Charlie Chaplin's epic 1930s movie on the modern workplace, poignantly illustrates the travails of a workplace bereft of autonomy. Echoes of such workplaces are depicted in recent movies on call centers such as *Call Center Movie* and *Outsourced*.

But autonomy in the workplace has lofty origins. For close to a century, the International Labor Organization (ILO) has explicitly promoted the cause of freedom, equity, security, and dignity. Autonomy, after all, is how individual rights to freedom and dignity, enshrined in the ILO constitution, manifest in the workplace. Autonomy figured as key ingredient of modern organizations in the writings of early management scholars including Chester Barnard (1938), Mary Parker Follett (1926), and Elton Mayo (1933). Even Frederick Taylor (1911) considered the father of scientific management, emphasized that scientific management was not an efficiency fad but a "mental revolution" on part of workers that would come about when management and worker interests were aligned. Through the years, therefore, theorists have highlighted autonomy as a critical interest for employees that organizations need to address (Budd, 2004; Hirschman, 1970). Evidence abounds for the importance of autonomy to employees. Spector (1986) showed in a meta-analysis of over a hundred North American samples that perceptions of job control, often considered a form of work autonomy, were associated with higher job satisfaction, commitment, involvement, performance, and motivation and with lower physical symptoms, emotional distress, role stress, absenteeism, turnover intentions, and actual turnover. Whether it is in discussions of job design or leadership, autonomy is

---

M. Gagné (✉)
Department of Management, John Molson School of Business, Concordia University, Montreal, QC, Canada H3G 1M8
e-mail: mgagne@jmsb.concordia.ca

often at the heart of heated debates in management—some researchers argue that it is an essential ingredient to employee engagement, while others say it is peripheral.

In this chapter, we first review theories, primarily from industrial–organizational psychology and organizational behavior perspectives that include autonomy as a key construct. Next, we illustrate empirical results in support of these theories, drawing particular attention to cross-cultural findings. To examine cross-cultural evidence, we adopt Hofstede's (2001) values framework because it has been the most popular one in management. When evaluating these cultural results, we try to take into account the possible effects of organizational characteristics (e.g., industry, job type, size) that could be confounded with cultural effects. We also draw on empirical evidence based on self-determination theory (Deci & Ryan, 1985). Because I/O psychology research has not drawn from self-determination theory much, our job here is to integrate these independent literatures and attempt to find future avenues for I/O psychology research based on self-determination theory. We next integrate empirical findings with the variety of organizational practices that draw upon concepts and theories related to autonomy. Finally, we present an organizing framework based on self-determination theory (Deci & Ryan, 1985) to guide future cross-cultural research on autonomy in the workplace.

Conceptualizations of Autonomy

Organizational behavior research has studied autonomy by examining how workplace practices that affect experienced autonomy, such as job design and participative management, influence the performance and engagement of employees (Evans & Fischer, 1992). Conceptualizations of autonomy reflect the historical and economic environment of organizations. For instance, in the 1970s most developed economies were predominantly based on manufacturing with employees working on traditional assembly lines. Hackman and Oldham's (1975) job characteristics model (discussed below) therefore conceptualized autonomy as the extent to which the job provided employees with freedom and independence over their work schedules and work processes. In the succeeding decades, the advent of new manufacturing technologies such as flexible manufacturing systems, total quality management practices, just-in-time inventory management, and others, highlighted that a more nuanced view of autonomy was required—these new manufacturing technologies relied increasingly on integration across work units and employees (Jackson, Wall, Martin, & Davids, 1993). Considering this shift in manufacturing technologies, Wall, Corbett, Clegg, Jackson, and Martin (1990) presented several forms of control (a term that represents one conceptualization of experienced autonomy) that can be designed into manufacturing work, namely timing control (work schedules and machine-pacing), method control (discretion in undertaking work tasks), and boundary control (control over secondary activities, such as maintenance, modifications, ordering supplies, and quality assurance).

Recent economic trends include globalization, increased competition, and the transition to a services-based economy. Employee empowerment practices, centered on giving decision-making control to employees, spawned in such an environment (Spreitzer, 1995). The current thinking in organizational behavior research draws on these developments and considers three distinct but complimentary perspectives on employee autonomy: work scheduling autonomy, work methods autonomy, and decision-making autonomy (Morgeson & Humphrey, 2006).

There are other related conceptualizations of autonomy. For example, Breaugh (1985) separated autonomy into several subcomponents, including method autonomy, scheduling autonomy, and criterion autonomy (i.e., choice in how to measure job performance), all of which have been associated with positive work outcomes, such as work satisfaction, job involvement, absenteeism, and performance quality. Sadler-Smith, El-Kot, and Leat (2003) even found support for Breaugh's multi-dimensional work autonomy scale in an Egyptian sample of employees. Another conceptualization of autonomy is the Maastricht Autonomy List, which purports to assess actual job autonomy by examining *opportunities* to exercise control. It differentiates autonomy into subcomponents of work tempo, work method, and job evaluation (de Jonge, Landeweerd, & Van Breukelen, 1994). Finally, other conceptualizations of autonomy include task-related and context-related autonomy (Gomez-Mejia, 1986) and the High Involvement Work Practices model (Lawler, 1986), which includes the power to act and make decisions. The latter has been positively related to organizational return on equity, employee commitment and satisfaction, and also negatively related to turnover in a North American sample of 3,500 employees (Vandenberg, Richardson, & Eastman, 1999). Gomez-Mejia (1986) has shown the validity of his conceptualization in a sample of over 5,000 employees from 20 countries on the 5 continents.

In addition, and consistent with the broader theme of this book, research based on self-determination theory (Deci & Ryan, 1985) has also provided strong evidence of the importance of autonomy in the workplace. In self-determination theory, autonomy means "to endorse one's actions to the highest level of reflection" (Deci & Ryan, 2007, http://www.psych.rochester.edu/SDT/index.php). When people feel autonomous, they feel free to choose to do things that are interesting or personally meaningful to them. Self-determination theory argues for the existence of three basic psychological needs, one of which is the need for autonomy. Compared to the other conceptualizations of autonomy mentioned above, self-determination theory makes a strong claim that autonomy is a need that must be satisfied in order for humans to function optimally. It has been related to better work motivation, productivity, and well-being (see Gagné & Deci, 2005 for a review).

We can see from the above review that autonomy has been discussed at great lengths in the field of organizational behavior. In this chapter we use the term "job autonomy" throughout except when referring to the specific forms of autonomy outlined above. Because autonomy has been examined from many more perspectives, its effects in the domain of work have been studied in research about concrete organizational practices aimed at improving employee performance and engagement. For this reason, the rest of the chapter focuses on research about these practices so that we can extract what we know about the importance of autonomy in the work domain. But first we turn to the theories that underlie these practices.

Theoretical Frameworks

Because autonomy, as conceptualized above, is at the heart of how work is structured, organized, designed, and managed, we organize the review of empirical research that pertains to autonomy in the workplace around theories of job design. Job design is one of the most well-studied organizational behavior topics and has generated a large body of literature from around the world. Therefore, it offers compelling cross-cultural evidence for the importance of autonomy in the workplace. Early views of job design came from a backlash against Taylorism, an early industrial approach to structuring work in organizations that included job specialization and standardization, and the use of performance-contingent pay systems (Taylor, 1911). This technique was soon found to create monotonous jobs where people could not exercise any discretion, and where they felt dissatisfied and alienated (e.g., Fay & Kamps, 2006).

Early job design approaches recommended the use of job enlargement (giving people varied tasks) and job enrichment (decision-making power) to motivate workers. Later on, more refined models of job design were developed. The most popular one was developed by Hackman and Oldham (1975), and proposed five core job characteristics to motivate employees: skill variety, task identity, task significance, job autonomy, and feedback. According to these authors, job autonomy is what makes employees feel responsible and accountable for work outcomes, and has been linked to intrinsic motivation, job satisfaction performance, and employee retention (Hackman & Oldham, 1975). Morgeson and Humphrey (2006) validated a revised and expanded job characteristics scale where they exploded the job autonomy scale intro three subscales based on Breaugh's (1985) typology discussed earlier.

There is substantial evidence validating the Job Characteristics Model (e.g., Fried & Ferris, 1987; Lawler & Hall, 1970). Employee perceptions of job characteristics are related with objective measures of job complexity derived from the Dictionary of Occupational Titles (Gerhart, 1988). In a comparative study of business owners and employed workers, Prottas and Thompson (2006) reported that although business owners experience greater stress than employed workers, they feel more autonomous in their work. This can be explained through the enriched job design of business owners relative to employed workers. Self-employed workers in the UK (business owners and independent contractors) reported higher levels of job autonomy than employees, but overall, perceptions of autonomy were equally associated with positive outcomes in all three groups of workers (Prottas, 2008). Using a repeated measures design in a South African organization, Orpen (1979) found that clerical employees who underwent job enrichment showed increases in work motivation, job satisfaction and involvement, lower absenteeism and turnover. In a recent meta-analysis of over 250 publications, mostly with Western samples, job characteristics explained between 24 and 34% of the variance in many work outcomes (Humphrey, Nahrgang, & Morgeson, 2007).

The job characteristics model is totally compatible with self-determination theory. Like the JCM, SDT argues that task design and job context can influence intrinsic motivation, and that this can be explained as the satisfaction of needs. While the JCM argues for three psychological states as mediators, namely meaningfulness, responsibility, and knowledge of results, SDT argues for the importance of satisfying needs for competence, autonomy, and relatedness. Indeed, enriched job designs have been associated with greater intrinsic work motivation in both employed and voluntary Canadian workers (Gagné, Senécal, & Koestner, 1997; Millette & Gagné, 2008).

Autonomy in the design of jobs has been shown to be important in different cultures. Vlerick and Goeminne (1994) found higher job autonomy in Belgian nurses whose work was organized around patient cases than in nurses whose work was organized around assigned tasks. In a study of 13,795 workers from Canada, China, Finland, France, and Sweden, lack of job autonomy and work complexity were related to functional incapacity, and this impact was stronger in China than in less collectivistic countries (Vaananen et al., 2005). These findings contradict what some authors have argued, which is that job autonomy is less important in collectivitistic and high power-distance cultures than it is in individualistic and low power-distance cultures (Iyengar & Lepper, 1999). Indeed, a study of Chinese and US information technology recruits shows that they hold similar beliefs regarding employer–employee obligations, including the obligation to provide job autonomy (King & Bu, 2005). Discussions between Chinese senior managers working in Chinese public organizations and the first author support this belief. These senior managers argued that feeling autonomous is essential to employee engagement in Chinese organizations.

There are still some contradictory findings related to job autonomy highlighted in the broader job design literature. Among Indian textile mill workers, perceptions of job characteristics were not associated with job involvement (Naaz, 1999), and in a Taiwanese sample working in high technology, job specialization (i.e., low job enrichment) was positively associated with self-efficacy and negatively with burnout (Hsieh & Chao, 2004). However, job design was associated with hotel performance in India (Chand & Katou, 2007), and job autonomy was related to skill utilization in Kuwait (Abdalla, 1988). More research is needed to understand these discrepant findings and find some possible cultural or organizational moderators (such as the type of work being done) of the relations between job autonomy and outcomes.

Besides the Job Characteristics Model, other job design models have been developed. Campion and Thayer's (1985) Multimethod Job Design Model includes motivational subcomponents (including job autonomy), mechanistic subcomponents, biological and perceptual/motor subcomponents. Campion (1988) showed that motivational designs are linked to satisfaction outcomes, while mechanical designs are linked to efficiency outcomes, biological designs are linked to comfort outcomes, and perceptual/motor designs are linked to reliability outcomes. Some research has shown that it is not easy to have a design that is sound motivationally *and* mechanically (Campion, 1988), and this is likely because designs that are mechanically sound probably limit the amount of discretion employees have in their job. Indeed, the introduction of just-in-time methods (which increases process control) has been shown to decrease individual autonomy (Klein, 1991). The introduction of lean production practices (lean teams, assembly lines and workflow formalization) is associated with decreased perceptions of job autonomy, which in turn is associated with reduced organizational commitment, self-efficacy, and depression (Parker, 2003). Hackman and Oldham's (1975) job characteristics differ significantly in jobs that use different technologies, and these design differences impact satisfaction and motivation (Rousseau, 1977). However, more recent research shows that there are ways to design jobs so that they are sound both motivationally and mechanically (Morgeson & Campion, 2002). For instance, Wall, Corbett, Martin, Clegg, and Jackson (1990) found that giving computer-numerical-control machine operators in UK manufacturing environments control over the maintenance and programming to rectify operational problems (in addition to loading, monitoring and unloading tasks), improved their productivity, their job satisfaction, and lowered perceived job pressure.

Warr's Vitamin model (1995) proposes yet another framework for examining job autonomy. Warr proposed that certain job attributes (for e.g., job autonomy, job demands, etc.) function like "vitamins"—they are desirable up to specific levels but are harmful or ineffective at excessive levels. Thus, Warr hypothesized curvilinear relationships between the "vitamins" and employee outcomes. Some research has shown curvilinear effects, but not always in the expected direction. Champoux (1992) found that under different levels of supervisor satisfaction or growth need strength, the curvilinear relationship could be U-shaped or inversely U-shaped. However, Xie and Johns (1995) found U-shaped relationships between some of the job characteristics and burnout, but the relationship with autonomy was linear. But in two samples of Dutch healthcare workers, job autonomy was linearly related to burnout (de Jonge & Schaufeli, 1998; Jeurissen & Nyklicek, 2001). Perhaps some variables, such as expertise level or supervisor behaviors, moderate the positive impact of job autonomy on outcomes, such that autonomy remains positive as long as it is coupled with other support mechanisms, or has more impact coupled with them.

The broader literature on job design has examined how certain contextual factors can impact the effect of job design on outcomes. Peters and O'Connors (1980) argued that situational constraints, such as technology, budgets, and time, can limit the impact of job redesign on employee motivation. However, Phillips and Freedman (1984) found that although situational constraints lead to negative affective reactions, they do not limit the effects of job design on outcomes. Organizational climate has also been shown to enhance the effects of job design on the job satisfaction of US nurses (Ferris & Gilmore, 1984). In a recent study drawing on self-determination theory, Bellerose and Gagné (2009) found that a motivational job design can actually compensate for poor leadership and help maintain motivation levels (the opposite was also true). So, if employees feel in control of the situation (through job autonomy) constraints do not necessarily have debilitating effects on their motivation. What remains to be tested in the cross-cultural generalizability of these findings? Next, we examine the effects associated with job autonomy for important outcomes for employees and organizations: employee engagement, employee performance, and employee well-being.

Employee Engagement

Employee engagement has been alternatively defined as involvement, commitment, passion, enthusiasm, effort, and energy (Macey & Schneider, 2008). Engagement has been operationalized both in cognitive terms, such as vitality, absorption, involvement, commitment, and empowerment, and in behavioral terms, such as extra-role behavior, proactivity, initiative, and adaptation. It has also been equated with autonomous motivation (Meyer & Gagné, 2008). Employee engagement has been shown in a meta-analysis to relate moderately to job autonomy (Brown, 1996). Research based on self-determination theory also shows that satisfaction of the need for autonomy is associated with greater work engagement (Baard, Deci, & Ryan, 2004; Deci et al., 2001). One popular work engagement measure, the Utrecht Work Engagement Scale, includes subscales for vigor, dedication, and absorption (Schaufeli, Martinez, Pinto, Salanova, & Bakker, 2002; Schaufeli, Salanova, González-Romá, & Bakker, 2002), which have been related to the amount of control one felt he or she had on the job (Schaufeli, Taris, & vanrhenen, 2008; Sonnentag, 2003). This model is highly compatible with Ryan and Frederick's (1997) conceptualization and empirical evidence for subjective vitality, which is based on self-determination theory.

The concept of empowerment has also been used to examine employee engagement. Structural empowerment, like job autonomy, refers to having decision-making power and adequate resources to work autonomously. Kakabadse (1986) has shown that centralized and formalized organizational structures lead employees to feel powerless, which is related to job dissatisfaction, decreased organizational commitment, and over time to a greater need for rule enforcement. Psychological empowerment refers to the feelings associated with having power over one's work situation. Thomas and Velthouse (1990) put autonomy at the heart of the experience of empowerment itself, by including it among the four key psychological factors associated with empowerment (along with meaning, competence, and impact). Empowerment has been positively related to work effectiveness and satisfaction, and negatively to strain (Spreitzer, Kizilos, & Nason, 1997). Similar results were found in a large sample of Filipino service workers (Hechanova, Alampay, & Franco, 2006). The five core job characteristics from Hackman and Oldham's theory have been related to feelings of empowerment, which in turn were associated with intrinsic work motivation, in a sample of technicians and telemarketers of a Canadian telecommunications company (Gagné et al., 1997).

Job autonomy has been linked to many other behavioral and attitudinal engagement indicators. Job autonomy is positively related to role breadth (how broadly you view your organizational role), self-efficacy, flexibility, organizational commitment, and feelings of ownership (Aubé, Rousseau, & Morin, 2007; Morgeson, Delaney-Klinger, & Hemingway, 2005; Parker & Axtell, 2001). Naus, van Iterson, and Roe (2007) found that perceptions of job autonomy in a sample of Dutch workers were associated with decreased organizational cynicism, and Parish, Cadwallader, and Busch (2008) found that role autonomy was related to commitment to organizational change. Because these findings are mostly from Western samples, cross-cultural research is needed to validate them in non-Western cultures.

The opposite of engagement has been studied under different labels: burnout and powerlessness, for instance. González-Romá, Schaufeli, Bakker, and Lloret (2006) argued that burnout is the opposite of work engagement. However, Schaufeli and Bakker (2004), and Schaufeli, Taris and vanrhenen (2008) also found in samples of Dutch workers that burnout and engagement are not always related to the same antecedents and outcomes, although job autonomy was related to both (see the section on well-being below for more results). Lack of engagement has also been called powerlessness. For instance, Ashforth (1989) defined powerlessness as lack of autonomy and participation, and found that it can generate reactance, helplessness, and alienation. Powerlessness has also been associated with lowered efforts, performance, and tardiness (Cummings & Manring, 1977).

Individual Performance

Job autonomy is related to individual performance and to other work behaviors. Satisfaction of the need for autonomy has been related to US bankers' performance evaluation scores (Baard et al., 2004). Claessens, Van Eerde, Rutte, and Roe (2004) found job autonomy to be a significant predictor of performance in a sample of Dutch employees. Interestingly, having high job autonomy also enhances the relationship between one's personality (as assessed through the Big 5) and job performance (Barrick & Mount, 1993) and extra-role performance (Gellatly & Irving, 2001). Millette and Gagné (2008) found that the five core job characteristics were associated with greater autonomous work motivation and better performance in a sample of French Canadian volunteer workers. Parker, Axtell, and Turner (2001) showed that job autonomy was positively associated with safe working behaviors in a UK sample. Job autonomy has been an important factor for proactive work behavior (proactive idea implementation and problem solving), and innovative work behaviors (Parker, Williams, & Turner, 2006; Ramamoorthy, Flood, Slattery, & Sardessai, 2005).

The satisfaction of the need for autonomy was related to positive training intentions in a Spanish sample of workers (Roca & Gagné, 2008). Cabrera, Collins, and Salgado (2006) found in a Spanish sample that job autonomy was essential to the motivation of knowledge sharing in the workplace. Gagné (2009) argues that this is because autonomy fosters the internalization of the value for sharing knowledge. Would sharing these findings be even stronger in a collectivistic culture and would autonomy be as important in this context? Morrison (2006) found that job autonomy was related to pro-social rule breaking (breaking a rule to promote the welfare of an organization or a stakeholder) in a US sample. Would we find pro-social rule breaking behavior in a culture high in power-distance or uncertainty avoidance?

Well-Being

Job autonomy has been linked to employee well-being across many cultures. Self-determination theory research clearly shows such a link between satisfaction of the need for autonomy and well-being (e.g., Baard et al., 2004; Deci et al., 2001). In a US sample of over 3,000 workers, job autonomy was related to higher satisfaction, and lower work–family conflict, turnover intentions and stress (Thompson & Prottas, 2006). A study of over 9,000 Netherland workers in 28 professions found that job autonomy was negatively related to burnout (Taris et al., 2002). Several studies of service and welfare workers (many in the US but also some from European countries and Japan) have found that the negative effect of work autonomy on burnout because it buffers against job stress (Daniels & Guppy, 1994; Grandey, Fisk, & Steiner, 2005; Hall et al., 2006; Lee & Ashforth, 1993; Peiro, Gonzalez-Roma, & Lloret, 1994; Stalker, Mandell, Frensch, Harvey, & Wright, 2007; Van Yperen & Hagedoom, 2003). Karasek's (1979) study of Swedish and American employees showed that job control can buffer employees against stress-caused high job demands. Interestingly, this effect was only found in people with high autonomous motivation in a sample of French-Canadian university professors (Fernet, Guay, & Senécal, 2004); and Tai and Liu (2007) found in a Taiwanese sample that the buffering effects of job autonomy were particularly important for neurotic people. Moreover, Van den Broeck, Vansteenkiste, De Witte, and Lens (2008) found that the satisfaction of the need for autonomy was a strong mediator of the effects of job control on burnout and engagement.

Are the effects of job autonomy limited to psychological health? Sprigg, Stride, Wall, Holman, and Smith (2007) found no main or moderating effect of job autonomy on musculoskeletal disorders in call center employees (although they were influenced by stress). However, Liu, Spector, and Jex (2005) found that US university employees who reported high job autonomy also reported less frustration, anxiety, turnover intentions, physical symptoms, and doctor visits. One question is whether in some cultures where people express psychological distress more physically, and whether the effects of strain would be more highly related to physical health in these groups. For example, in a German sample of male public service workers, Rau (2004) found that high job scope was related to higher diastolic blood pressure during work hours, and lower diastolic blood pressure during the night. The author interprets these results to mean that high job scope is healthy to employees. Would we find the same results in China or Latin countries?

Based on the above theoretical framework of job design, we next examine organizational practices, such as autonomous work groups and workplace monitoring, and also new work arrangements such as telecommuting and workplace monitoring.

Organizational Practices

Autonomous Work Groups

Related research from the field of organizational development (out of which quality circles and sociotechnical systems became popular; Emery, 1959) also provide much evidence for the importance of autonomy in the workplace. This work led to new ways of structuring and organizing work done by teams in organizations. Wall et al. (1990) talk about 4 key constructs that define "advanced manufacturing technology": control, cognitive demands, production responsibility, and social interaction, which they say can be promoted through the use of autonomous work groups. Autonomous work groups typically do not have a supervisor and have the following responsibilities: allocate jobs among themselves, reach production targets while meeting quality standards, solve production problems, record production data, organize schedules, order raw materials, deliver finished goods to the client, call for engineering support, and select and train new recruits (Kemp, Wall, Clegg, & Cordery, 1983). These authors found that employees working in autonomous work groups in a UK plant reported higher job satisfaction and also perceived greater work role complexity compared to workers in another industrial organization using traditional design. Similarly, in the US, Ward (1997) found that autonomous work groups reported higher receptivity to change, trust in management, and organizational commitment. Parker, Wall, and Jackson (1997) undertook a rigorous study comparing three types of work groups: work groups that were not redesigned, work groups where Just-in-Time (JIT) and Total-Quality-Management (TQM) methods were introduced, and work groups where JIT and TQM methods were introduced in conjunction with establishing autonomous work groups. The authors observed that the latter group cognitively redefined their role in the organization more than the other two groups: employees in this group developed a more strategic orientation (i.e., endorsing the organization's key strategies) and a broader role orientation (i.e., changed views of their own work responsibilities). Parker et al. argued that it was the addition of job autonomy in this group that made the difference. Other research demonstrates that the positive effects of autonomous work groups are long-lasting, especially on intrinsic work motivation (Wall, Kemp, Jackson, & Clegg, 1986).

Autonomous work groups arguably enrich the design of tasks (Campion, Medsker, & Higgs, 1993; Campion, Papper, & Medsker, 1996; Griffin, Patterson, & West, 2001). Some researchers have integrated notions from team and job design research to develop, for example, a Team Characteristics Model (Strubler & York, 2007). Cohen, Ledford, and Spreitzer (1996) found in a US sample that autonomous work groups demonstrated better group management, such as stability, clear norms, better coordination, more expertise and innovation, because of the enriched design this form of work organization creates. Members of these groups were also more involved in their work and reported more job satisfaction, commitment, and trust. Finally, they performed better (in terms of quality, productivity, costs, and safety) and were less absent.

Although more research is needed to examine how autonomous work groups would fare in other cultures, there is some cross-cultural research that addresses this issue. For example, Jin (1993) demonstrated that teams that were voluntarily formed in Chinese manufacturing plants evidenced higher motivation and performance quality (but not quantity) than teams formed through assignments. Cordery, Mueller, and Smith (1991) found that employees in autonomous work groups in a minerals processing plant in Australia reported more positive attitudes than employees in traditionally designed jobs. In an Israeli sample, Meier (1984) found that a team approach to organizing work was related to feeling autonomous. Autonomous work groups in the Netherlands evidenced more motivating task design, higher quality relationships among team members, decreased work load, and increased well-being (van Mierlo, Rutte, Seinen, & Kompier, 2000).

Participative Management

Early organizational behavior researchers discovered that when employees were allowed to participate in decision-making, they seemed to be more engaged, to put more effort into their work, and to feel less strain (Coch & French, 1948; Kornhauser & Reid, 1965; Likert, 1967; Lowin, 1968). Participative management can take many forms. Hackman (1986) discusses the implications of giving people the authority to (1) execute their work the way they want to; (2) monitor and manage the work process; (3) design and distribute work; and (4) set goals for the unit or organization. Sashkin (1976) offers four forms of participative approaches, including (1) participation in setting goals; (2) participation in decision-making; (3) participation in solving problems; and (4) participation in the development and implementation of change in the organization, and describes when each should be used.

Cotton, Vollrath, Froggatt, Lengnick-Hall, and Jennings (1988) showed in their meta-analysis how six forms of participation (i.e., work decisions, consultative, short-term, informal, employee ownership, and representative) lead to different performance and satisfaction outcomes. Scott-Ladd, Travaglione, and Marshall (2006) found in an Australian sample that task variety fosters participation in decision making, which in turn promotes job satisfaction and commitment. Cassar (1999) found that participation is especially related to job satisfaction when used at a tactical level (task decisions). Similarly, Sagie, Elizur, and Koslowsky (1995) found that strategic change decisions made by management coupled with participation in tactical decisions (how to conduct the change) increases acceptance of the change. Black and Gregersen (1997) found in a US sample that participation in planning and evaluation was related to satisfaction, while participation in planning was related only to productivity.

Hodson (1996) found in US manufacturing firms that autonomy mediated the effects of worker participation on job satisfaction and the willingness to train co-workers (a form of prosocial behavior). Mikkelsen and Gundersen (2003) demonstrated that a participative management implementation in a Norwegian postal service yielded higher levels of perceived job autonomy, as well as improvements in stress and subjective health. Meta-analyses show that the effect of participation on satisfaction and performance is mediated by the experience of control and autonomy (Miller & Monge, 1986; Sagie, 1994). This is supportive of the self-determination theory perspective, which demonstrates that giving employees choice, a good rationale, and perspective taking is related to greater feelings of autonomy (Baard et al., 2004; Deci, Connell, & Ryan, 1989; Deci et al., 2001). Coye and Belohlav (1995) surveyed 326 US CEOs to find that the use of participative management was related to employee engagement. Overall, Western research shows that the positive effects of participative management are attributable to increased experienced autonomy.

Given these favorable effects associated with participative management, some researchers argue that employee participation is an ethical imperative (Sashkin, 1984). However, other researchers contend that too much importance is assigned to participation for employee motivation (e.g., Locke, Schweiger, & Latham, 1986), that it does not always yield desired productivity outcomes and is onerous to manage (Locke & Schweiger, 1979). For instance, Latham, Winters, and Locke (1994) found in a lab study that subjects in participative goal setting conditions felt more self-efficacious but did not perform better than subjects in assigned goal conditions. However, Latham, Erez, and Locke (1988) found that it may not be the participation itself that leads to greater acceptance and performance. In a study where they compared experimental subjects in a participatively set goals condition to those in a condition where goals were assigned along with a strong rationale for the goal, there were no performance differences. Deci, Eghrari, Patrick, and Leone (1994) indeed showed that offering a good rationale for asking someone to work on a task can lead to increased feelings of autonomy and greater internalization of the importance of the task, leading to greater intrinsic motivation and performance. Therefore, participative management may work because it increases experienced autonomy, but there may be other ways to increase this experience. Sagie's (1994) meta-analysis supports this conclusion, showing that a "tell and sell" approach to goal setting is as strongly associated with performance as is a participative method. Perhaps the need for participative management (for engaging employees) may depend on task and other structural characteristics.

The little cross-cultural research that exists shows that different forms of participative management are used in some non-western cultures with positive outcomes. Deci et al. (2001) showed, for example, that support of the need for autonomy was related to positive outcomes in both US and Bulgarian organizations. Sagie and Aycan (2003) found that two cultural dimensions, individualism-collectivism and power distance were predictively related to specific participative management approaches, such as face-to-face participative management, collective participative management, pseudo-participative management, and paternalistic participative management. In Europe, Cabrera, Ortega, and Cabrera (2003) found that two forms of participative management prevail: consultative and delegative. Pradhan, Kumar, Singh, and Mishra (2004) examined the types of prevailing organizational climates in Indian organizations, and concluded that public organizations emphasize participative management. Vardi, Shirom, and Jacobson (1980) found that Israeli managers have positive attitudes toward participative management, and Tzafrir (2006) found in 104 Israeli firms that human resource management practices that enhance employee decision-making power exhibit higher organizational performance. Lam, Chen, and Schaubroeck (2002) found that perceived participative decision making was equally related to employee performance in comparable samples of bank employees from Hong Kong and the US (controlling for the values of allocentrism and idiocentrism).

What is painfully lacking from the above review is more compelling cross-cultural evidence of the effects of participative management on feelings of autonomy and outcomes. Is participative management used at all in some cultures, such as those high power-distance or uncertainty avoidance? Would participative management yield the same positive outcomes in these cultures? These questions need to be addressed by future research.

New Work Arrangements

A number of new work arrangements have recently appeared in organizational life. These work arrangements reflect differences in job design and have been linked to differential autonomy levels and differential outcomes. We discuss two of them, namely telecommuting and electronic monitoring.

Telecommuting has been argued to increase job autonomy (Feldman & Gainey, 1997), and to require that employees be more self-regulated in their work behavior (Raghuram, Wiesenfeld, & Garud, 2003). Although the use of telecommuting has been linked to firm performance in Spain (Sánchez, Pérez, de Luis Carnicer, & Jimenez, 2007), very little research actually tests whether telecommuting increases job autonomy and requires more self-regulation than regular jobs. No research to our knowledge even looks at the design of telecommuting jobs. Research on telecommuting should compare the design of these types of jobs to the design of more traditional and equivalent work arrangements (i.e., same job done on organizational premises). Job autonomy may actually vary across different telecommuting jobs, depending on the rules that are established for these workers, the technology they need to use, and the type of work they do from home. Golden, Veiga, and Simsek (2006) found that job autonomy levels mitigate the negative impact that telecommuting sometimes has on work–family conflict. Similarly, Senécal, Vallerand, and Guay (2001) found that management support of the need for autonomy increased work autonomous motivation, and decreased work–family conflict and the resulting exhaustion in a sample of physical therapists and psychologists.

Workplace electronic monitoring is a relatively recent trend that often limits job autonomy. Although supervisory micro-management may have been the way to monitor employee behavior before, today this is also done through technology. Employees often work from remote office locations, knowledge work is more prevalent and more difficult to monitor, and today's managers are typically overwhelmed with paperwork and meetings, preventing close monitoring of employee behavior. The last decades have seen increases in the use of card swipe systems, physiological monitoring equipment (eye and fingerprint detectors), location sensing technologies such as global positioning systems (GPS), as well as computer monitoring and the use of cameras to monitor employee behaviors. A 2007 Electronic Monitoring and Surveillance Survey (American Management Association, 2008) revealed that 66% of the surveyed US employers reported using Internet monitoring, 43%

reported using email monitoring, 45% reported using telephone monitoring, 48% reported using video surveillance, and 8% reported using GPS to monitor company vehicles.

Besides concerns over invasion of privacy (Ambrose, Alder, & Noel, 1998), early writings on performance monitoring argued that performance monitoring increases stress levels and can lead to health problems (Aiello, 1993; Carayon, 1993; Smith, Carayon, Sanders, Lim, & LeGrande, 1992). This perspective is compatible with self-determination theory research on the negative effects of surveillance on intrinsic motivation (Enzle & Anderson, 1993). Although some research shows that employee monitoring increases work performance (Canoni, 2004; Komaki, 1986; Komaki, Desselles, & Bowman, 1989; Larson & Callahan, 1990), possibly because of the social facilitation it causes (Aiello & Kolb, 1995), others have shown that it can decrease performance on complex tasks (Aiello & Svec, 1993). These decreases in performance and increases in stress have been argued to be caused by the effect that monitoring systems have on job autonomy (Carayon, 1994). A study indeed showed that a computer-based performance monitoring system was less stressful when it was done in conjunction with increased job autonomy (Ball & Wilson, 2000). Other research shows that using monitoring to give feedback to employees leads to more positive outcomes (Aiello & Shao, 1993; Griffith, 1993; Wells, Moorman, & Werner, 2007). Stone and Stone (1990) argued that these positive effects occur because such use of a monitoring system does not decrease feelings of autonomy. Ways to restore feelings of autonomy have also included employee input into the design of the monitoring system (De Tienne & Abbott, 1993), and control over the monitoring system (Stanton & Barnes-Farrell, 1996). Spitzmuller and Stanton (2006) argue that control over monitoring enhances the relationship between attitudes toward monitoring systems and intentions to comply with it.

Research on monitoring, however, has not only concentrated on the mere usage of these technologies, but also on company and managerial motives for their utilization. Lyon (2006), for example, presented a model to show different types of monitoring, ranging from soft (passive) to sharp (active utilization). Ambrose et al. (1998) state that monitoring can range from work-related (e.g., computer monitoring) to work and non-work related (e.g., video surveillance), and that non-work related monitoring is perceived to be much more controlling and even unethical by some employees. This was supported by a recent study (McNall & Roch, 2007). It would be important for future research to further examine the impact of these characteristics of monitoring systems and organizational motives on experienced autonomy.

The use of these technologies is likely to increase globally. However, there is limited research evaluating the role of autonomy and monitoring from a cross-cultural perspective, and this should be one focus of future research in this field. There is clearly a need for more cross-cultural research on autonomy and its relationship with these particular new work arrangements and with other ones not discussed herein, such as virtual teams, job sharing, and flexible work schedules.

Future Avenues

We can conclude from this review that autonomy is a crucial element of employee motivation and engagement. We can also conclude that the empirical results reviewed above strongly support self-determination theory (Deci & Ryan, 1985). Autonomy in the workplace can take many forms that can be examined through the study of specific organizational practices that influence it. Throughout the chapter, we have shown how these practices create opportunities or barriers to experienced autonomy. By focusing research on how practices influence autonomy, we can use rigorous and systematic methods to examine the effects of these practices on employee outcomes. Self-determination theory would serve as a useful framework to explain many of these characteristics' effects on employee motivation and outcomes. Because self-determination theory predicts how situational and personal factors influence the satisfaction of basic psychological needs, including autonomy, it can significantly help develop tests of different workplace practices. New tools, such as the Need Satisfaction at Work Scale (Van den Broeck, Vansteenkiste, De Witte, Soenens, & Lens, in press) and the Motivation at Work Scale (Forest et al., 2010), both already available in multiple languages, will hopefully encourage organizational behavior researchers to use self-determination theory to expand our knowledge on job autonomy.

Many cross-cultural questions remain about job design. In an interesting study of 7,000 jobs in 7 countries, similar jobs were found to carry different levels of job autonomy (Dobbin & Boychuk, 1999). Although the authors argue that differences were attributable to differences in national employment systems, could these differences be caused by cultural values? In a study of over 4,000 companies from 14 European countries, national culture influenced the type of flexible work arrangements chosen by companies (Raghuram, London, & Larsen, 2001). For example, power distance and individualism were related to using part-time work; uncertainty avoidance and individualism were related to using contract work and shift work; feminity was related to using telecommuting. However, another study conducted across 42 countries found that the intra-cultural variation in job autonomy was associated with positive outcomes beyond mean differences in job autonomy across the countries (Au & Cheung, 2004); although job autonomy may vary across countries, there is still significant within-culture variation, and autonomy level has the same impact across cultures.

What we know much less about is how to foster autonomy in the workplaces of the world. Can we use the same practices in the same way in every culture? It is doubtful. How should current practices be applied or adapted for different cultures? Should new practices be developed for particular cultures? We clearly need more research to answer these questions. We also need more research to examine other work-related issues. For example, how can we enhance the experience of autonomy in simple/monotonous jobs if we cannot redesign these jobs? What are the job design characteristics for people who work in virtual teams (i.e., people working remotely together)? In matrix structures, where people are managed by more than one person? In unionized versus non-unionized environments? For example, one study showed that unionized US employees were found to have less job autonomy than non-unionized employees (Kirmeyer & Shirom, 1986). Finally, contingent work (e.g., part-time temporary work, summer work, contract work) is becoming more and more common. The conditions underlying these types of jobs can affect their design, especially in the area of decision-making power, thereby affecting the experience of autonomy.

We need to remember that examining cross-cultural generalizability of methods to improve feelings of autonomy in the workplace is not an easy feat. Several contextual factors other than cultural values could influence the success or failure of practices. Johns (2006) provides a useful framework to organize our research methods and interpretation of results around categories of contextual variables, including job design and culture. Moreover, when we conduct meta-analyses, we should consider culture as a potential moderator.

In conclusion, discussions of autonomy in the workplace are as relevant as ever. Complexity in organizational structures, changes in employment practices, the globalization of business, among other trends, all make incorporating autonomy in organizational practices increasingly critical. More rigorous research, especially cross-cultural, is imperative to guide practitioners on the mechanisms to do so.

References

Abdalla, I. A. (1988). Work environment, job structure, and behavior orientation as predictors of skill utilization in Kuwait: The moderating effect of ability. *Genetic, Social, and General Psychology Monographs, 114*, 173–189.

Aiello, J. R. (1993). Computer-based work monitoring: Electronic surveillance and its effects. *Journal of Applied Social Psychology, 23*, 499–499.

Aiello, J. R., & Kolb, K. J. (1995). Electronic performance monitoring and social context: Impact on productivity and stress. *Journal of Applied Psychology, 80*, 339–353.

Aiello, J. R., & Shao, Y. (1993). Electronic performance monitoring and stress: The role of feedback and goal setting. In M. J. Smith & G. Salvendy (Eds.), *Human-computer interaction: Applications and case studies* (pp. 1011–1016). Amsterdam: Elsevier Science Publishers B.V.

Aiello, J. R., & Svec, C. M. (1993). Computer monitoring of work performance: Extending the social facilitation framework to electronic presence. *Journal of Applied Social Psychology, 23*, 537–548.

Ambrose, M. L., Alder, G. S., & Noel, T. W. (1998). Electronic monitoring and ethics: A consideration of employer and employee rights. In M. Schminke (Ed.), *Managerial ethics: Morally managing people and processes* (pp. 61–80). Hillsdale, NY: Erlbaum.

American Management Association. (2008). *The 2007 Electronic monitoring and surveillance survey from the American Management Association and the ePolicy Institute*. New York: American Management Association. http://www.amanet.org/research/

Ashforth, B. E. (1989). The experience of powerlessness in organizations. *Organizational Behavior and Human Decision Processes, 43*, 207–242. DOI: 10.1016/0749-5978(89)90051-4.

Au, K., & Cheung, M. W. L. (2004). Intracultural variation and job autonomy in 42 countries. *Organization Studies, 8*, 1339–1362.

Aubé, C., Rousseau, V., & Morin, E. M. (2007). Perceived organizational support and organizational commitment. *Journal of Managerial Psychology, 22*, 479–495. DOI: 10.1108/02683940710757209.

Baard, P. P., Deci, E. L., & Ryan, R. M. (2004). Intrinsic need satisfaction: A motivational basis of performance and well-being in two work settings. *Journal of Applied Social Psychology, 34*, 2045–2068.

Ball, K., & Wilson, D. C. (2000). Power, control and computer-based performance monitoring: Repertoires, resistance and subjectivities. *Organization Studies, 21*, 539–565. DOI: 10.1177/0170840600213003.

Barnard, C. I. (1938). *The functions of the executive*. Cambridge, MA: Harvard University Press.

Barrick, M. R., & Mount, M. K. (1993). Autonomy as a moderator of the relationships between the big five personality dimensions and job performance. *Journal of Applied Psychology, 78*, 111–118. DOI: 10.1037/0021-9010.78.1.111.

Bellerose, J., & Gagné, M. (2009, June). *The combined effects of leadership and work design on work motivation*. Poster presented at the Canadian Psychological Association, Montreal, CA.

Black, J., & Gregersen, H. (1997). Participative decision-making: An integration of multiple dimensions. *Human Relations, 50*, 859–878. DOI: 10.1023/A:1016968625470.

Breaugh, J. A. (1985). The measurement of work autonomy. *Human Relations, 38*, 551–570. DOI: 10.1177/001872678503800604.

Brown, S. P. (1996). A meta-analysis and review of organizational research on job involvement. *Psychological Bulletin, 120*, 235–255. DOI: 10.1037/0033-2909.120.2.235.

Budd, J. W. (2004). *Employment with a human face: Balancing efficiency, equity, and voice*. Ithaca, NY: Cornell University Press.

Cabrera, Á., Collins, W. C., & Salgado, J. F (2006). Determinants of individual engagement in knowledge sharing. *The International Journal of Human Resource Management, 17*, 245–264. DOI: 10.1080/09585190500404614.

Cabrera, E. F., Ortega, J. & Cabrera, A. (2003). An exploration of the factors that influence employee participation in Europe. *Journal of World Business, 38*, 43–54.

Campion, M. A. (1988). Interdisciplinary approaches to job design: A constructive replication with extensions. *Journal of Applied Psychology, 73*, 467–481.

Campion, M. A., Medsker, G. J., & Higgs, A. C. (1993). Relations between work group characteristics and effectiveness: Implications for designing effective work groups. *Personnel psychology, 46*, 823–823.

Campion, M. A., Papper, E. M., & Medsker, G. J. (1996). Relations between work team characteristics and effectiveness: A replication and extension. *Personnel psychology, 49*, 429–452.

Campion, M. A., & Thayer, P. W. (1985). Development and field evaluation of an interdisciplinary measure of job design. *Journal of Applied Psychology, 70*, 29–43. DOI: 10.1037/0021-9010.70.1.29.

Canoni, J. D. (2004). Location awareness technology and employee privacy rights. *Employee Relations Law Journal, 30*, 26–31.

Carayon, P. (1993). Effect of electronic performance monitoring on job design and worker stress: Review of the literature and conceptual model. *Human Factors: The Journal of the Human Factors and Ergonomics Society, 35*, 385–395.

Carayon, P. (1994). Effects of electronic performance monitoring on job design and worker stress: Results of two studies. *International Journal of Human-Computer Interaction, 6*, 177–190.

Cassar, V. (1999). Can leader direction and employee participation co-exist? Investigating interaction effects between participation and favourable work-related attitudes among Maltese middle managers. *Journal of Managerial Psychology, 14*, 57–68.

Champoux, J. E. (1992). A multivariate analysis of curvilinear relationships among job scope, work context satisfactions and affective outcomes. *Human Relations, 45*, 87–111.

Chand, M., & Katou, A. A. (2007). The impact of hrm practices on organisational performance in the Indian hotel industry. *Employee Relations, 29*, 576–594. DOI: 10.1108/01425450710826096.

Claessens, B. J., Van Eerde, W., Rutte, C. G., & Roe, R. A. (2004). Planning behavior and perceived control of time at work. *Journal of Organizational Behavior, 25*, 937–950. DOI: 10.1002/job.292.

Coch, L., & French, J. R., Jr. (1948). Overcoming resistance to change. *Human Relations, 1*, 512.

Cohen, S. G., Ledford, G. E., & Spreitzer, G. M. (1996). A predictive model of self-managing work team effectiveness. *Human Relations, 49*, 643–676. DOI: 10.1177/001872679604900506.

Cordery, J. L., Muller, W. S., & Smith, L. M. (1991). Attitudinal and behavioral effects of autonomous group working: A longitudinal field study. *Academy of Management Journal, 34*, 464–476.

Cotton, J. L., Vollrath, D. A., Froggatt, K. L., Lengnick-Hall, M. L., & Jennings, K. R. (1988). Employee participation: Diverse forms and different outcomes. *The Academy of Management Review, 13*, 8–22.

Coye, R. W., & Belohlav, J. A. (1995). An exploratory analysis of employee participation. *Group and Organization Management, 20*, 4–17.

Cummings, T. G., & Manring, S. L. (1977). The relationship between worker alienation and work-related behavior. *Journal of Vocational Behavior, 10*, 167–179.

Daniels, K., & Guppy, A. (1994). Occupational stress, social support, job control, and psychological well-being. *Human Relations, 47*, 1523–1544. DOI: 10.1177/001872679404701205.

de Jonge, J., Landeweerd, J. A., & Van Breukelen, G. J. (1994). De maastrichtse autonomielijst: Achtergrond, constructie en validering. [The Maastricht autonomy questionnaire: Background, construction and validation]. *Gedrag en Organisatie, 7*, 27–41.

de Jonge, J. D., & Schaufeli, W. B. (1998). Job characteristics and employee well-being: A test of Warr's vitamin model in health care workers using structural equation modelling. *Journal of Organizational Behavior, 19*, 387–407.

De Tienne, K. B., & Abbott, N. T. (1993). Developing an employee-centered electronic monitoring system. *Journal of Systems Management, 44*, 12–12.

Deci, E. L., Connell, J. P., & Ryan, R. M. (1989). Self-determination in a work organization. *Journal of Applied Psychology, 74*, 580–590.

Deci, E. L., Eghrari, H., Patrick, B. C., & Leone, D. (1994). Facilitating internalization: The self-determination theory perspective. *Journal of Personality, 62*, 119–142.

Deci, E. L., & Ryan, R. M. (1985). *Intrinsic motivation and self-determination in human behavior*. New York: Plenum Publishing Co.

Deci, E. L., Ryan, R. M., Gagné, M., Leone, D. R., Usunov, J., & Kornazheva, B. P. (2001). Need satisfaction, motivation, and well-being in the work organizations of a former eastern bloc country. *Personality and Social Psychology Bulletin, 27*, 930–942.

Dobbin, F., & Boychuk, T. (1999). National employment systems and job autonomy: Why job autonomy is high in the Nordic Countries and low in the United States, Canada, and Australia. *Organization Studies, 20*, 257–291. DOI: 10.1177/0170840699202004.

Emery, F. E. (1959). *Characteristics of socio-technical systems*. London: Tavistock.

Enzle, M. E., & Anderson, S. C. (1993). Surveillant intentions and intrinsic motivation. *Journal of Personality and Social Psychology, 64*, 257–266.

Evans, B. K., & Fischer, D. G. (1992). A hierarchical model of participatory decision-making, job autonomy, and perceived control. *Human Relations, 45*, 1169–1189. DOI: 10.1177/001872679204501103.

Fay, D., & Kamps, A. (2006). Work characteristics and the emergence of a sustainable workforce: Do job design principles matter? *Gedrag & Organisatie, 19*, 184–203.

Feldman, D. C., & Gainey, T. W. (1997). Patterns of telecommuting and their consequences: Framing the research agenda. *Human Resource Management Review, 7*, 369–388. DOI: 10.1016/S1053-4822(97)90025-5.

Fernet, C., Guay, F., & Senécal, C. (2004). Adjusting to job demands: The role of work self-determination and job control in predicting burnout. *Journal of Vocational Behavior, 65*, 39–56. DOI: 10.1016/S0001-8791(03)00098-8.

Ferris, G. R., & Gilmore, D. C. (1984). The moderating role of work context in job design research: A test of competing models. *Academy of Management Journal, 27*, 885–892.

Forest, J., Gagné, M., Vansteenkiste, M., Van den Broeck, A., Crevier-Braud, L., Bergeron, E., et al. (2010). *International validation of the "revised motivation at work scale": Validation evidence in five different languages (French, English, Italian, Spanish, & Dutch)*. Paper presentation at the 4th international conference on Self-Determination Theory, Belgium, Ghent.

Fried, Y., & Ferris, G. R. (1987). The validity of the job characteristics model: A review and meta-analysis. *Personnel Psychology, 40*, 287–322.

Gagné, M. (2009). A model of knowledge sharing motivation. *Human Resource Management, 48*, 571–589.

Gagné, M., & Deci, E. L. (2005). Self-determination theory as a new framework for understanding organizational behavior. *Journal of Organizational Behavior, 26*, 331–362.

Gagné, M., Senécal, C., & Koestner, R. (1997). Proximal job characteristics, feelings of empowerment, and intrinsic motivation: A multidimensional model. *Journal of Applied Social Psychology, 27*, 1222–1240.

Gellatly, I. R., & Irving, P. G. (2001). Personality, autonomy, and contextual performance of managers. *Human Performance, 14*, 231. DOI: 10.1207/S15327043HUP1403_2.

Gerhart, B. (1988). Sources of variance in incumbent perceptions of job complexity. *Journal of Applied Psychology, 73*, 154–162.

Golden, T. D., Veiga, J. F., & Simsek, Z. (2006). Telecommuting's differential impact on work-family conflict: Is there no place like home? *Journal of Applied Psychology, 91*, 1340–1350. DOI: 10.1037/0021-9010.91.6.1340.

Gomez-Mejia, L. R. (1986). The cross-cultural structure of task-related and contextual constructs. *Journal of Psychology, 120*, 5–19.

González-Romá, V., Schaufeli, W. B., Bakker, A. B., & Lloret, S. (2006). Burnout and work engagement: Independent factors or opposite poles? *Journal of Vocational Behavior, 68*, 165–174. DOI: 10.1016/j.jvb.2005.01.003.

Grandey, A. A., Fisk, G. M., & Steiner, D. D. (2005). Must "service with a smile" be stressful? The moderating role of personal control for American and French employees. *Journal of Applied Psychology, 90*, 893–904. DOI: 10.1037/0021-9010.90.5.893.

Griffin, M. A., Patterson, M. G., & West, M. A. (2001). Job satisfaction and teamwork: The role of supervisor support. *Journal of Organizational Behavior, 22*, 537–550. DOI: 10.1002/job.101.

Griffith, T. L. (1993). Monitoring and performance: A comparison of computer and supervisor monitoring. *Journal of Applied Social Psychology, 23*, 549–572. DOI: 10.1111/j.1559-1816.1993.tb01103.x.

Hackman, J. R. (1986). The psychology of self-management in organizations. In M. S. Pallack & R. O. Perloff (Eds.), *Psychology and work: Productivity, change and employment*. Washington, DC: American Psychological Association.

Hackman, J. R., & Oldham, G. R. (1975). Development of the job diagnostic survey. *Journal of Applied Psychology, 60*, 159–170. DOI: 10.1037/h0076546.

Hall, A. T., Royle, M. T., Brymer, R. A., Perrewé, P. L., Ferris, G. R., & Hochwarter, W. A. (2006). Relationships between felt accountability as a stressor and strain reactions: The neutralizing role of autonomy across two studies. *Journal of Occupational Health Psychology, 11*, 87–99. DOI: 10.1037/1076-8998.11.1.87.

Hechanova, M. R. M., Alampay, R. B. A., & Franco, E. P. (2006). Psychological empowerment, job satisfaction and performance among Filipino service workers. *Asian Journal of Social Psychology, 9*, 72–78. DOI: 10.1111/j.1467-839X.2006.00177.x.

Hirschman, A. O. (1970). *Exit, voice and loyalty*. Cambridge, MA: Harvard University Press.

Hodson, R. (1996). Dignity in the workplace under participative management: Alienation and freedom revisited. *American Sociological Review, 61*, 719–738.

Hofstede, G. (2001). *Culture's consequences, comparing values, behaviors, institutions, and organizations across nations*. Thousand Oaks, CA: Sage Publications.

Hsieh, A.-T., & Chao, H.-Y. (2004). A reassessment of the relationship between job specialization, job rotation and job burnout: Example of Taiwan's high-technology industry. *International Journal of Human Resource Management, 15*, 1108–1123.

Humphrey, S. E., Nahrgang, J. D., & Morgeson, F. P. (2007). Integrating motivational, social, and contextual work design features: A meta-analytic summary and theoretical extension of the work design literature. *Journal of Applied Psychology, 92*, 1332–1356. DOI: 10.1037/0021-9010.92.5.1332.

Iyengar, S. S., & Lepper, M. R. (1999). Rethinking the value of choice: A cultural perspective on intrinsic motivation. *Journal of Personality and Social Psychology, 76,* 349–366.

Jackson, P. R., Wall, T. D., Martin, R., Davids, K. (1993). New measures of job control, cognitive demand, and production responsibility. *Journal of Applied Psychology, 78,* 753–762.

Jeurissen, T., & Nyklicek, I. (2001). Testing the Vitamin Model of job stress in Dutch health care workers. *Work & Stress, 15,* 254–264. DOI: 10.1080/02678370110066607.

Jin, P. (1993). Work motivation and productivity in voluntarily formed work teams: A field study in China. *Organizational Behavior and Human Decision Processes, 54,* 133–155.

Johns, G. (2006). The essential impact of context on organizational behavior. *Academy of Management Review, 31,* 386–408.

Kakabadse, A. (1986). Organizational alienation and job climate: A comparative study of structural conditions and psychological adjustment. *Small Group Research, 17,* 458–471. DOI: 10.1177/104649648601700406.

Karasek, R. A. (1979). Job demands, job decision latitude, and mental strain: Implications for job design. *Administrative Science Quarterly, 24,* 285–308.

Kemp, N. J., Wall, T. D., Clegg, C. W., & Cordery, J. L. (1983). Autonomous work groups in a green field site: A comparative study. *Journal of Occupational psychology, 56,* 271–288.

King, R. C., & Bu, N. (2005). Perceptions of the mutual obligations between employees and employers: A comparative study of new generation IT professionals in China and the United States. *International Journal of Human Resource Management, 16,* 46–64. DOI: 10.1080/0958519042000295948.

Kirmeyer, S. L., & Shirom, A. (1986). Perceived job autonomy in the manufacturing sector: Effects of unions, gender, and substantive complexity. *The Academy of Management Journal, 29,* 832–840.

Klein, J. A. (1991). A reexamination of autonomy in light of new manufacturing practices. *Human Relations, 44,* 21–38. DOI: 10.1177/001872679104400102.

Komaki, J. L. (1986). Toward effective supervision: An operant analysis and comparisons of managers at work. *Journal of Applied Psychology, 71,* 270–279.

Komaki, J. L., Desselles, M. L., & Bowman, E. D. (1989). Definitely not a breeze: Extending an operant model of effective supervision to teams. *Journal of Applied Psychology, 74,* 522–529.

Kornhauser, A., & Reid, O. M. (1965). *Mental health of the industrial worker: A Detroit study.* New York: Wiley.

Lam, S. S., Chen, X. P., & Schaubroeck, J. (2002). Participative decision making and employee performance in different cultures: The moderating effects of allocentrism/idiocentrism and efficacy. *The Academy of Management Journal, 45,* 905–914.

Larson, J. R., & Callahan, C. (1990). Performance monitoring: How it affects work productivity. *Journal of Applied Psychology, 75,* 530–538.

Latham, G. P., Erez, M., & Locke, E. A. (1988). Resolving scientific disputes by the joint design of crucial experiments by the antagonists: Application to the Erez-Latham dispute regarding participation in goal setting. *Journal of Applied Psychology, 73,* 753–772.

Latham, G. P., Winters, D. C., & Locke, E. A. (1994). Cognitive and motivational effects of participation: A mediator study. *Journal of Organizational Behavior, 15,* 49–63.

Lawler, E. E., III. (1986). *High involvement management.* San Francisco: Jossey-Bass.

Lawler, E. E., & Hall, D. T. (1970). Relationship of job characteristics to job involvement, satisfaction, and intrinsic motivation. *Journal of Applied psychology, 54,* 305–312.

Lee, R. T., & Ashforth, B. E. (1993). A longitudinal study of burnout among supervisors and managers: Comparisons between the Leiter and Maslach (1988) and Golembiewski et al. (1986) models. *Organizational Behavior and Human Decision Processes, 54,* 369–398. DOI: 10.1006/obhd.1993.1016.

Likert, R. (1967). *The human organization: Its management and value.* New York: McGraw-Hill.

Liu, C., Spector, P. E., & Jex, S. M. (2005). The relation of job control with job strains: A comparison of multiple data sources. *Journal of Occupational & Organizational Psychology, 78*, 325–336. DOI: 10.1348/096317905X26002.

Locke, E. A., & Schweiger, D. M. (1979). Participation in decision-making: One more look. *Research in Organizational Behavior, 1*, 265–339.

Locke, E. A., Schweiger, D. M., & Latham, G. P. (1986). Participation in decision making: When should it be used? *Organizational Dynamics, 14*, 65–79. DOI: 10.1016/0090-2616(86)90032-X.

Lowin, A. (1968). Participative decision making: A model, literature critique, and prescriptions for research. *Organizational Behavior and Human Performance, 3*, 68–106. DOI: 10.1016/0030-5073(68)90028-7.

Lyon, D. (2006). The search for surveillance theories. In D. Lyon (Ed.), *Theorizing surveillance: The panopticon and beyond* (pp. 1–20). Devon, UK: Willan Publishing.

Macey, W. H., & Schneider, B. (2008). The meaning of employee engagement. *Industrial and Organizational Psychology, 1*, 3–30.

Mayo, E. (1933). *The human problems of an industrial civilization*. London, UK: Routledge.

McNall, L. A., & Roch, S. G. (2007). Effects of electronic monitoring types on perceptions of procedural justice, interpersonal justice, and privacy. *Journal of Applied Social Psychology, 37*, 658–682. DOI: 10.1111/j.1559-1816.2007.00179.x.

Meier, R. B. (1984). The impact of the structural organization of public welfare offices on the psychosocial work and the treatment environments. *Journal of Social Service Research, 7*, 1–18.

Meyer, J. P., & Gagné, M. (2008). Employee engagement from a self-determination theory perspective. *Industrial and Organizational Psychology, 1*, 60–62.

Mikkelsen, A., & Gundersen, M. (2003). The effect of a participatory organizational intervention on work environment, job stress, and subjective health complaints. *International Journal of Stress Management, 10*, 91–110. DOI: 10.1037/1072-5245.10.2.91.

Miller, K. I., & Monge, P. R. (1986). Participation, satisfaction, and productivity: A meta-analytic review. *Academy of Management Journal, 29*, 727–753.

Millette, V., & Gagné, M. (2008). Designing volunteers' tasks to maximize motivation, satisfaction and performance: The impact of job characteristics on the outcomes of volunteer involvement. *Motivation and Emotion, 32*, 11–22.

Morgeson, F. P., & Campion, M. A. (2002). Minimizing tradeoffs when redesigning work: Evidence from a longitudinal quasi-experiment. *Personnel Psychology, 55*, 589–612.

Morgeson, F. P., Delaney-Klinger, K., & Hemingway, M. A. (2005). The importance of job autonomy, cognitive ability, and job-related skill for predicting role breadth and job performance. *Journal of Applied Psychology, 90*, 399–406. DOI: 10.1037/0021-9010.90.2.399.

Morgeson, F. P., & Humphrey, S. E. (2006). The work design questionnaire (WDQ): Developing and validating a comprehensive measure for assessing job design and the nature of work. *Journal of Applied Psychology, 91*, 1321–1339. DOI: 10.1037/0021-9010.91.6.1321.

Morrison, E. W. (2006). Doing the job well: An investigation of pro-social rule breaking. *Journal of Management, 32*, 5–28. DOI: 10.1177/0149206305277790.

Naaz, H. (1999). Job characteristics and demographic variables as predictor of job involvement of textile mill workers. *Journal of the Indian Academy of Applied Psychology, 25*, 75–78.

Naus, F., van Iterson, A., & Roe, R. A. (2007). Value incongruence, job autonomy, and organization-based self-esteem: A self-based perspective on organization cynicism. *European Journal of Work and Organizational Psychology, 16*, 195–219. DOI: 10.1080/13594320601143271.

Orpen, C. (1979). The effects of job enrichment on employee satisfaction, motivation, involvement, and performance: A field experiment. *Human Relations, 32*, 189–217. DOI: 10.1177/001872677903200301.

Parish, J. T., Cadwallader, S., & Busch, P. (2008). Want to, need to, ought to: Employee commitment to organizational change. *Journal of Organizational Change Management, 21,* 32. DOI: 10.1108/09534810810847020.

Parker Follet, M. (1926). The Psychological Foundations. In H.C. Metcalf (Ed.), *Scientific foundations of business administration.* Baltimore, MD: Williams & Williams Co.

Parker, S. K. (2003). Longitudinal effects of lean production on employee outcomes and the mediating role of work characteristics. *Journal of Applied Psychology, 88,* 620–634. DOI: 10.1037/0021-9010.88.4.620.

Parker, S. K., & Axtell, C. M. (2001). Seeing another viewpoint: Antecedents and outcomes of employee perspective taking. *Academy of Management Journal, 44,* 1085–1100.

Parker, S. K., Axtell, C. M., & Turner, N. (2001). Designing a safer workplace: Importance of job autonomy, communication quality, and supportive supervisors. *Journal of Occupational Health Psychology, 6,* 211–228. DOI: 10.1037/1076-8998.6.3.211.

Parker, S. K., Wall, T. D., & Jackson, P. R. (1997). "That's not my job": Developing flexible employee work orientations. *Academy of Management Journal, 40,* 899–929.

Parker, S. K., Williams, H. M., & Turner, N. (2006). Modeling the antecedents of proactive behavior at work. *Journal of Applied Psychology, 91,* 636–652. DOI: 10.1037/0021-9010.91.3.636.

Peiró, J. M., González-Romá, V., & Lloret, S. (1994). Role stress antecedents and consequences in nurses and physicians working in primary health care teams: A causal model. *European Review of Applied Psychology, 44,* 105–116.

Peters, L. H., & O'Connors, E. J. (1980). Situational constraints and work outcomes: The influences of a frequently overlooked construct. *Academy of Management Review, 5,* 391–397.

Phillips, J. S., & Freeman, S. M. (1984). Situational performance constraints and task characteristics: Their relationship to motivation and satisfaction. *Journal of Management, 10,* 321–331.

Prottas, D. (2008). Do the self-employed value autonomy more than employees? *Career Development International, 13,* 33–45. DOI: 10.1108/13620430810849524.

Prottas, D. J., & Thompson, C. A. (2006). Stress, satisfaction, and the work-family interface: A comparison of self-employed business owners, independents, and organizational employees. *Journal of Occupational Health Psychology, 11,* 366–378. DOI: 10.1037/1076-8998.11.4.366.

Raghuram, S., London, M., & Larsen, H. H. (2001). Flexible employment practices in Europe: Country versus culture. *International Journal of Human Resource Management, 5,* 738–753.

Raghuram, S., Wiesenfeld, B., & Garud, R. (2003). Technology enabled work: The role of self-efficacy in determining telecommuter adjustment and structuring behavior. *Journal of Vocational Behavior, 63,* 180–198. DOI: 10.1016/S0001-8791(03)00040-X.

Ramamoorthy, N., Flood, P. C., Slattery, T., & Sardessai, R. (2005). Determinants of innovative work behaviour: Development and test of an integrated model. *Creativity and Innovation Management, 14,* 142–150. DOI: 10.1111/j.1467-8691.2005.00334.x.

Rau, R. (2004). Lern-und gesundheitsforderliche arbeitsgestaltung: Eine empirische studie. [Job design promoting personal development and health: An empirical study]. *Zeitschrift fur Arbeits- und organisationspsychologie, 48,* 181–192. DOI: 10.1026/0932-4089.48.4.181.

Roca, J. C., & Gagné, M. (2008). Understanding e-learning continuance intention in the workplace: A self-determination theory perspective. *Computers in Human Behavior, 24,* 1596–1604.

Rousseau, D. M. (1977). Technological differences in job characteristics, employee satisfaction, and motivation: A synthesis of job design research and sociotechnical systems theory. *Organizational Behavior and Human Performance, 19,* 18–42. DOI: 10.1016/0030-5073(77)90052-6.

Ryan, R. M., & Frederick, C. M. (1997). On energy, personality and health: Subjective vitality as a dynamic reflection of well-being. *Journal of Personality, 65,* 529–565.

Sadler-Smith, E., El-Kot, G., & Leat, M. (2003). Differentiating work autonomy facets in a non-western context. *Journal of Organizational Behavior, 24,* 709–731. DOI: 10.1002/job.200.

Sagie, A. (1994). Participative decision making and performance: A moderator analysis. *Journal of Applied Behavioral Science, 30,* 227–246. DOI: 10.1177/0021886394302006.

Sagie, A., & Aycan, Z. (2003). A cross-cultural analysis of participative decision-making in organizations. *Human Relations, 56,* 453–473.

Sagie, A., Elizur, D., & Koslowsky, M. (1995). Decision type, participative decision making (PDM), and organizational behavior: An experimental simulation. *Human Performance, 8*, 81–94.

Sánchez, A. M., Pérez, M. P., de Luis Carnicer, P., & Jiménez, M. J. (2007). Teleworking and workplace flexibility: A study of impact on firm performance. *Personnel Review, 36*, 42–64. DOI: 10.1108/00483480710716713.

Sashkin, M. (1976). Changing toward participative management approaches: A model and methods. *Academy of Management Review, 1*, 75–86.

Sashkin, M. (1984). Participative management is an ethical imperative. *Organizational Dynamics, 12*, 5–22. DOI: 10.1016/0090-2616(84)90008-1.

Schaufeli, W. B., & Bakker, A. B. (2004). Job demands, job resources, and their relationship with burnout and engagement: A multi-sample study. *Journal of Organizational Behavior, 25*, 293–315. DOI: 10.1002/job.248.

Schaufeli, W. B., Martinez, I. M., Pinto, A. M., Salanova, M., & Bakker, A. B. (2002). Burnout and engagement in university students: A cross-national study. *Journal of Cross-Cultural Psychology, 33*, 464–481. DOI: 10.1177/0022022102033005003.

Schaufeli, W. B., Salanova, M., González-romá, V., & Bakker, A. B. (2002). The measurement of engagement and burnout: A two sample confirmatory factor analytic approach. *Journal of Happiness Studies, 3*, 71–92. DOI: 10.1023/A:1015630930326.

Schaufeli, W., Taris, T., & vanrhenen, W. (2008). Workaholism, burnout, and work engagement: Three of a kind or three different kinds of employee well-being? *Applied Psychology-An International Review, 57*, 173–203. DOI: 10.1111/j.1464-0597.2007.00285.x.

Scott-Ladd, B., Travaglione, A., & Marshall, V. (2006). Causal inferences between participation in decision making, task attributes, work effort, rewards, job satisfaction and commitment. *Leadership and Organization Management, 27*, 399–414.

Senécal, C., Vallerand, R. J., & Guay, F. (2001). Antecedents and outcomes of work-family conflict: Toward a motivational model. *Personality and Social Psychology Bulletin, 27*, 176–186.

Smith, M. J., Carayon, P., Sanders, K. J., Lim, S., & LeGrande, D. (1992). Employee stress and health complaints in jobs with and without electronic performance monitoring. *Applied Ergonomics, 23*, 17–27. DOI: 10.1016/0003-6870(92)90006-H.

Sonnentag, S. (2003). Recovery, work engagement, and proactive behavior: A new look at the interface between non-work and work. *Journal of Applied Psychology, 88*, 518–528.

Spector, P. E. (1986). Perceived control by employees: A meta-analysis of studies concerning autonomy and participation at work. *Human Relations, 39*, 1005–1016. DOI: 10.1177/001872678603901104.

Spitzmuller, C., & Stanton, J. M. (2006). Examining employee compliance with organizational surveillance and monitoring. *Journal of Occupational and Organizational Psychology, 79*, 245–272.

Spreitzer, G. M. (1995). An empirical test of a comprehensive model of intrapersonal empowerment in the workplace. *American Journal of Community Psychology, 23*, 601–629.

Spreitzer, G. M., Kizilos, M. A., & Nason, S. W. (1997). A dimensional analysis of the relationship between psychological empowerment and effectiveness satisfaction, and strain. *Journal of Management, 23*, 679–704. DOI: 10.1177/014920639702300504.

Sprigg, C. A., Stride, C. B., Wall, T. D., Holman, D. J., & Smith, P. R. (2007). Work characteristics, musculoskeletal disorders, and the mediating role of psychological strain: A study of call center employees. *Journal of Applied Psychology, 92*, 1456–1466. DOI: 10.1037/0021-9010.92.5.1456.

Stalker, C. A., Mandell, D., Frensch, K. M., Harvey, C., & Wright, M. (2007). Child welfare workers who are exhausted yet satisfied with their jobs: How do they do it? *Child & Family Social Work, 12*, 182–191. DOI: 10.1111/j.1365-2206.2006.00472.x.

Stanton, J. M., & Barnes-Farrell, J. L. (1996). Effects of electronic performance monitoring on personal control, task satisfaction, and task performance. *Journal of Applied Psychology, 81*, 738–745. DOI: 10.1037/0021-9010.81.6.738.

Stone, E. F., & Stone, D. L. (1990). Privacy in organizations: Theoretical issues, research findings, and protection mechanisms. In G. R. Ferris & K. M. Rowland (Eds.), *Research in personnel and human resource management* (Vol. 8, pp. 349–411). Greenwich, CT: JAI.

Strubler, D. C., & York, K. M. (2007). An exploratory study of the team characteristics model using organizational teams. *Small Group Research, 38*, 670–695. DOI: 10.1177/1046496407304338.

Tai, W., & Liu, S. (2007). An investigation of the influences of job autonomy and neuroticism on job stressor-strain relations. *Social Behavior & Personality: An International Journal, 35*, 1007–1019.

Taris, T. W., Stoffelsen, J. M., Bakker, A. B., Schaufeli, W. B., & van Dierendonck, D. (2002). Verschillen in burnoutrisico tussen functies en individuen: Wat is de rol van regelmogelijkheden?. [Differences in burnout risk between jobs and individuals: About the role of job autonomy]. *Gedrag & Gezondheid: Tijdschrift voor Psychologie en Gezondheid, 30*, 17–29.

Taylor, F. W. (1911). *The principles of scientific management*. New York: Harper Bros.

Thomas, K. W., & Velthouse, B. A. (1990). Cognitive elements of empowerment: An "Interpretive" model of intrinsic task motivation. *Academy of Management Review, 15*, 666–681.

Thompson, C. A., & Prottas, D. J. (2006). Relationships among organizational family support, job autonomy, perceived control, and employee well-being. *Journal of Occupational Health Psychology, 11*, 100–118. DOI: 10.1037/1076-8998.10.4.100.

Tzafrir, S. S. (2006). A universalistic perspective for explaining the relationship between HRM practices and firm performance at different points in time. *Journal of Managerial Psychology, 21*, 109–130.

Väänänen, A., Pahkin, K., Huuhtanen, P., Kivimäki, M., Vahtera, J., Theorell, T., et al. (2005). Are intrinsic motivational factors of work associated with functional incapacity similarly regardless of the country? *Journal of Epidemiology and Community Health, 59*, 858–863. DOI: 10.1136/jech.2004.030106.

Van den Broeck, A., Vansteenkiste, M., De Witte, H., & Lens, W. (2008). Explaining the relationships between job characteristics, burnout and engagement: The role of basic psychological need satisfaction. *Work & Stress, 22*, 277–294.

Van den Broeck, A., Vansteenkiste, M., De Witte, H., Soenens, B., & Lens, W. (in press). Capturing autonomy, competence, and relatedness at work: Construction and initial validation of the Work-Related Basic Need Satisfaction Scale. *Journal of Occupational and Organizational Psychology*.

van Mierlo, H., Rutte, C., Seinen, B., & Kompier, D. (2000). Autonomous team work, individual task characteristics and psychological well-being: A pilot study. *Gedrag en Gezondheid, 28*, 159–171.

van Yperen, N. W. V., & Hagedoorn, M. (2003). Do high job demands increase intrinsic motivation or fatigue or both? The role of job control and job social support. *Academy of Management Journal, 46*, 339–348.

Vandenberg, R. J., Richardson, H. A., & Eastman, L. J. (1999). The impact of high involvement work processes on organizational effectiveness: A second-order latent variable approach. *Group Organization Management, 24*, 300–339. DOI: 10.1177/1059601199243004.

Vardi, Y., Shirom, A., & Jacobson, D. (1980). A study on the leadership beliefs of Israeli managers. *Academy of Management Journal, 23*, 367–374.

Vlerick, P., & Goeminne, D. (1994). Onderzoek naar de gevolgen van verpleegkundige functieontwerpen op de arbeidsbeleving. [Research on the impact of job design on nursing work experience]. *Gedrag & Organisatie, 7*, 101–113.

Wall, T. D., Corbett, J. M., Clegg, C. W., Jackson, P. R., & Martin, R. (1990). Advanced manufacturing technology and work design: Towards a theoretical framework. *Journal of Organizational Behavior, 11*, 201–219.

Wall, T. D., Corbett, J. M., Martin, R., Clegg, C. W., & Jackson, P. R. (1990). Advanced manufacturing technology, work design, and performance: A change study. *Journal of Applied Psychology, 75*, 691–697.

Wall, T. D., Kemp, N. J., Jackson, P. R., & Clegg, C. W. (1986). Outcomes of autonomous workgroups: A long-term field experiment. *Academy of Management Journal, 29,* 280–304.

Ward, E. A. (1997). Autonomous work groups: A field study of correlates of satisfaction. *Psychological Reports, 80,* 60–62.

Wells, D. L., Moorman, R. H., & Werner, J. M. (2007). The impact of the perceived purpose of electronic performance monitoring on an array of attitudinal variables. *Human Resource Development Quarterly, 18,* 121–138. DOI: 10.1002/hrdq.1194.

Xie, J. L., & Johns, G. (1995). Job scope and stress: Can job scope be too high? *Academy of Management Journal, 38,* 1288–1309.

Part III
Human Autonomy in Modern Economy, Democracy Development, and Sustainability

Chapter 9
Capitalism and Autonomy

Tim Kasser

Since its inception, self-determination theory has insisted that the dynamics of personal autonomy play out in a relational context because the extent to which people can experience interest, enjoyment, and freedom depend mightily on how well other people in their social surround support their efforts to be autonomous, self-determined individuals. People's feelings of autonomy can be undermined in a multitude of ways by a variety of social actors: Experimenters giving rewards for playing games, teachers providing gold stars and instructing on the basis of standardized tests, employers and managers making mandates to their workers, doctors ignoring their patients' perspectives, coaches focusing on wins at all costs, and parents stifling their young child's emerging imagination and vitality. These are among the many ways that the empirical literature on self-determination theory has documented that authority figures often fail to support people's autonomy, at the costs of long-term motivation, optimal performance, and personal well-being (see Deci & Ryan, 2002).

As can be gathered from this list of controlling social environments, the vast majority of this research literature has focused on rather proximal interpersonal interactions: The parent and the child; the teacher and the student; the boss and the worker, etc. While such a research focus is not atypical of most psychological approaches, and while such interpersonal interactions are certainly crucial determinants of people's experience of autonomy, it is important to note that such interactions make up only a part of the social world which people inhabit. That is, humans are not only relational creatures, but are also *cultural* creatures, existing in broader social entities composed of political, religious, and economic systems. As such, aspects of one's culture can also affect people's experience of autonomy, and thus their motivation, performance, and well-being. For example, living under a totalitarian dictatorship likely provides fewer opportunities for self-determination than does living in a democracy, and being surrounded by religious fundamentalist ideology that insists upon conformity to certain tenets and practices will similarly

---

T. Kasser (✉)
Department of Psychology, Knox College, Galesburg, IL 61401, USA
e-mail: tkasser@knox.edu

prove less autonomy-supportive than living among religious ideologies more open to spiritual inquiry and variations in beliefs.

Just as cultures vary with regard to religious and political features, they also vary economically, i.e., in how the material bases of life are produced, distributed, and consumed. Indeed, a variety of forms of economic organization have existed throughout humanity's pre- and written history. Early humans seem to have lived primarily in egalitarian bands that gathered, hunted, and shared most of their possessions with other tribe members. A later economic system, feudalism, concentrated most wealth in the hands of a relatively few landowners. The highly bureaucratic, state-run economies of the late twentieth century Soviet Bloc placed most decision making about economic issues in the hands of the government and claimed to distribute goods more or less equally across the people (though often times at rather low levels).

In the twenty-first century, the vast majority of nations on Earth practice the economic system of *capitalism*. This form of economic organization prioritizes private ownership of property (as opposed to collective ownership) and attempts to maximize people's opportunity to use this property (i.e., capital) in the service of purchasing what they desire (i.e., consuming) or of investing that capital (e.g., in the stock market) in the hopes of attaining more capital (i.e., a profit). The particular variety of capitalism that has taken strong hold in Anglo-cultures derives in large part from the thinking of the eighteenth century moral philosopher Adam Smith (1776/1976). Smith's formulation of capitalism places front and center two concepts particularly relevant to freedom and autonomy. The first concept is *self-interest*, which concerns people's desires to do what they want to do. The second concept is the *free market*, which is the economic locale in which people pursue their self-interest. Smith's remarkably influential proposal was that the ideal economic system maximizes individuals' opportunities to pursue their own self-interest in a free market largely unregulated by the government but instead guided by the "invisible" hand of competition between and among individuals. Smith proposed that such systems yield the most desirable psychological and material results. Psychologically, people living under this form of capitalism should feel relatively free, for they can work to get what they want, be it profit, widgets, or leisure, unencumbered by the dictates of government. Materially, this system should produce the best products at the lowest prices via the competition between and amongst entrepreneurs, laborers, and consumers.

In terms of its material promises, capitalism can undoubtedly be said to have been quite successful in generating remarkable wealth and in creating a vast panoply of products and services; that said, a couple of billion people still languish in poverty and squalor under capitalist economic systems, and the economic system's mandate for high levels of consumption threatens the ecological health of our only home planet (Jackson, 2009; Speth, 2008). But the purpose of this essay is to focus not on capitalism's material promises, but on its psychological claim that freedom is maximized when people are encouraged to pursue their own self-interest and when social actors compete with each other with minimal governmental restraint. Such ideology has become enormously influential in the US and other Anglo-cultures since

Smith's time, having captured the thought of many (if not most) Anglo-economists and politicians. Like many other widely accepted cultural ideas, it can happen that those living within the culture remain rather unaware of quite how much the notion has become the water through which they swim. For this reason, let me briefly describe how two of the most well-known advocates of capitalism suggest that it promotes the optimal experience of autonomy.

First we can consider the Nobel-winning economist Milton Friedman (an interesting surname in the context of this chapter), known of course for important economic papers but also for his book *Capitalism and Freedom* (Friedman, 1962/2002) and his 1980 10-part television special *Free to Choose*. These works, created to reach large popular audiences, insisted that maximum personal and political freedom could be attained only through laissez-faire capitalism (i.e., the minimum intervention of the government in the free market)—the polar opposite of the state-run, hegemonic bureaucracies that ruled the Soviet Union and China at the time these works were released. Consider, for example, the following three quotes from Friedman:

> History suggests that capitalism is a necessary condition for political freedom.
>
> I think that nothing is so important for freedom as recognizing in the law each individual's natural right to property, and giving individuals a sense that they own something that they're responsible for, that they have control over, and that they can dispose of.
>
> Underlying most arguments against the free market is a lack of belief in freedom itself.

Second, we have Ayn Rand, who wrote both philosophical works (on Objectivism) and extremely popular novels (i.e., *The Fountainhead* and *Atlas Shrugged* (Rand, 1943, 1957)) expounding the usefulness of free-market capitalism for providing people with freedom. Consider for example Rand's reply to a request to summarize her philosophy while standing on one foot:

> The ideal political-economic system is *laissez-faire* capitalism. It is a system where men deal with one another, not as victims and executioners, nor as masters and slaves, but as *traders*, by free, voluntary exchange to mutual benefit (emphasis in original). Copyright © 1962 by Times-Mirror Co.

Or consider this description of a 2008 lecture by Yaron Brook, current president of the Ayn Rand Institute:

> Two centuries ago the Founding Fathers established a nation based on the individual's rights to life, liberty, property—and the selfish pursuit of his own happiness. But neither the Founders nor their successors could properly defend self-interest and the profit motive in the face of moral denunciation. The result has been a slow destruction of freedom in America, leading us to today's economic mess.

For both of these thinkers, as well as for many others, freedom is understood as best occurring via the pursuit of self-interest in a free market. Given the enormous influence this neo-liberal capitalist ideology has had on economic and governmental policy both nationally (e.g., Ronald Reagan, Margaret Thatcher) and internationally (e.g., NAFTA, WTO, the World Bank), it seems crucial for psychologists interested in autonomy, motivation, and well-being to consider the merit of these claims. Said differently, in addition to examining the characteristics that lead children and students and athletes to feel autonomous (or not) in their interactions with parents and teachers and coaches, psychology can also begin to examine how well certain forms of economic organizations support people's autonomy. The kinds of claims that have been summarized above clearly suggest that the experience of freedom is maximized under the form of capitalism proposed by Smith, supported by Friedman and Rand, and practiced by millions of economists, entrepreneurs, politicians, and ordinary citizens. Is that actually the case?

Value Conflicts

Kasser, Cohn, Kanner, and Ryan (2007) recently set out to examine some of the psychological dynamics that occur when people live under the highly competitive, laissez-faire form of capitalism dominant in the United States. Their argument was premised on the assumption that capitalism is like any other social system in that it can only function smoothly if the people living under it care about and prioritize the aims in life that are consistent with its ideology and institutions. That is, just as a religious systems needs people to value spirituality so that they are more likely to come to places of worship, to practice the tenets of the religion, and to behave in ways consistent with the religion's rules, economic systems such as capitalism also depend on citizens caring about a particular set of values that will help to guide their attitudes and behaviors. Different economic systems will of course require different values to be prioritized by their citizens. Given the description of laissez-faire capitalism provided above, it is hopefully clear that this form of capitalism depends on people believing that it is important to pursue their own self-interest, that economic activity should be ruled by the free market rather than by the government, that the accumulation of capital and other forms of private property is a crucial aim in life, and that competition between people is necessary and good. Beyond these basic features are several other practices key to Anglo-capitalism that also depend on people's assent and values. These include the ideas that corporations should attempt to maximize their profit in the service of shareholder interest; that economic growth is a key goal of a nation; that globalization is beneficial because it creates new markets for products to be bought and sold; and that advertising is an important tool for informing consumers about goods and services which they may desire to purchase in the pursuit of their own self-interest (see Kasser et al., 2007, for a more in-depth description of these features of Anglo-capitalism).

As can be seen, Anglo-capitalism rests on a certain set of values that its citizens must care about if it is to maintain itself. Kasser et al. (2007) argued that this set of values is easily recognizable in psychological cross-cultural research on people's values and goals. Specifically, the primary values required by Anglo-capitalism are quite consistent with certain values identified in the seminal research of Shalom Schwartz (1992), conducted in dozens of nations around the world. Schwartz's work has demonstrated that one of the personal values that consistently emerges across cultures is the *self-enhancing* value of Power (which involves "dominance over people and resources"), and that one of the basic cultural value orientations is Hierarchy (an orientation that "relies on differential, hierarchical allocation of roles and resources to groups and individuals as the legitimate, desirable way to regulate interdependencies" (Schwartz, 2007, p. 54)). Both types of values emphasize aims such as wealth, social power, and competition. Research from the self-determination theory tradition similarly identifies a set of *extrinsic* aspirations (Grouzet et al., 2005; Kasser & Ryan, 1996) consistent with these primary aims of Anglo-capitalism. These aims in life are focused on the attainment of rewards and praise, and include specific concerns for financial success, popularity/status, and image.

These cross-cultural studies also make it clear that no particular value is an island to itself within a person's psyche. Instead, values are organized psychologically into *systems*, such that some values are psychologically consistent with each other whereas others tend to stand in psychological conflict (Grouzet et al., 2005; Schwartz, 1992). For example, it is relatively easy to simultaneously care about one's image and one's status, for both of these aims require attitudes and behaviors that are similar to each other; liking and purchasing a Prada bag or a BMW work both to enhance one's image and one's status in contemporary American consumer culture. In contrast, it is typically difficult to simultaneously pursue the aims of spirituality and hedonism, for they propose quite different attitudes toward a variety of social objects and quite different ways to spend one's time; pursuing a life of spiritual meaning tends not to be consistent with participation in alcohol-infused orgies.

The extent of consistency or conflict between values has been statistically represented through the creation of circumplex models such as those shown in Figs. 9.1 and 9.2. In each of these models, which have together been validated on thousands of people in dozens of nations, values that people experience as psychologically compatible are adjacent to each other on the circle, whereas values that are in psychological conflict are on opposite sides of the circle. Kasser et al. (2007) noted that examination of these circumplex models suggests that the values and goals most relevant to the aims of Anglo-capitalism lay across from the aims most supportive of autonomy. Specifically, in Schwartz's individual values circumplex (Fig. 9.1), the value of Power stands in opposition to the value of *Self-direction*, which includes specific aims such as "creativity," "freedom," and "choosing own goals." Similar results occur in Schwartz's cultural values model (not pictured here), where Hierarchy stands in relative opposition to *Intellectual Autonomy*, which is a cultural orientation that "encourages individuals to pursue their own ideas and intellectual directions independently" (Schwartz, 2007, p. 54). And in the Grouzet et al. (2005) model (Fig. 9.2), the extrinsic goals stand in relative opposition to *self-acceptance* goals, which include aims such as "I will choose what I do, instead of being pushed along by life" and "I will feel free."

Kasser et al. (2007) thus suggested that to the extent a culture encourages the self-enhancing, hierarchical, extrinsic values required for the smooth functioning of neo-liberal, highly competitive, laissez faire capitalist economic systems, it will be relatively difficult for citizens to place a strong priority on values that promote

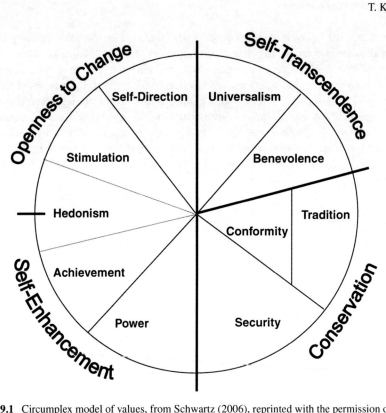

Fig. 9.1 Circumplex model of values, from Schwartz (2006), reprinted with the permission of the publisher

freedom and autonomy. The reason for this is that there tends to be an inherent conflict between the two sets of aims, as attested to by the circumplex models presented in Figs. 9.1 and 9.2. In a commentary on the Kasser et al. (2007) piece, Schwartz (2007) set out to test this hypothesis by correlating archival nation-level value data with an economic index developed by Hall and Gingerich (2004) that assessed the extent to which each of 20 wealthy capitalistic nations pursued a more laissez-faire, "competitive" approach vs. a more governmental-involved "strategic" approach in its particular variety of capitalism. (Notably, in support of the contention that Anglo-forms of capitalism are particularly laissez-faire, the six Anglo nations in the sample (USA, UK, Canada, New Zealand, Ireland, & Australia) scored as the most competitively oriented of the 20 nations on Hall & Gingerich's index). Schwartz then correlated each nation's score on this index with the extent to which citizens in these nations rated a variety of cultural and individual values as important. Regarding the results most relevant to the argument being developed here, the correlations revealed that citizens living in nations more oriented toward the competitive form of capitalism rated Hierarchy and Power values as relatively *more* important; thus, it appears that such forms of capitalism do indeed encourage people to prioritize such self-enhancing, extrinsic values at relatively high levels. What's

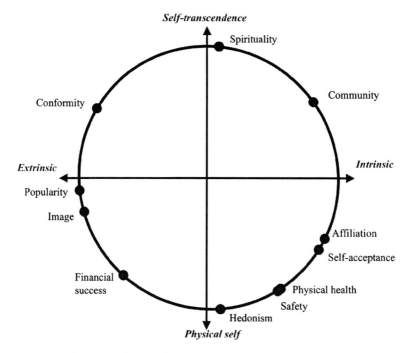

Fig. 9.2 Circumplex model of values, from Grouzet et al. (2005), reprinted with the permission of the publisher

more, findings also revealed that people living under more competitive, laissez-faire economic systems rated Intellectual Autonomy and Self-direction values as relatively *less* important than did citizens living in nations with a more cooperative, strategic form of capitalism. Thus, these Anglo-economic systems appear to interfere with people's autonomy and freedom values, supporting Kasser et al.'s hypothesis.

For the purposes of this chapter, I attempted to conceptually replicate Schwartz's (2007) findings with a different measure of national economic organization. Specifically, I used the *Index of Economic Freedom*, developed by the Wall Street Journal and the Washington, DC think-tank, The Heritage Foundation. According to its authors, this index "has brought Smith's theories about liberty, prosperity and economic freedom to life." Economic freedom is defined by the authors of this index as:

> the fundamental right of every human to control his or her own labor and property. In an economically free society, individuals are free to work, produce, consume, and invest in any way they please, with that freedom both protected by the state and unconstrained by the state. In economically free societies, governments allow labor, capital and goods to move freely, and refrain from coercion or constraint of liberty beyond the extent necessary to protect and maintain liberty itself. (http://www.heritage.org/index/FAQ.aspx)

In the current context, I used the 1998 index, a year that falls approximately midway between the years during which Schwartz's (2007) value data were collected.

The 1998 version of the Index of Economic Freedom gives each of dozens of nations a score ranging from 0 to 100 on nine different measures of economic freedom: Business Freedom, Trade Freedom, Fiscal Freedom, Government Size, Monetary Freedom, Investment Freedom, Financial Freedom, Property Rights, and Freedom from Corruption. All of these nine scores are composed of numerous sub-indicators, but they are ultimately averaged together to form a single Index of Economic Freedom, with high scores indicate greater economic freedom, i.e. a more free-market, neo-liberal, laissez-faire variety of capitalism. (As with the Hall & Gingerich, 2004 measure used by Schwartz, 2007, Anglo-nations appear to be among the most "economically free" of the 20 nations studied here, as five of the Anglo-nations score among the six most economically free nations (the anomalies being Switzerland coming in second and Canada missing the top six, being instead in ninth position)).

I next computed correlations between the Index of Economic Freedom and the four value variables derived from Schwartz's (1992, 2007) work, controlling for 1998 national GDP. As expected, national economic freedom was positively correlated with how much citizens valued Power ($pr = 0.45, p = 0.05$) and Hierarchy ($pr = 0.59, p < 0.01$). In contrast, as national economic freedom increased, there were significant declines in the extent to which citizens valued Intellectual Autonomy ($pr = -0.48, p < 0.05$) and Self-direction ($pr = -0.47, p < 0.05$). (Degrees of freedom for all analyses were 17).

Combined with Schwartz's (2007) findings, these results provide strong support for Kasser et al.'s (2007) analysis of value conflicts under Anglo-forms of capitalism, but are rather difficult to reconcile with the claims of Smith, Friedman, Rand, and the many others who propose that neo-liberal, laissez-faire, Anglo forms of capitalism produce maximum individual freedom. For if freedom is something everyone wants (a point upon which Rand, Friedman, and self-determination theory would of course agree), why would citizens who live in wealthy nations that have the economic system that supposedly maximizes freedom place relatively *high* value on aims that emphasize the acceptance of status hierarchies and of social control, but place relatively *low* emphasis on the expression of their own ideas, freedom, and choice?

The answer, I think, lies in dynamics long described by self-determination theory and reflected in the circumplex models of values and goals described above. Self-interest under the laissez-faire, neo-liberal form of capitalism typical of Anglo-nations has come to mean wealth and status and praise for one's image, and the free market has come to mean a system that prizes competition and economic growth and profit and consumption. The result is an emphasis on self-enhancing, extrinsic values and goals. And because such extrinsic motivations have the long-documented power to undermine intrinsic motivations (Deci, Koestner, & Ryan, 1999) and because it is difficult to think about and pursue self-enhancing, extrinsic goals like financial success and power while also thinking about and pursuing goals like self-direction and self-acceptance (Figs. 9.1 and 9.2), autonomy becomes "crowded out," to use Bruno Frey's (Frey & Jegen, 2001) wonderfully descriptive phrase.

Controlled, Non-autonomous Regulation of ACC's Ideology

It is also worth mentioning a second set of findings based in self-determination theory that supports the idea that the values dominant in Anglo-capitalism's laissez-faire ideology stand in opposition to the experience of autonomy. Specifically, empirical research suggests that people have some difficulty freely choosing to believe some of the key tenets of capitalistic ideology. Put into SDT parlance, some of the beliefs central to Anglo-capitalism appear to be often regulated for controlled, non-autonomous reasons (such as guilt, anxiety, or external coercion and the promise of rewards) rather than for autonomous reasons (such as interest or personal value).

For example, research typically finds that the importance people place on extrinsic, materialistic goals is positively correlated with controlled regulations and negatively correlated with autonomous regulations for pursuing one's goals (Carver & Baird, 1998; Sheldon & Kasser, 1995, 1998, 2001; Sheldon, Ryan, Deci, & Kasser, 2004; Srivastava, Locke, & Bortol, 2001). Similarly, it appears difficult for people to autonomously internalize beliefs about the benefits of competition. For example, Chirkov, Ryan, Kim, and Kaplan (2003) found that US, South Korean, Russian, and Turkish subjects reported more controlled and less autonomous reasons for "vertical individualistic" beliefs such as thinking it is important to strive "to work in situations involving competition with others," for wanting to express the idea that "competition is the law of nature" and for believing that "without competition, it is impossible to have a good society." Even beliefs about self-interest can be difficult to internalize, as Miller (1999) and his colleagues have shown. When people act under "the norm of self-interest," placing their own concerns ahead of others, they also often report feeling a sense of pressure to conform in situations where they may otherwise want to act in a non-self-interested manner. This pressure typically involves a worry about being censured or thought "strange" by others for acting altruistically; such descriptions clearly reflect what SDT would consider a controlled, non-autonomous type of regulation.

This body of findings suggests that beliefs in materialism, competition, and self-interest (all core components of the ideology of laissez-faire, Anglo-capitalism) tend to be associated with feelings of pressure and coercion rather than experienced as freely chosen. Once again, then, such results suggest that people find it difficult to reconcile autonomy with a strong endorsement of the values and beliefs that are key to laissez-faire, Anglo-capitalism.

Behaviors and Institutions

In the preceding sections I have tried to establish that the experience of autonomy can be undermined by the highly competitive, laissez-faire form of capitalism especially common in Anglo-cultures. Thus far, my arguments have primarily focused on the ideological aspects of Anglo-capitalism. That is, I have primarily been suggesting that the ideas, values, and beliefs necessary for the smooth functioning of Anglo-capitalism are (a) typically experienced as conflicting with values that prioritize freedom; and (b) difficult to autonomously internalize.

Cultural systems, however, are more than ideology: They also include the behaviors that people emit and the institutions that they create. For example, a religion requires not just a set of ideas about gods and the after life, but also a set of behaviors (e.g., praying/meditating, reading holy books) and institutions (churches, training institutions for religious leaders) in order to support the system. Or to take a political example, consider a typical dictatorship in which a cult of personality is built around the leader, with the support of citizen behaviors (e.g., writing songs uplifting the leader) and institutions (e.g., laws restricting criticism of the leader). Such behaviors and institutions should not be seen as separate from the cultural system's ideology, but instead as concrete manifestations of the ideology that help to reinforce the cultural system. Essentially, as more and more people in a culture take on the ideology of a particular social system, the relevant values and beliefs of the ideology come to increasingly inform the ways that people work and consume and interact and raise their children, as well as the types of institutions, laws, and policies that people create and support or dismantle and oppose. Through such processes, we can see both how culture influences people's values and how people's values help to create the culture.

In the case of laissez-faire, neo-liberal capitalism, what this means is that once people begin to prioritize the self-enhancing, extrinsic values required for the maintenance of the economic system, they become more likely to act in ways that bolster the system and they become more likely to support the creation of the kinds of social institutions (e.g., laws, governmental organizations) that perpetuate the system. As we shall see next, it appears that the behaviors and institutions associated with Anglo-capitalism can also interfere with people's experience of autonomy.

Personal Behaviors

Many specific behaviors are encouraged by the self-enhancing, materialistic values of Anglo-capitalism, but three in particular are especially noteworthy with regard to autonomy. These are working, watching television, and shopping.

Individuals living under Anglo-capitalism enter the labor market in an attempt to earn wages from employers. The logic of Anglo-capitalism suggests that it is in the self-interest of both workers and employers for workers to work relatively long hours: Doing so maximizes income that can be spent by the worker (purchasing cell phones and corn chowder or paying the plumber and the massage therapist) and profit for both the employer and for other businesses that sell the products and services to the workers. Research suggests, however, that the long work hours typical of this form of capitalism (Schor, 1993) tend not to promote autonomy. For example, people who work long hours and feel more "time poverty" report feeling that their psychological needs (including for autonomy) are less well-satisfied, with consequent reductions in their well-being (Kasser & Sheldon, 2009). What's more, people tend to report lower well-being on weekdays than weekends, largely because they experience lower levels of autonomy at work in comparison to during their leisure time (Ryan, Bernstein, & Brown, 2010). Thus, in working the long hours required for accumulating the wages so necessary to the smooth functioning of Anglo-capitalism, people seem to give up some experience of autonomy.

When they aren't working, people in consumer capitalist cultures spend many of their hours in the conjoined activities of watching television and shopping. While people may engage in these behaviors to de-stress after long work hours, both behaviors ultimately support the economic system: Watching television exposes people to the advertising messages that entice them to spend their wages on products and services (increasingly without even having to leave their homes). Neither watching television nor shopping seem to promote strong satisfaction of autonomy needs, however. For example, Delle Fave and Bassi (2000) asked subjects to report the experiences that provide feelings of "flow," a psychological state characterized by intrinsic motivation, challenge, and feelings of enjoyment. Very rarely were either shopping or watching television mentioned (Delle Fave, 2000, Personal communication). Further, Kubey and Csikszentmihalyi's (1990) experience-sampling studies document that when people are watching television, they typically report feeling zoned out or apathetic, rather than in the highly challenged and engaged states typical of the experience of autonomy.

Research also suggests that the more that people prioritize the self-enhancing, materialistic values of Anglo-capitalism, the more likely they are to behave in ways that undermine the autonomy of the people with whom they interact. For example, stronger materialistic values are associated with being less empathic, nurturant, and unconditionally accepting (Kasser, Ryan, Zax, & Sameroff, 1995; Sheldon & Kasser, 1995), with acting in more competitive and less cooperative ways during resource-dilemma games (Sheldon, Sheldon, & Osbaldiston, 2000), and with having more Machiavellian, manipulative, and socially dominant attitudes toward interpersonal interactions (Duriez, Vansteenkiste, Soenens, & De Witte, 2007; McHoskey, 1999). Further, some research demonstrates that materialistic values are associated with more authoritarian and racist attitudes (Duriez et al., 2007), and with engaging in more antisocial activities that violate the rights of others (Cohen & Cohen, 1996; Kasser & Ryan, 1993; McHoskey, 1999). Thus, it seems that self-enhancing, materialistic values seep into people's social behaviors, coloring them in ways that likely undermine *other* people's experience of autonomy.

Institutional Dynamics

While people's behaviors can be seen as individualized representations of the ideology of a particular social system, institutions such as laws, customs, policies and governmental, educational, and business organizations can be seen as the manifestation of the ideologies in the social structures that compose a culture. For example, in the case of Anglo-capitalism, laws have been passed that protect private property, that give corporations the same rights as individual people, and that make money spent on advertising a tax deduction; these influence the rules under which people live their lives. Organizations also exist to help keep the wheels of Anglo-capitalism well oiled; these range from local Chambers of Commerce to national organizations such as the Treasury Department to pan-national organizations such as the World Trade Organization and the International Monetary Fund; again, these organizations set policies, influence laws, and have powers that influence people's actual experience, including their experience of autonomy, as we shall see next.

For-pay work is one arena of life in which Anglo-capitalism has created a certain set of laws, customs, and organizations that can influence people's felt autonomy. For example, while part of the reason that some people work long hours is no doubt to make the money so valued under the economic system (see above), a variety of laws also increase the likelihood that people must work relatively long hours. For instance, the United States, one of the most laissez-faire of the Anglo-capitalist nations, has no laws that mandate paid vacations or paid parental leave (whereas most nations offer at least some of each) and relatively little recourse for workers if their employer demands that they work over-time (see de Graaf, 2003). Such laws (or lack of laws) not only limit people's options with regards to work, but place them in situations that force them to work more hours, often to the detriment of their autonomy (as shown above).

Other aspects of work life under Anglo-capitalism can also interfere with people's experience of autonomy in the workplace. For example, under the dominant approach to organizing people's experience in the workplace, known as Taylorism (Taylor, 1914), "expert" bosses and consultants, rather than the employees themselves, hold the ultimate power for deciding the specific activities of workers (e.g., physical motions on factory lines, scripts of telemarketers, protocols of lawyers and paralegals). The goal, of course, is to shape workers' behaviors in ways that maximize profit for the business, even if that interferes with workers' sense of having an influence on the way their job is constructed. Another example of how little input most workers have in their workplaces is that the boards that run most large corporations very rarely include representation from non-administrative employees (see Kelly, 2001); as such, most workers are disenfranchised from the decision-making processes that influence their work lives. Such institutional factors might help explain why Deci et al. (2001) found that, compared to Bulgarian workers, American workers reported less autonomy on the job, feeling that they have little say in the workplace or input to supervisors.

Another type of institutional feature of Anglo-capitalism that can interfere with people's experience of autonomy includes the pan-national treaties and organizations that govern global capitalism. A classic example is the North American Free Trade Agreement (NAFTA), which opened up "free trade" (note the ideology) across the US, Canada, and Mexico. One result of this treaty has been the flooding of inexpensive US corn (grown by huge, agricultural corporations) into Mexico, depressing the price of Mexican corn so greatly that thousands of farmers have had little choice but to leave the rural areas where their families have often lived for generations and to seek wages in the slums outside of large cities; it seems a stretch to believe that all the affected farmers undertook this decision to abandon their homesteads out of true choice. Or consider the power of the World Trade Organization

(WTO), which can insist that laws passed by democratically elected legislatures of participating nations be overturned if those laws are perceived as "barriers to free trade," i.e. if they interfere with the profit-making ability of a corporation (Danaher & Burbach, 2000). Similarly, the International Monetary Fund and the World Bank have the power to insist that nations applying for loans or attempting to enter into trade agreements change the ways that they regulate industries, protect the environment, and spend portions of their revenue on public services (Cavanagh, Welch, & Retallack, 2001) if those practices are seen as interfering with opportunities to enhance the nation's economic growth or corporations' profit-making ability. What hopefully stands out to the reader from these examples is how the institutional practices of capitalism, focused as they are on self-enhancing, extrinsic values, can interfere with the ability of people to govern themselves, which of course is a key expression of autonomy.

A final way that autonomy is limited by the institutions of Anglo-capitalism concerns the fact that while a remarkable number of certain types of freedoms and options do exist under the system, the system also limits particular options, especially those that are less consistent with the logic of capitalism. Kasser et al. (2007) referred to this as the distinction between *micro*-options and *macro*-options. For example, while people in the US can choose from a bewildering array of types of used or new cars with seemingly limitless variations in features (multiple micro-options), most Americans do not have a choice between private ownership of a vehicle and using a sound, reliable, safe public transportation system (limited macro-option). Or while Americans have thousands of choices of advertisements that they can examine as they go about their day (multiple micro-options), they do not have the option of avoiding advertisements (limited macro-option). Or while there are hundreds of television channels one might watch (multiple micro-options), the vast majority are owned by a handful of for-profit corporations (McChesney, 1997), with non-commercial television quickly fading into oblivion (limited macro-option). Like any social system, Anglo-capitalism delimits the types of choices that are available to people, supporting those options that are most consistent with the system and restricting those that are either unsupportive of the system or opposed to it.

Perhaps the most insidious reflection of how macro-options can be limited under Anglo-capitalism is the widely-cited acronym introduced by Margaret Thatcher, prime minister of the UK during the 1980s: TINA, or *There Is No* Alternative (http://en.wikipedia.org/wiki/TINA). No alternative to Anglo-capitalism, that is. Clearly, when people are told that they have no choice but to live under a particular economic system, and that no other options are feasible than the one that those in authority endorse, feelings of autonomy are likely to be undermined.

Conclusion

This chapter has argued that just as people's experience of autonomy can be affected by their interactions with social actors in their homes, schools, and workplaces, it can also be affected by the broader cultural environment in which they exist. While this observation could potentially be explored for a variety of aspects of broader cultural environments, including their political or religious arrangements, in this chapter I examined how people's experience of autonomy is affected by a particular form of economic organization, namely the kind of highly competitive, laissez-faire capitalism found in Anglo-cultures. In contrast to the strong claims by some proponents that such economic organizations are the best ways to promote autonomy and freedom, I presented a variety of types of evidence suggesting that some features of Anglo-capitalism stand in the way of people's experience of autonomy and self-determination; such evidence has clear implications for their optimal motivation, performance, and well-being.

Such an analysis suggests that SDT can be useful in understanding and critiquing various forms of economic organizations in particular, and of cultural systems in general. That is, just as SDT has demonstrated can occur in the workplace, on the sports field, and in the classroom, it appears that autonomy can be undermined by Anglo-capitalism's focus on the self-enhancing, extrinsic values embodied in the priority this economic system places on profit, consumption, and economic growth.

And while it has not been the focus of this chapter, it seems to me that this lens can also be used to inform the development of other types of economic systems that might better support people's need for autonomy, and thus their well-being. Some hints about the directions these alternative systems might take are, I think, provided by the analyses reported above suggesting that autonomy may be more strongly valued in more co-operatively oriented economic systems that do not turn most problems over to the free-market's competitive, profit-making machine. Other ways to help people and society shift from self-enhancing, extrinsic values include encouraging lifestyles such as voluntary simplicity, more closely regulating advertising messages (especially to children), and developing policies that promote time affluence and other, less materialistic means of assessing national progress (Kasser, 2005, 2006, 2009).

Clearly, far more theoretical and empirical work is necessary to bring such ideas to fruition, and many roadblocks stand in the way. But my hope nonetheless is that the current chapter might spur others to begin to more deeply consider the various ways that insights from SDT can be applied to economics so as to promote higher levels of autonomy and well-being for citizens.

References

Carver, C. S., & Baird, E. (1998). The American dream revisited: Is it what you want or why you want it that matters? *Psychological Science, 9*, 289–292.

Cavanagh, J., Welch, C., & Retallack, S. (2001). The IMF formula: Prescription for poverty. *International Forum on Globalization (IFG): Special Poverty Report, 1*(3), 8–10.

Chirkov, V., Ryan, R. M., Kim, Y., & Kaplan, U. (2003). Differentiating autonomy from individualism and independence: A self-determination theory perspective on internalization of cultural orientations and well-being. *Journal of Personality and Social Psychology, 84*, 97–109.

Cohen, P., & Cohen, J. (1996). *Life values and adolescent mental health*. Mahwah, NJ: Lawrence Erlbaum.

Danaher, K., & Burbach, R. (Eds.). (2000). *Globalize this! The battle against the world trade organization and corporate rule*. Monroe, ME: Common Courage Press.

Deci, E. L., Koestner, R., & Ryan, R. M. (1999). A meta-analytic review of experiments examining the effects of extrinsic rewards on intrinsic motivation. *Psychological Bulletin, 125*, 627–668.

Deci, E. L., & Ryan, R. M. (Eds.) (2002). *Handbook of self-determination research*. Rochester, NY: University of Rochester Press.

Deci, E. L., Ryan, R. M., Gagné, M., Leone, D. R., Usunov, J., & Kornazheva, B. P. (2001). Need satisfaction, motivation, and well-being in the work organizations of a former Eastern bloc country: A cross-cultural study of self-determination. *Personality and Social Psychology Bulletin, 27*, 930–942.

de Graaf, J. (Ed.). (2003). *Take back your time: Fighting overwork and time poverty in America*. San Francisco, CA: Berrett-Koehler.

Delle Fave, A., & Bassi, M. (2000). The quality of experience in adolescents' daily life: Developmental perspectives. *Genetic, Social, and General Psychology Monographs, 126*, 347–367.

Duriez, B., Vansteenkiste, M., Soenens, B., & De Witte, H. (2007). The social costs of extrinsic relative to intrinsic goal pursuits: Their relation with social dominance and racial and ethnic prejudice. *Journal of Personality, 75*, 757–782.

Frey, B. S., & Jegen, R. (2001). Motivation Crowding Theory. *Journal of Economic Surveys, 15*, 589–611.

Friedman, M. (1962/2002). *Capitalism and freedom* (40th Anniversary ed.). Chicago: University of Chicago Press.

Grouzet, F. M. E., Kasser, T., Ahuvia, A., Fernandez-Dols, J. M., Kim, Y., Lau, S., et al. (2005). The structure of goal contents across 15 cultures. *Journal of Personality and Social Psychology, 89*, 800–816.

Hall, P. A., & Gingerich, D. W. (2004). *Varieties of capitalism and institutional complementarities in the macroeconomy: An empirical analysis* (MPIfG Discussion Paper 04/5). Cologne, Germany: Max Planck Institute for the Study of Societies.

Jackson, T. (2009). *Prosperity without growth: Economics for a finite planet*. London: Earthscan Publications Ltd.

Kasser, T. (2005). Personal aspirations, the "good life," and the law. *Deakin Law Review, 10*, 33–47.

Kasser, T. (2006). Materialism and its alternatives. In M. Csikszentmihalyi & I. S. Csikszentmihalyi (Eds.), *A life worth living: Contributions to positive psychology* (pp. 200–214). Oxford: Oxford University Press.

Kasser, T. (2009). Values and ecological sustainability: Recent research and policy possibilities. In S. R. Kellert & J. G. Speth (Eds.), *The coming transformation: Values to sustain human and natural communities* (pp. 180–204). New Haven, CT: Yale School of Forestry & Environmental Studies.

Kasser, T., Cohn, S., Kanner, A. D., & Ryan, R. M. (2007). Some costs of American corporate capitalism: A psychological exploration of value and goal conflicts. *Psychological Inquiry, 18*, 1–22.

Kasser, T., & Ryan, R. M. (1993). A dark side of the American dream: Correlates of financial success as a central life aspiration. *Journal of Personality and Social Psychology, 65*, 410–422.

Kasser, T., & Ryan, R. M. (1996). Further examining the American dream: Differential correlates of intrinsic and extrinsic goals. *Personality and Social Psychology Bulletin, 22*, 280–287.

Kasser, T., Ryan, R. M., Zax, M., & Sameroff, A. J. (1995). The relations of maternal and social environments to late adolescents' materialistic and prosocial values. *Developmental Psychology, 31*, 907–914.

Kasser, T., & Sheldon, K. M. (2009). Time affluence as a path towards personal happiness and ethical business practices: Empirical evidence from four studies. *Journal of Business Ethics, 84*(2), 243–255.

Kelly, M. (2001). *The divine right of capital: Dethroning the corporate aristocracy*. San Francisco, CA: Berrett-Koehler Publishers.

Kubey, R., & Csikszentmihalyi, M. (1990). *Television and the quality of life*. Hillsdale, NJ: Erlbaum.

McChesney, R. W. (1997). *Corporate media and the threat to democracy*. New York: Seven Stories Press.

McHoskey, J. W. (1999). Machiavellianism, intrinsic versus extrinsic goals, and social interest: A self-determination theory analysis. *Motivation and Emotion, 23*, 267–283.

Miller, D. T. (1999). The norm of self-interest. *American Psychologist, 54*, 1053–1060.

Rand, A. (1943). *The fountainhead*. Indianapolis, IN: Bobbs-Merrill Company.

Rand, A. (1957). *Atlas shrugged*. New York: Random House.

Ryan, R. M., Bernstein, J. H., & Brown, K. W. (2010). Weekends, work, and well-being: Psychological need satisfactions and day of the week effects on mood, vitality, and physical symptoms. *Journal of Social and Clinical Psychology, 29*, 95–122.

Schor, J. B. (1993). *The overworked American*. New York: Basic Books.

Schwartz, S. H. (1992). Universals in the content and structure of values: Theory and empirical tests in 20 countries. In M. Zanna (Ed.), *Advances in experimental social psychology* (Vol. 25, pp. 1–65). New York: Academic Press.

Schwartz, S. H. (2006). Les valeurs de base de la personne : théorie, mesures et applicationshe. *Revue française de sociologie, 47*(4), 929–968.

Schwartz, S. H. (2007). Cultural and individual value correlates of capitalism: A comparative analysis. *Psychological Inquiry, 18*, 52–57.

Sheldon, K. M., & Kasser, T. (1995). Coherence and congruence: Two aspects of personality integration. *Journal of Personality and Social Psychology, 68*, 531–543.

Sheldon, K. M., & Kasser, T. (1998). Pursuing personal goals: Skills enable progress, but not all progress is beneficial. *Personality and Social Psychology Bulletin, 24*, 1319–1331.

Sheldon, K. M., & Kasser, T. (2001). "Getting older, getting better": Personal strivings and psychological maturity across the life span. *Developmental Psychology, 37*, 491–501.

Sheldon, K. M., Ryan, R. M., Deci, E. L., & Kasser, T. (2004). The independent effects of goal contents and motives on well-being: It's both what you do *and* why you do it. *Personality and Social Psychology Bulletin, 30*, 475–486.

Sheldon, K. M., Sheldon, M. S., & Osbaldiston, R. (2000). Prosocial values and group assortation in an N-person prisoner's dilemma. *Human Nature, 11*, 387–404.

Smith, A. (1776/1976). *An inquiry into the nature and causes of the wealth of nations*. New York: Random House.

Speth, J. G. (2008). *The bridge at the edge of the world: Capitalism, the environment, and crossing from crisis to sustainability*. New Haven, CT: Yale University Press.

Srivastava, A., Locke, E. A., & Bortol, K. M. (2001). Money and subjective well-being: It's not the money, it's the motives. *Journal of Personality & Social Psychology, 80*, 959–971.

Taylor, F. W. (1914). *The principles of scientific management*. New York: Harper.

Chapter 10
Economy, People's Personal Autonomy, and Well-Being

Maurizio Pugno

Introduction

The idea that the usual measures of welfare, such as national income or even individual income, do not properly reflect people's overall well-being has increasingly gained consensus both within and outside the community of economists.[1] In particular, it has been increasingly recognized that people's command over resources is not a sufficient metric with which to determine how well-off people are, because it ignores the fact that people with different characteristics will have different capacities to transform income or wealth into actual well-being. People with fewer abilities for achievement in valuable domains of life may be worse-off even if they command more economic resources.

This problem has been recently approached in economics by studying the subjective dimension in the evaluation of people's well-being or "happiness," including self-reported life satisfaction. The new research field of "happiness economics" has thus arisen on the basis of surveys of very large samples of people, and of countries, and over fairly long periods of time; and it asks very simple questions with which to self-score the level of happiness or life satisfaction.[2]

One of the main findings of happiness economics is that people's well-being does not necessarily grow with national income over time. In some countries it has

---

M. Pugno (✉)
Department of Economic Sciences, University of Cassino, Cassino, FR I-03043, Italy
e-mail: m.pugno@unicas.it

[1] A notable example is the initiative by the President of the French Republic Nicholas Sarkozy to create a Commission, including Joseph Stiglitz, Amartya Sen and Jean Paul Fitoussi, to identify the limits of Gross Domestic Product as an indicator of economic performance and social progress, and to consider what additional information might be required for a more satisfactory evaluation of economic performance, quality of life, and the sustainability of development and environment (www.stiglitz-sen-fitoussi.fr/documents/rapport_anglais.pdf).

[2] Typical questions, taken from the Word Value Survey, are: "All considered you would say that you are very happy; pretty happy; not too happy; not at all happy?"; "All considered are you satisfied or unsatisfied with your current life?". The answer to this second question can be given on a scale from 1 to 10.

declined although national income has increased. The most striking example is the USA since WWII, while the other advanced countries generally show a lagging or no trend in happiness (Easterlin & Angelescu, 2009; Layard, Mayraz, & Nickell, 2009; Stevenson & Wolfers, 2008). In West Germany, for which country there is one of the few data-sets available on happiness for a same sample of individuals who have been followed for a fairly long time (since 1985), the happiness indicator shows a slightly declining trend even if individual income, on average, has substantially increased (Di Tella, Haisken-De New, & McCulloch, 2007).[3]

These findings, which regard trends over time, are surprising because they contrast with cross-sectional findings. In samples of countries at a given time, in fact, happiness appears positively correlated to national income, and in samples of individuals within the same country, happiness appears positively correlated to household income (Easterlin, 1974, 1995).

This chapter intends to provide an original answer to why people's well-being may diverge from both national and individual income over time and thus not conform to the cross-sectional pattern. The arguments, which are based on psychology, and especially self-determination theory, on economics and sociology, run as follows. First, people's well-being has been negatively affected by the deterioration of their autonomy, which is the basic psychological need to maintain volitional control over one's life, and by the compensatory need for financial success and status (Koestner & Losier, 2006; Ryan & Deci, 2001). Secondly, some important factors that promote economic growth in the advanced countries and especially in the USA, also hamper the development of people's personal autonomy. In fact, the increasing competitions of production and commercialization on global markets on the one hand make people vulnerable to strain, insecurity, and stress, and on the other, induce them to gain a momentary satisfaction by consuming market goods.

This explanation of the income/well-being gap is composed of some analytical components, each of them based on specific and often interdisciplinary evidence. The concept of autonomy, which is a psychology concept, will be related to the rational choice framework, which is conventional in economics, so that both very micro dimensions, such as the individual's motivations, and macro dimensions, such as aggregate economic growth, can be considered.

The concept of well-being, also in the economic reformulation of happiness, appears to be an hedonic concept, i.e. an affective state of mind. However, the approach of this chapter is eudaimonic, since the analysis concentrates on what matters most in people's lives for their well-being (Ryan, Huta, & Deci, 2008). In particular, it will be shown that income is important for well-being, but only if conditioned by a variety of factors, while personal autonomy may be not less important. For example, an economic study has found that the related concepts of locus of

---

[3] Studies on less developed countries show that these are not immune to this phenomenon. For example, in Peru and Russia around half of the workers with the greatest upward income mobility reported that their economic situation was negative, or very negative, compared to 10 years previously, with deteriorating effects on their perceived well-being (Graham & Pettinato, 2002).

control and freedom to choose are the most important correlates with people's self-reported life satisfaction over a sample covering more than 20 years in 84 countries (Verme, 2009).[4]

Furthermore, the explanation of the income/well-being gap as based on personal autonomy both integrates and strengthens the explanations most popular in happiness economics: the one based on comparing own income with that of others, which links individuals' behaviors to aggregate outcomes; the one based on hedonic adaptation to rising standards of income; and the one based on people's deteriorating social lives, which argues that an individual's choice to relate with others is constrained by whether the others make similar choices, with the consequence that s/he may prefer less satisfying options.

The chapter finally shows that the concept of personal autonomy paves the way for some interesting forms of policy intervention. The explanations based on income comparisons, in fact, leave little and questionable room for policy intervention because incentives and taxes for redistribution are at risk of paternalism, and of counterproductive consequences. Enhancing personal autonomy, instead, implies interventions on skills formation, specifically through parenting and early education, and on the removal of frustrating socio-economic conditions.

The chapter is organized as follows. Section "The Divergence Between Economic Growth and People's Well-Being" gives a brief account of both the facts and the most popular explanations in economics concerning the divergence between national income and people's well-being over a long period of time. Section "Personal Autonomy: Placing a Psychological Concept into Economics" introduces the concept of personal autonomy into economics. Section "Economic Growth, the Erosion of Personal Autonomy, and Well-Being" uses this concept to explain the income/well-being divergence, also accounting for why people's autonomy has been deteriorating, and it discusses how these arguments integrate and strengthen the other economic explanations of the income/well-being divergence. Section "Policy" concludes by drawing some policy implications.

The Divergence Between Economic Growth and People's Well-Being

The Facts

The problem of the divergence between national income and people's well-being over time has been studied in happiness economics by using surveys on self-reported well-being. Despite the apparent elusiveness of the survey question (see footnote 2), people's answers have proved to convey valuable information. A variety of studies,

---

[4]The exact wording of the survey questions is "how much freedom of choice and control [do] you feel you have over the way your life turns out" (World Value Survey).

in fact, have shown that self-reported well-being, or a similar measure, is significantly correlated with the duration of so-called Duchenne smiles (Ekman, Davidson, & Friesen, 1990), physical health indicators (Shedler, Mayman, & Manis, 1993), measures of specific cerebral activity (Sutton & Davidson, 1997), and well-being as reported by the interviewees' friends and family members (see Diener & Lucas, 1999; Sandvik, Diener, & Seidlitz, 1993).

Different versions of the problem of divergence between income and people's well-being over time have been put forward. The most widely accepted version is that the increase in well-being tends to substantially *lag behind* economic growth, especially in the richest countries. This result is now entering basic economic textbooks, although the most frequently cited evidence concerns the cross-country concave relationship between per-capita income and self-reported well-being (e.g. Blanchard, 2005).

However, Easterlin (2005a) points out that cross-country evidence cannot be used to predict change over time, and he states the second version of the problem thus: "over time happiness *does not increase* when a country's income increases [although] at a point in time happiness varies directly with income" (Easterlin & Angelescu, 2009, p. 2). This has been called the "Easterlin paradox" from his seminal paper (Easterlin, 1974), and it has been at the centre of heated debate (Deaton, 2008; Stevenson & Wolfers, 2008). However, very recently the Easterlin paradox has been confirmed by the insignificant relationship between the improvement in happiness and the long-term rate of growth of GDP per capita for three groups of countries: 17 developed, 9 developing, and 11 transition countries (Easterlin & Angelescu, 2009).

The strongest version of the problem states that the trend of happiness has *decreased* in the USA since WWII, although to a small extent (Blanchflower & Oswald, 2004; Layard et al., 2009; Stevenson & Wolfers, 2008). Also other advanced countries seem to exhibit a decreasing trend in happiness, but available data are not sufficient to prove this fact.[5]

Note that the trend of happiness is usually studied in the economic literature as a change of the proportion of the happiest people over large samples of interviews, which are different from year to year but are controlled for demographic characteristics. When the same samples of people are available, however, as in the case of the German Socio-Economic Panel and the British Household Panel Study, the results are similar (Clark & Oswald, 2002; Di Tella et al., 2007). Note, moreover, that the problem of the divergence between national or individual income and people's well-being is considered here as a bivariate correlation over a long period of time. Only in the next subsection will the impact of national income or individual income on people's well-being, while taking many other conditions as constant, be discussed. Not surprisingly, the impact is usually found to be positive in this case.

---

[5]Easterlin and Angelescu's (2009) graphs show that Belgium, Austria, Canada, Portugal, and Greece have negative happiness trends. According to Layard et al.'s (2009) graph, Italy exhibits a break in the trend, from positive until the early 1990s to negative or no trend afterwards. Di Tella and McCulloch (2008) find a slightly negative trend for Europe as a whole. However, also some developing countries, China and Chile, exhibit a negative trend in happiness (Layard et al., 2009).

Objective measures of well-being seem to confirm the worst case of the USA. High blood pressure, which is regarded as a good (inverted) proxy for well-being (Blanchflower & Oswald, 2008; Mojon-Azzi & Sousa-Poza, 2007), rose in the US adult population from 1988 to 2004 (Ostchega, Dillon, Hughes, Carroll, & Yoon, 2007). The suicide rate increased in the USA from the mid-1960s until the mid-1980s, then declined until the end-1990s. Since then it has been stable, but at a greater rate than the initial one, despite the massive use of antidepressants (Cutler, Glaeser, & Norberg, 2001; CDC; McKeown, Cuffe, & Schulz, 2006; Kessler, Berglund, Borges, Nock, & Wang, 2005).

A variety of other evidence points in the same worrying direction for the USA and other advanced countries. For example, the suicide rate also increased for the EU and Japan from the mid-1960s until the 1980s (Chishti, Stone, Corcoran, Williamson, & Petridou, 2003; Levi, La Vecchia, & Saraceno, 2003, p. 111),[6] while the suicide rate among adolescents and young adults rose even more dramatically from the 1950s to the 1990s in all the developed nations except Japan (Eckersley & Dear, 2002). Mental health in the UK is apparently gradually worsening, if measured with the General Health Questionnaire (Oswald & Powdthavee, 2007). Several studies report that depression has significantly increased in the USA and other major developed countries since WWII (Hodiamont, Rijnders, Mulder, & Furer, 2005; Klerman, 1988, 1993; Lavori, Warshaw, Klerman, & Mueller, 1993; Layard & Dunn, 2009; Olfson, Marcus, Weissman, Jensen, & Peter, 2002; Rutter & Smith, 1995; Sacker & Wiggins, 2002). Again, the phenomenon is especially worrying in the case of children and adolescents, who also record a rise in anxiety and neuroticism, even if they belong to the more affluent classes (Collishaw, Maughan, & Goodman, 2004; Fombonne, Simmons, Meltzer, & Goodman, 2003; Luthar, 2003; Maughan, Iervolino, & Collishaw, 2005; Twenge, 2000).[7]

These are dramatic facts from the human and social point of view, but they also involve huge costs from the economic one. Quantitative evidence is very difficult to provide in this regard. However, the European Commission (2004) has attempted to estimate the economic costs of mental health for the EU, obtaining a figure of 2% of the total health care cost, which rises to 3–4% if the cost includes the effects

---

[6]Lester and Yang's (1997) survey of several studies shows that the correlation between income per head and suicide rates has been *positively* significant for the USA since WWII, and for a cross-section of the European countries. They also regress suicide rates against the unemployment rate and income per head for European countries, finding that only the latter variable is positively significant. Similar findings have been obtained by Jungeilges and Kirchgaessner (2002) and Huang (1996).

[7]Suicides and depression can be taken as reliable indicators of the well-being of the entire population because they show a significant inverse correlation with self-reported well-being (Di Tella et al., 2003, p. 812; van Hemert, van de Vijver, & Poortinga, 2002), because both suicides and well-being appear to be statistically well-explained by the same variables (Helliwell, 2007), and because the diffusion of clinical mental disorder is positively related to the mean number of the related symptoms in the population (Huppert, 2005). According to the epidemiologists Eckersley and Dear (2002), the tendencies of objective indicators of well-being like suicides and depression among young people are even more reliable than self-reported well-being, which in Europe exhibits a rising trend (Blanchflower & Oswald, 2000; Pichler, 2006).

on personal income, and on ability to work. Layard and Dunn (2009) report that a child with a conduct disorder costs the taxpayer £70,000 in crime, social care, and remedial costs by the time s/he is 28, compared to £7,000 for a child with no such problems.

The interest of economists in this kind of problem, however, is not simply due to these unexplored and unexpected huge economic costs; it is especially due to the scant effectiveness of economic policies generally, which mostly take national income as the key target variable. Even worse, pursuing economic growth as the final goal—this chapter will argue—may have perverse effects on people's well-being.

The Explanations in the Happiness Economics

Besides furnishing a great deal of evidence, happiness economics also provides an explanation as to why happiness tends to lag behind economic growth, or even declines, while the links with the other objective measures of well-being are still subject to careful study. More precisely, different explanations are proposed, but they are complementary rather than alternative. This subsection will briefly review this literature, while the explanation based on personal autonomy, and its integration with the other ones will be presented and discussed in the next subsection.

The most investigated explanation cites the human tendency to compare one's own situation with that of others (Kahneman, Wakker, & Sarin, 1997; Michalos, 1985), and to evaluate it accordingly. The relative economic situations of individuals change much more slowly with respect to their absolute situations because the benefits of economic growth are usually distributed over the population, although to a variable and different extent from country to country. Therefore, the rise of the incomes of all does not increase the happiness of all if relative income is what matters for happiness (Clark, Frijters, & Shields, 2008; Easterlin, 1995; Frank, 1999; Senik, 2009).

The empirical evidence on the existence of this relative income effect on happiness has been found to be robust (Ferrer-i-Carbonell, 2005; Luttmer, 2005). However, it does not emerge as an exhaustive explanation of the Easterlin paradox, mainly because it is heavily conditioned by at least two factors. Firstly, the chosen reference group for the income comparison changes the results, thus making the reference group as endogenous (Barrington-Leight & Helliwell, 2008; Knight, Song, & Gunatilaka, 2009). Secondly, the social context of income mobility may even change the negative sign of the relative income effect, because envy may turn into expectations of a possible future increase of income (Senik, 2008). Therefore, although comparison appears to be a natural tendency of individuals, it is heavily conditioned by their perception, and by the social context.[8]

---

[8]Consider, for example, the importance of the perception of immigrants in income comparisons (Knight & Gunatilaka, 2009).

The second popular explanation of the divergence between economic growth and happiness addresses the psychological mechanism of *hedonic adaptation*, generally defined as "a reduction in the affective intensity of favorable and unfavorable circumstances" (Frederick & Loewenstein, 1999, p. 302). A rise in income is a favorable circumstance for people, but they perceive that the initial benefit slows down as they become accustomed to the new level of income. A slightly different version of this explanation refers to *aspirations* concerning the future level of income (Easterlin, 2001). In this case, currently unrealized aspirations have a negative effect on individuals' well-being, but grow in line with income. Therefore, unrealized aspirations persist, and this negative effect may offset the positive effect of the actual rise in income. Both hedonic adaptation and aspirations are also consistent with the theory that personal traits fix the baseline for individuals' happiness, which may temporarily fluctuate because of external shocking events (Costa & McCrae, 1980).

Empirical investigation on adaptation in economic studies has scaled down the oft-cited results of Brickman, Coates, and Janoff-Bulman (1978), who found that lottery winners, and even paraplegics, completely adapt to their situations. By contrast, a more accurate analysis shows that medium-sized lottery winners adapt only partially (Gardner & Oswald, 2007), and large-sample longitudinal analyses also show a partial adaptation to rising individual income (Ferrer-i-Carbonell & Van Praag, 2008), although the adaptation may be substantial (Di Tella et al., 2007). Also the negative effects of rising aspirations on happiness have been found to partially offset the positive effects of rising individual income (Stutzer, 2004; Van de Stadt, Kapteyn, & de Geer, 1985).

The third economic explanation of the divergence between economic growth and people's well-being has been proposed by arguing for *deteriorating social relationships*. The idea is that income, whether of a country or an individual, maintains a positive net effect on happiness, but social relationships, which are also of great importance in people's well-being, have deteriorated in recent decades. Since relationships need the participation of the partners, this constrains individuals' actions, thus eroding their well-being.

The importance of social relationships in people's well-being has been widely confirmed by both psychology studies (Baumeister & Leary, 1995) and by happiness economics (Bruni & Stanca, 2008; Helliwell, 2006; Helliwell, Barringon-Leigh, Harris, & Huang, 2009). The deterioration of social relationships has been confirmed for the USA by various indicators. Some of them are included in "social capital," as studied by sociologists, like trust and civic participation in volunteer organizations (Bjørnskov, 2008; Costa & Kahn, 2003; McPherson, Smith-Lovin, & Brashears, 2006; Paxton, 1999; Putnam, 2000; Robinson & Jackson, 2001). The same worrying pattern is revealed by more specific indicators of family and social life, such as marriages (and their quality) in the USA (Amato, Johnson, & Booth, 2003; Crawford, Houts, Huston, & George, 2002; Glenn & Weaver, 1998; Rogers & Amato, 1997), cohabitations (Kamp Dush, Cohan, & Amato, 2003), infanticides (Pritchard & Butler, 2003), and violence among adolescents (Merrick, Kandel, & Vardi, 2003). Finally, a thorough test based on individual data has confirmed the importance of social capital indicators for well-being, their deterioration, and their correlation with the decline of happiness in the USA, after controlling for the relative income effect (Bartolini, Bilancini, & Pugno, 2008).

The dynamics of the quality of social relationships in other countries are much more difficult to investigate because of the scarcity of data. However, trust in people seems to have tendentially declined in the European countries, especially in the UK, while participation in volunteer organizations seems to have risen only in the Northern European countries (Sarracino, 2009).

According to this explanation, the deterioration of social relationships makes the preference of an individual for an extended social life more difficult simply because of a coordination problem with the partners in the relation (Bruni, 2005; Gui, 2005). Hence, every individual will be induced to substitute time for relationships with working time and time passed alone, thus substituting enjoyment from relationships with consumerism (Antoci, Sacco, & Vanin, 2007, 2008; Corneo, 2005). Indeed, the data on American households' time allocation confirm the increase in working time during the most recent decades (Alesina, Glaeser, & Sacerdote, 2005; Kuhn & Lozano, 2008).

The deterioration of social relationships can be explained, rather than being taken as exogenous, together with its effects on happiness, by recognizing that the geographic organization of production exerts negative externalities on social relationships. Cities are typically organized for production and consumption, rather than for meeting people during leisure time (Bartolini & Bonatti, 2002, 2006, 2008; Hirsch, 1976; Polanyi 1968). The production structure requires the geographical mobility of individuals, thus disrupting social networks (Routledge & von Amsberg, 2003). Therefore, a vicious circle from economic growth to social relationships through negative externalities, and from social relationships to economic growth through substitution of time allocation, may explain both a growing material opulence and social poverty, with the consequence that people's happiness may change little.

This explanation of the possible divergence between economic growth and people's well-being neatly clarifies the effect of the aggregation of individual decisions, and, more precisely, how social constraints force individuals in their decision making along a suboptimal path for their well-being.

Personal Autonomy: Placing a Psychological Concept into Economics

This section introduces the concept of autonomy into economics so that the next section can base the new explanation of the divergence between economic growth and people's well-being on the deterioration of their personal autonomy. A preliminary theoretical discussion is necessary because the concept of autonomy, which is commonly used in psychology—especially where it plays a key role in self-determination theory—is completely ignored in economic theory. Psychology and economics can thus contribute to an analysis which relates very micro dimensions, such as the individuals' motivations, to macro dimensions, such as aggregate economic growth.

The concept of autonomy in self-determination theory can be defined on the basis of the following quotations. "The autonomy orientation is characterized by the awareness of one's organismic and integrated needs and feelings" (Deci & Ryan, 1985, p. 156). "Autonomy refers to volition—the organismic desire to self-organize experience and behavior and to have activity be concordant with one's integrated sense of self" (Deci & Ryan, 2000, p. 231). "Autonomy-oriented individuals displayed a strong positive relation among behaviors and self-reports of traits and attitudes" (Deci & Ryan, 2000, pp. 241–242). "The very concept of well-being, which has been associated with experiences of autonomy, competence, and relatedness, bespeaks an evolved preferences for functioning in ways that are consistent with the satisfaction of psychological needs" (Deci & Ryan, 2000, p. 255), which is conceived as a process of "extending, assimilating, bringing meaning and coherence to life experiences" (Ryan & Brown, 2003, p. 71).

Autonomy thus implies a feeling of the body, an experience. Specifically, it is an experience of volition, of concordance between what one has chosen to do, and how one feels the self. Autonomous behavior appears to be the outcome of a person's preferences, since these are well-integrated with her/his self. Such experience satisfies a basic psychological need, so that well-being ensues as a growing self.

By contrast, economics represents people's behavior by means of the theoretical model of *homo economicus*, who is a processor of information and a producer of solutions. Information consists of the available given resource constraints and options, as well as preferences that characterize *homo economicus*. The solutions are the options which maximize his utility drawn from given resources. *Homo economicus* pursues maximization by learning from past errors of his own or of others, by impartially updating information, and by improving his predictions about the consequences of his decisions (see, e.g., McFadden, 1999).

Homo economicus thus does not know autonomy, because he cannot feel concordance with the self, he cannot experience well-being and the process of the growing self. He is a sophisticated goal achiever, but without really choosing, because he does not experience the sense of freedom in his behavior (Deci & Ryan, 1985, p. 155).

This theoretical model has proved extremely powerful in economics when dealing with a variety of problems of both interpretation and prediction. This model may be useful in this chapter as well, but for a different reason, i.e. for studying the gap between *homo economicus*' behavior and people's behavior as characterized by different degrees of autonomy. In fact, autonomy-oriented and non autonomy-oriented individuals can be distinguished not only by their different type of motivations, but also by the different patterns of their decisions over similar bundles of options. Autonomy-oriented individuals place relatively more weight, by means of a mixture of intuition and cognition, on the options that bring them more well-being. Therefore, a special capacity to choose, i.e. to experience an enduring advantage from given resources, can be identified in autonomy-oriented individuals, and it can be evaluated against *homo economicus*' decision-making (Pugno, 2008b).

The first step in recognizing that people may have limits in drawing utility, or personal advantage from given material resources has been taken by the economics Nobel prize winner Amartya Sen, and by the capability approach more generally (Alkire, 2008; Bruni, Comim, & Pugno, 2008; Nussbaum, 2000; Sen, 1985, 1999a). Sen first criticized the conventional model of *homo economicus* because, among other shortcomings, it ignores that real persons may have some internal constraint on their decision making due to possible lacks in specific abilities. Sen's typical example refers to nutritional problems in less developed countries, where illnesses thwart the absorption of nourishing substances from food. In this case, the availability of material goods, and more generally of several options, does not necessarily make individuals free to choose, because they are subject to an internal constraints, in that they lack a bodily functioning. Physical health is a good example, but Sen also extends these constraints to include the social and cultural pressure on individuals, and especially on women, deriving from communitarian and religious traditions (Sen, 1999b).

Sen thus argues that each person is endowed with a variety of functionings and capabilities. The former can be defined as a collection of the observable achievements, e.g. being able to digest properly; the latter is the person's freedom to choose and to exercise these functionings, e.g. fasting for religious reasons. Sen stresses that an individual's real advantage should be substantive or positive freedom, that is, freedom to achieve valued outcomes. If the person lacks functionings or capabilities, s/he has internal constraints on achieving advantage and well-being.

The philosopher Martha Nussbaum (2003) has even proposed a list of central human capabilities. Some items on the list are psychological functionings and abilities such as "being able to use the senses, to imagine, think and reason", "to love those who love and care for us," "to show concern for other human beings," "to laugh and play," and, finally, what most resembles personal autonomy, i.e. "control over one's environment." Nussbaum is especially concerned with defining the requirements of human dignity and rights to construct a conception of social justice, while Sen has been more concerned with defining freedom and advantage in opposition to the economic theory of rational choice.[9]

Sen comes close to the concept of personal autonomy as a special capability when he cites the case of those individuals, who, after following some external prescriptions or conventions, change their mind after reasoning and self-scrutiny, realize that they have been externally constrained, and conclude that better lines of conduct are possible. Sen relies on collective decision-making processes based on public discussions and democratic participation in order to help these individuals

---

[9]Both Sen and Nussbaum stress the importance of the objective evaluation of individuals' conditions, rather than the self-evaluations of own well-being. Sen (1985), in particular, is generally skeptical of the subjective evaluations of well-being, because adaptation would induce individuals to be content with their current material state, thus biasing the evaluation of their real conditions (see section "The Explanations in the Happiness Economics"). While empirical research shows that adaptation does not completely deprive subjective information on well-being of valuable content, recent theoretical research attempts to find synergies between the capability approach with happiness economics (*Review of Social Economy* 63(2), 2005; Bruni, Comim, & Pugno, 2008).

change their minds and escape from the constraints of social and cultural backward rules, thus increasing their personal autonomy (Pugno, 2008a; Sen, 1999a).

Self-determination theory goes a step further by arguing that "social controls, evaluative pressures, rewards, and punishments can powerfully constrain or entrain behavior, sometimes outside awareness," so that "people can easily lose sight of important values and needs," among which is the basic psychological need of autonomy (Ryan & Deci, 2006, p. 1566).

The key point where self-determination theory departs from the *homo economicus* model is that external constraints such as social controls, or even economic incentives, may induce individuals to "lose sight" of something important for the development of their self, for their personal growth (see also Ryff & Singer, 1998), thus losing autonomy, and hence the ability to evaluate the available options. The experience of those external constraints work as a prime on individuals which may trigger negative self-reinforcing consequences on their inner functioning, and, eventually, on their well-being.

The typical prime occurs during infancy and adolescence. Self-determination theory and other psychology research show that family background, both economic and educational, is of great importance in shaping personal autonomy during childhood and adolescence (Kasser, Ryan, Zax, & Sameroff, 1995; Williams, Cox, Hedberg, & Deci, 2000). In particular, inadequate parenting, such as the use of conditional regard, which can be worsened by deteriorated socio-economic conditions, may thwart children's autonomy (Assor, Roth, & Deci, 2004; Gronlick, 2003; Roth, Assor, Niemiec, Ryan, & Deci, 2009; Soenens, Vansteenkiste, Duriez, & Goossens, 2006).

Self-determination theory further departs from the *homo economicus* model by providing an interesting argument against the assumption that people tend to resume personal autonomy after the prime of controlling experiences. Instead of learning how to increase their autonomy from others—the argument runs—people develop, as a defensive reaction, need substitutes that do not really satisfy autonomy but provide temporary compensating satisfaction.

As Deci and Ryan (1985, pp. 238–241) put it in an example: "when a child does not receive adequate love, s/he may develop a need for food, one that is over and above the organismic hunger need. The substitute need for food would be conscious, but the original need for love would be nonconscious and would be the real motivator of the behavior." In this example, the deprivation of a basic psychological need induces the individual to seek an immediate gratification through material means, thus failing to obtain nutriment for her/his psychological growth. This failure may become even stronger over time because it is based on learning the immediate effectiveness of substituting needs satisfaction, like money, material possessions, and image-oriented goals, so that substitute needs are preferred even when options for satisfying basic psychological need become available (Deci & Ryan, 2000, p. 249).[10]

---

[10]This possible change of direction in the tastes for different kinds of needs is consistent with studies in neuroscience which report the particular plasticity of the brain during infancy, childhood and adolescence, with respect to adulthood (e.g. Siegel, 2001).

This self-reinforcing change in the preferred option which diverts individuals from the possibility to enjoy the best outcomes can be seen as a self-reinforcing bias in decision making. Self-reinforcement springs from an updating of information which is not impartial, since it draws from experiences of the immediate gratification of substitute needs while "losing sight" of the possible experience of autonomy need satisfaction.

This argument is consistent with the perspective put forward by the economist Scitovsky in an oft-cited book (Scitovsky, 1976).[11] He distinguished two main sources of satisfaction for individuals: the stimulating and interesting activities which can engage individuals in an ever-growing process of learning and developing their faculties, and the comfort activities which provide the temporary satisfaction of reducing excessive stimulations arising from inner needs, such as hunger and the need for warmth and safety, or from external social pressures, such as the need for status. The goods associated with comfort activities are also called "defensive goods," the purpose being to underline their compensatory role when the necessary ability to appreciate stimulating and interesting activities is lacking.

Self-determination theory departs even further from the *homo economicus* model by distinguishing between pursuing utility as the main goal and pursuing the full functioning of one's own potential, and specifically autonomy, as a process desirable in itself and from which the experience of well-being emerges as a side effect (Ryan et al., 2008). The difference between the two approaches lies primarily in the concept of utility as an abstract quantity vs. the concept of well-being as the evaluation of a feeling. A second difference is that ignoring autonomy impedes *homo economicus* from considering the possible detrimental feedback effects from pursuing utility as the main goal on autonomy and well-being itself.

Economic Growth, the Erosion of Personal Autonomy, and Well-Being

The Explanation Based on the Deterioration of Personal Autonomy

The concept of personal autonomy can play a key role in an original explanation of the divergence between economic growth and people's well-being. This can be shown by integrating some analytical components and references to the empirical underpinnings available in both the psychology and the economic literature.

The first analytical components regard the individual level, as they were briefly discussed in the previous section. According to self-determination theory, "individual differences in autonomy predict well-being," and more precisely "controlling contexts yield negative effects on wellness, whereas those that are autonomy supportive enhance it" (Ryan & Deci, 2006, p. 1565). More precisely, the negative

---

[11] Scitovsky's *The Joyless Economy* has been classified as one of "The Hundred Most Influential Books Since World War II" (Times Literary Supplement, Oct. 6, 1996).

effect on self-reported well-being is due to the non-satisfaction of the basic psychological need for autonomy, which entails developing need substitutes like money and material possessions (Deci & Ryan, 2000).[12]

It can thus be argued that if the context becomes more and more controlling, then people's autonomy may be expected to deteriorate, while people's aspirations for greater wealth may be expected to rise, with negative consequences for the well-being of most individuals. This may help explain the fact discussed in section "The Divergence Between Economic Growth and People's Well-Being" that the self-reported well-being of large samples of individuals in the USA and other advanced countries has been slightly changing, if not declining, during the most recent decades, despite economic growth.

Some empirical studies are consistent with this claim. Two meta-analyses on college students and child samples of the USA between 1960 and 2002 find that young people increasingly believe that their lives are controlled by outside forces rather than by their own efforts (Twenge, Zhang, & Im, 2004). Another study on a large sample of American college freshpersons has found that the importance as a life goal of personal self-fulfilment declined sharply from the early seventies until the eighties, while private materialism increased greatly (Easterlin & Crimmins, 1991), and it does not seem to have declined in the following two decades (Pryor, Hurtado, Sharkness, & Korn, 2007). People's orientation toward money and material possessions, often called materialism, has also been found to have strengthened— according to a number of works (Kasser, 2002; Putnam, 2000; Schor, 1998)—with the expansion of the market production.

This link that goes from the deterioration of people's autonomy to the strengthening of their materialistic orientation as a compensatory need at the individual level can be complemented with reverse links that go from the expansion of market economic activity to the deterioration of people's autonomy at the aggregate level. Adult individuals, in fact, express a demand for products and supply labor to finance it, but they are conditioned at the aggregate level by both the quantity and the quality of the supply of products and demand for labor.

Two main reverse links can in fact be identified. Both of them start from the expansion of market competition and commercialization, and from the necessity of persistent production reorganization. One link passes mainly through the product market and the striving for higher sales, through the psychological pressure on the family, to thwarting needs in children and adolescents. The other link mainly extends through the labor market, and greater flexibility in hiring and firing, to inequality, insecurity, and stress.

Market production and commercialization have raised unfair competition against parents in their relating with children and adolescents. Usually, only the bright side of the increase in economic production for children and adolescents is considered, i.e. more comfort, more technology, more market services. However, the

---

[12]It has also been found that experiential avoidance fully mediated the association between materialistic values and emotional well-being (Kashdan & Breen, 2007).

dark side of this production is its aim to give these very young consumers strong but unhealthy sensations: from hyper-caloric and salted food, to thrilling and violent fictions and games. The debate on the effects of advertising and violent media products on children and adolescents ranges from seriously negative to negligible negative but usually very significant (Anderson and Bushman, 2001; Chamberlain, Wang, & Robinson, 2006; Ferguson, 2007; Gentile, Saleem, & Anderson, 2007; Robinson, Saphir, Kraemer, Varady, & Haydel, 2001; Schmitt, Wagner, & Kirch, 2007; Bhattacharya & Munasib, 2007). The bottom line of the debate is whether advertising and violent media products causally affect actual behaviors like overeating and aggression, or only criminal aggression (Savage, 2004). However, the autonomy of children and adolescents may be largely eroded without these specific behavioral consequences through the diverting of their attention to models of consumption and social competition (Schor, 2004), and, in the case of violence, through desensitization (Carnagey, Anderson, & Bushman, 2007).

By contrast, parents are often ill-equipped to evaluate, anticipate, or even avoid the undesirable effects of advertising and products for children and adolescents (Buijzen & Valkenburg, 2003, 2005; Buijzen, van der Molen, & Sondij, 2007; Weintraub, 2000). In fact, parents' time is increasingly scarce, information is relatively insufficient in a world which becomes ever more complex. But children must put up with their parents and accept them as allocated to them by chance. Children cannot choose their parents like they can choose market products. Nor can they induce their parents to learn the necessary ability because they develop substitute needs which are very easily satisfied with market goods.

Therefore, the competition of productive and commercial organizations with parents in satisfying children's needs is unfair because sales failures are sanctioned by the market, whereas parenting inadequacies are not necessarily self-correcting. Parents' inadequacies can persist and even cumulate across generations.

Market production requires labor time, and economic growth requires increasing skills that households must provide. Again, the bright side of the gender division of labor in households, and of increased women's education, undoubtedly lies in their greater self-determination. However, reconciling the demands made by children, marriage, and work requires greater ability, especially for women, with the risk of increasing their stress and affecting their parenting ability (Ford, Heinen, & Langkamer, 2007; Grönlund, 2007).

Moreover, also the context of the competition between parents and market production in satisfying children's needs tends to be unfair. Cities and, more generally, space and mobility are organized around economic production and consumption rather than around caring for children. Space is a scarce resource, and its scarcity is signaled by a price which embodies rent. If space is employed for market production, it yields a more immediate and certain reward than if it is employed for children's healthy development. Family mobility follows work requirements more than community ties. Therefore, children have fewer open safe spaces in which to gain autonomous experiences, while market production is able to equip their rooms with amusing gadgets and high-tech consumption. This implies that children's relations tend to shift from long-term friends to simple contacts through virtual social networks (Layard & Dunn, 2009). Their implicit demand for satisfaction of their basic psychological needs is thus especially restricted to their parents, who may even find themselves in a less socially friendly environment.

Public resources devoted to children are available in greater quantities in richer countries, so that they may offset the negative effects of the "privatisation" of space and time. However, an iron law of economic growth, also called "Baumol's law," runs counter to this trend (Baumol, 1967). The law states that personal services, or more generally labor-intensive products, are subject to lower labor productivity growth than the other market products. The music of a Mozart quartet requires exactly the same time today as it did when it was originally performed, i.e. labor productivity growth is zero. Consequently, whilst pay levels are similar among the different lines of production, the costs of personal services relatively to the costs of the other market products tend to rise. Childcare is a highly labor-time-consuming activity, so that it is subject to Baumol's law, and it becomes increasingly more costly than, for example, public utilities, which are much more technology intensive. Hence costs compression in education tends to ration the quantities of the services offered, and to reduce the pay of the personnel, thereby deteriorating the quality of education.

In conclusion, economic growth and the expansion of market activities make parenting an increasingly difficult task. In fact, the ability required adequately to satisfy children's autonomy and their other basic psychological needs becomes ever greater, and the market goods to satisfy their substitute needs increase in quantity and quality. Social life outside the family, and at school in particular, does not seem to offer a way out of this impasse, because children's friendships appear to be more superficial than they were in the past, and school less authoritative.

The other link between the expansion of market competition and the reduction of people's autonomy passes through the rise of inequality, insecurity, and stress in the adult population.[13]

The expansion of the market on the international scale has increased income inequality within many advanced countries (Borghesi & Vercelli, 2003; OECD, 2008). In the USA, for example, the Gini coefficient, which is a common measure of income inequality, increased from 0.403 in 1980 to 0.469 in 2005 (Miringoff & Opdyke, 2008, p. 234). One of the main reasons for this phenomenon is the fierce competition raised by less developed but high-growth countries for medium-skilled and unskilled labor (Jagannathan, Kapoor, & Schaumburg, 2009). It is thus unsurprising that job insecurity has been found to be significantly rising (Blanchflower & Oswald, 1999), while working hours become longer (Bell & Freeman, 2001). A poll conducted in 1982, when unemployment reached 10%, found that 12% of workers were "frequently concerned about being laid off." In 2005, with unemployment at about 5%, over 30% expressed this concern (Hacker, 2006, p. 18).

---

[13]"Chronic stress can be defined as a pathologic state of prolonged threat to homeostasis by persistent or frequently repeated stressors and is considered a significant contributing factor in pathophysiology of manifestations that characterize a wide range of diseases and syndromes" (Kyrou, Chrousos, & Tsigos, 2006, p. 78).

Job insecurity has increased in Germany as well (Green & Tsitsianis, 2005), together with a rise in work effort (Green & Gallie, 2002). Also in Britain work effort has increased, while task discretion has diminished (Green, 2007).

Although these findings should be further deepened and confirmed, they are surprising, because greater wealth, technical progress, and the shift to services would instead predict improvements in the labor conditions. The often-cited prediction by John Maynard Keynes was that working long hours would be unnecessary within some decades.

The worsening of job security and other labor conditions are stressing factors. Some surveys have confirmed the increase in anxiety due to job insecurity (Hertzenberg, Alic, & Wial, 1998; Mishel, Bernstein, & Schmitt, 1999). From a biological point of view, "a considerable number of studies have shown that various strains during work, particularly when demands are larger than decision latitude, and in situations with monotonous type of work and lack of control, are followed by elevated secretion of cortisol," which is often called the "stress hormone" (Björntorp, 2001, p. 75).

Inequality, insecurity, and stress also involve social relationships. Income inequality and trust are found to be inversely correlated in the USA (Kawachi, Kennedy, Lochner, & Prothrow-Stith, 1997; Uslaner, 2002). Income inequality seems also correlated to homicides in the USA, both over time and across states, after controlling for state income (Mellor & Milyo, 2001). More generally, income inequality and crime appear correlated across developed countries (Fajnzylber, Lederman, & Loayza, 2000). The emergence of stress in social contexts has been studied by biologists, who find that low-ranked positions in comparison with others produce stress (McEwen, 1998; Sapolsky, 1993), while many studies on the effects of inequality on health agree that social comparison and social support play an important role in regulating stress-related diseases (Deaton, 2002).[14]

The rise of stress has also been found by specific studies. By using the GHQ index, which includes questions on good sleeping, self-confidence, cheerfulness, and other symptoms, it has been shown that stress has risen in the UK (Sacker & Wiggins, 2002), in the Netherlands (Verhaak, Hoeymans, & Westert, 2005), and even among 15-year-olds in Scotland (Sweeting, Young, & West, 2009).

Insecurity and stress make people passive and vulnerable to controlling conditions, thus putting their autonomy under strain. In the case of adults in modern economies, this means vulnerability to commercial pressures and to social

---

[14]Inequality promotes [survival] strategies that are more self-interested, less affiliative, often highly anti-social, more stressful and likely to give rise to higher levels of violence, poorer community relations, and worse health. In contrast, the less unequal societies tend to be much more affiliative, less violent, more supportive and inclusive, and marked by better health....more unequal societies tend to have higher rates of violent crime and homicide, and...people living in them feel more hostility, are less likely to be involved in community life, and are much less likely to trust each other; in short, they have lower levels of social capital. (Wilkinson, 2005, p. 24).

conformism, which make the substitute needs of consuming for its own sake and social competition more and more attractive.

The increase in passivity in decision making can be detected by the diffusion of mental depression, as mentioned in section "The Facts," and by decline in the locus of control in American students, as mentioned above (Twenge et al., 2004). The pressure applied by advertisements for adults to consume more has been widely documented (Kasser, Ryan, Couchman, & Sheldon, 2004; Schor, 1998). Also the negative effects of a relatively strong consumption orientation on autonomy and well-being has been investigated in psychology (Kasser, 2002; Kasser, Cohn, Kanner, & Ryan, 2007).

Economics still resists considering consumerism or materialism as a relevant concept, because in this case the individual would be represented as choosing to consume over and above what is worthwhile for her/him, which is not rational. This case, however, seems to apply in one important instance investigated in the economic literature. This is the case of overweight and obesity, which has been recognized as being very costly in terms not only of illnesses and unhappiness (Katsaiti, 2009; Oswald & Powdthavee, 2007) but also of lower earnings (Brunello, Michaud, & Sanz-de-Galdeano, 2009; Cawley, 2004), and less skill accumulation (Cawley & Spiess, 2008).

The economic debate on the causes of the increase in overweight and obesity in recent decades, especially in the USA, recognizes that a lack of rationality has played a role in individuals' decision making, among other factors (Cutler, Glaeser, & Shapiro, 2003) such as, in particular, externalities in the family and among peers (e.g. Blanchflower, Oswald, & Van Landeghem, 2008). This means that overweight and obese individuals are recognized as failing in an autonomous decision because they fail to exercise self-control when consuming food (Brunello et al., 2009; Downs, Loewenstein, & Wisdom, 2009; Stutzer, 2007) because, in turn, their decision ability is eroded by stress (Offer, 2006; Wisman & Capehart, 2010).

In conclusion, economic growth and the expansion of market activities put adult people in difficult circumstances as far as exercising choice is concerned. On the one hand, their ability to evaluate the options available is put under strain by insecurity and stress; on the other, they are pressured to favor the options less conducive to enduring well-being.

The Integration Among Explanations

The proposed explanation of the divergence between income and people's well-being over time, which is based on the lack of personal autonomy, integrates, and at the same time strengthens, the other explanations reviewed in section "The Explanations in the Happiness Economics", which are based on relative income, hedonic adaptation, and social constraints. These explanations, in fact, are partial, and they reveal some weaknesses.

The first explanation assumes that the income of others negatively affects individuals' well-being. The underlying justification is that this is a typical psychological pattern of individuals (not only human individuals) that makes them rivals in social relationships. The evolutionary perspective would suggest that rivalry increases the survival probability in a scarce resources environment (Frank, 1999; Layard, 2005). However, this explanation is restricted to only one dimension of social relationships. Self-determination theory and other streams of research in psychology instead argue that humans are naturally designed with a tendency toward relatedness so that they can satisfy a need for social attachment (Baumeister & Leary, 1995; Deci & Ryan, 2000). People can thus shift time and effort from the dark side of social competition to the bright side of social relations, especially in the modern environment where resources are not as scarce as they were in the times of our ancestors. But why have people not sufficiently changed in that direction, with the consequence that they have actually eroded the enjoyment derived from their incomes?

The answer follows straightforwardly from the lack of personal autonomy, and the consequent onset of substitute needs. Since people may lack the ability to evaluate the capacity of available options to satisfy their basic psychological needs, perhaps because they have been controlled against external target-behaviors, they are induced to follow others, thus taking the others' conditions as references for comparison. The importance of relative income for appreciating own well-being is thus not given and fixed; rather, it depends on people's autonomy, and it may change accordingly. A different level of autonomy may change the reference group, so that this becomes, at least partly, endogenous. A greater level of autonomy may even turn the sign of the relative income effect from negative to positive, if the future realization of own possibilities thus appears more feasible.

The second explanation of the divergence between economic growth and people's well-being assumes hedonic adaptation, and the onset of the frustrating aspirations gap with material conditions. However, in these cases too, the psychological patterns considered are restricted. In fact, when hedonic adaptation is studied in regard to events that do not directly concern income, such as marriage, divorce, or unemployment, it emerges as being very partial, even when controlled for the economic consequences (Zimmermann & Easterlin, 2006; Frey & Stutzer, 2006; Clark, Georgellis, Lucas, & Diener, 2004; Ferrer-i-Carbonell & Van Praag, 2008). Adaptation also differs across individuals, especially in regard to marital status (Lucas, Clark, Georgellis, & Diener, 2003), and it is reduced if applied to positive activity rather than to positive circumstances (Sheldon & Lyubomirsky, 2009). Also aspirations differ according to the domain. In particular, unrealized aspirations are less frustrating if they are attached to social affiliation and personal growth (Kasser, 2002). Aspirations also differ according to people's mindfulness, which is the human capacity to be receptively attentive to and aware of present events and experience, so that it is associated with personal autonomy (Brown & Ryan, 2003). In fact, people with greater mindfulness seem to perceive a smaller gap between what they have and what they desire, and the gap they do perceive bothers them less (Brown, Kasser, Ryan, Linley, & Orzech, 2009). Obvious questions thus arise: why do people not devote more effort and time to experiences with more enduring effects? Why does the endeavor to increase income and consumption persist as a primary activity? (Easterlin, 2005b)

The autonomy argument is able to answer these questions. The lack of autonomy hampers people in self-determining their goals, and in particular in pursuing personal growth and affiliation. People are thus especially attracted by consumption and material possessions. Empirical studies show that relatively greater autonomy, less comparison striving, a narrower aspiration gap, and then higher well-being, are not abstract possibilities for people (Brown et al., 2009).

Also the explanation of the divergence between economic growth and people's well-being as based on deteriorating social relationships shows a weakness. It in fact assumes a uniform social constraint on all individuals. It is true that time and space for relationships are necessary for all partners, but the constraint usually binds them differently, because personal autonomy, and hence the ability to appreciate social relationships, differ across individuals. Therefore, people can relax the social constraint by properly allocating time across the preferred partners in relationships, thus satisfying their autonomy needs differently. For example, it is an established fact that more educated mothers spend more time with their children despite the fact that they work more (Guryan, Hurst, & Kearney, 2008). By contrast, a recent study shows that the reduction of working time in France due to the 1998 employment law did not result in more time devoted to relationships, whereas human capital emerged as much more important for relationships (Saffer & Lamiraud, 2008). Education, which is a rough proxy for personal autonomy, and not time seems to be the binding constraint.

In conclusion, considering the role of people's personal autonomy in the problem of the divergence between economic growth and people's well-being strengthens the existing explanations, besides proposing an original one. Moreover, integration among all the approaches can account for the problem in all relevant dimensions: from the individuals' motivations, through the externalities from parents to children, across peer relationships, and social competition, to the interaction between the productive organization of the economy and individuals as consumers and as workers. Therefore, a growth of individual income can have the expected positive effects on individuals' happiness, but other effects such as social comparison, expectation gap, deteriorated social relationships, and a lack of autonomy can work in the opposite direction, so that the final effect for some individuals, or for the whole community, may be significantly changed.

Policy

Arguing for policies in support of people's personal autonomy seems a novelty for economists, but it will prove helpful in the debate on economic policies to close the income/happiness gap. Economists usually think in terms of incentives and costs, disregarding any problem of personal autonomy in decision making. However, in the case of policies for happiness, the use of incentives and costs does not appear very convincing because of the risk of paternalism and of counterproductive consequences.[15] If instead autonomy is introduced into the analysis, not only the role of incentives and costs but also the role of happiness as a policy target can be considered in new light.

The discussion on the concept of autonomy in this and the previous chapters suggests that supporting people's autonomy implies improving their ability to evaluate and use information for more satisfactory choices, with a variety of positive consequences, including well-being. People should be primarily able to properly evaluate incentives and costs in order to draw advantage from material resources. Sen would say that policies should enhance people's capabilities to enjoy more freedom to choose, while self-determination theory reminds us that the use of incentives and costs may have perverse effects on autonomy (Sansone & Harackiewicz, 2000). Both Sen and self-determination theory share the eudaimonic approach to well-being, which regards well-being as a side-effect of proper support for persons' capabilities and need-satisfying ability (Ryan et al., 2008).

Policies should concentrate on the formation of people's autonomy, especially during their developmental ages, and on the removal of constraints on autonomy when this is lacking. Policies for children and for adults can thus be distinguished.

The primary line of intervention regards parenting, early education, and its socio-economic context. Economists have recently recognized that investing in children, rather than, e.g., in post-secondary education, has very high returns (Cascio, 2009; Sylva, Melhuish, Sammons, Siraj-Blatchford, & Taggart, 2010),[16] not only because children's abilities take longer to develop but also because the abilities are self-productive, cross-fertilizing, and often develop effectively only in specific ages (Berlinski, Galiani, & Manacorda, 2008, 2009; Blomeyer, Coneus, Laucht, & Pfeiffer, 2008; Borghans, Duckworth, Heckman, & ter Weel, 2008; Cunha & Heckman, 2009; Cunha, Heckman, Lochner, & Masterov, 2006; Frank & Meara, 2009; Huang, 2006). In particular, the Nobel prize winner Heckman and his co-authors recognize that family environments and investments in children (mainly represented by parental education and maternal ability) causally affect the development of their abilities of both cognitive and socio-emotional type, which prove to be crucial for a variety of outcomes, from dropping out of school to incarceration, from smoking to teenage pregnancy.

Policy should be directed to alleviating the conditions of disadvantaged children. But Heckman (2008, p. 16) warns that: "a substantial body of evidence suggests that a major determinant of child disadvantage is the quality of the nurturing environment rather than just financial resources available or presence or absence of parents. This evidence is supported by the evidence on the effects of early parenting enrichment programs."

---

[15] See Layard (2005) and Frank (1999) for happiness policies based on incentives and costs, and Sugden (2007) and Frey and Stutzer (2001) for skeptical views.
[16] Karoly, Kilburn, and Cannon (2003) estimate that early childhood interventions across the USA, working with children and parents to improve readiness for school, yield a rate of return for each dollar invested of 8.7 at age 27 and 17.1 at age 40.

Intervention in favor of children should be a policy priority also because both the material and human resources recently devoted to children are inadequate and unequally distributed, especially in the USA and the UK. In fact, the poverty rate among children in the early 2000s was 21.7% in the USA and 16.2% in the UK, while it was 2.4% in Denmark and 3.6% in Sweden. In the USA it had even risen since 1970, when it was 15.0%. Childcare fees, net of tax reductions, and of childcare benefits in 2003 amounted to 12.6% of family net income in the USA, and 32.7% in the UK, but only 7.8% in Denmark, and 6.2% in Sweden. Also parental leave varies greatly across countries. If its duration is multiplied by the percentage of salary paid in the early 2000s, the figure for the USA is 0 and for the UK 23, while for Denmark it is 53 and for Sweden 48. A similar pattern emerges for a dreadful phenomenon that mainly occurs within families: child maltreatment deaths exhibit the highest rate in the USA with respect to the other three countries considered, while the child neglect victimization rate even increased in the USA from 1990 to 2006 (US Department of Health and Human Services, 2008).

This evidence, although descriptive, is also consistent with the explanation proposed in this chapter concerning the divergence between economic growth and people's well-being. In fact, although the economies of the four above-mentioned countries grew at about the same average rate from 1973 to 2006, during the same period the USA exhibited a declining trend of self-reported well-being, the UK exhibited no trend, whereas Denmark and Sweden exhibited substantially positive ones.[17]

However, more abundant and more equally distributed material resources, both private and public, for children are not sufficient for a healthy development of their autonomy, since the type of parenting remains crucial. It is true that household income and parents' education may greatly improve the ability of parenting to support children's autonomy, but this is not a necessary outcome (see e.g. Luthar, 2003). Applying economic reasoning to parenting clarifies that it can remain indefinitely of suboptimal quality because it is not tradable, even intertemporally, i.e. children cannot exchange parenting on the market. This is well-known to commercial businesses, which in fact take children as one of their preferred targets in an attempt to bypass parent's educational monitoring.

The first policy suggested is to direct the focus of public opinion to the fact that inadequate parenting entails serious problems for children and for the future of everybody, that adequate parenting is under the threat of market economies, but also that investing in good parenting is possible. A large body of studies on parenting programs and support is available, and some robust results and prescriptions are slowly emerging (Layzer, Goodson, Bernstein, & Price, 2001; Mihalopoulos, Sanders, Turner, Murphy-Brennan, & Carter, 2007; Moran, Ghate, & van der Merwe, 2004). A policy that enlarged intervention to give more equal opportunities to children generally would have beneficial effects not only on well-being, but also on the aggregate

---

[17] The evidence in these paragraphs comes from different sources, mainly UNICEF, US-General Social Survey and Eurobarometer. See Pugno (2009) for more details.

efficiency of production, since more talented people would more easily reveal themselves on the market. This action would be also useful in the USA, which displays, contrary to a widespread belief, very low income mobility (Jäntti et al., 2006).[18]

Good practices in early education can be inspired by solid results in psychology research. "Attachment theory" (Ainsworth, Blehar, Waters, & Wall, 1978; Bowlby, 1969) can be complemented with the recent results on how the infant mind works, and in particular on how it needs an adequate response from adults (Gopnik, Meltzoff, & Kuhl, 2000). Good practices in the education of children and adolescents can be grounded on research into autonomy-supportive education (see the reviews by Guay, Chanal, & Ratelle, 2008; Reeve, 2006). In particular, information that gives structure to teacher's expectations and feedbacks to students is crucial for building self-confidence.

Families and schools are closely conditioned in their educational practices by commercial pressure. However, policies on regulating advertising and media products to children have been debated for decades, but without finding a convincing approach. Recognizing that advertising and media products are only potentially harmful to children, since the mediating role of parenting with children has been acknowledged as crucial, provides an easy escape from an awkward issue for governments. A guideline for a convincing approach may be derived from applying the informational role required of autonomy-supporting actions to advertising and media products. Scientific research should aid understanding of the extent to which advertising and media products exert control by diverting children's attention from the real content of the product advertised to sensation enjoyment. This should be the basis for both regulatory norms and proper information to parents (Gentile et al., 2007). This guideline, however imprecise, is distant from the current practice, which tends to divert even the parents' attention (Wooten, 2003).

The line of intervention in favor of adults should point to the aggravating socio-economic causes underlying the lack of their autonomy. The primary cause seems to be insecurity, which may stem from the labor market, and from society at large.

One of the strongest results of happiness economics is that the unemployed suffer much more than a loss of earnings (Clark & Oswald, 1994; Di Tella, McCulloch, & Oswald, 2003); a further result is that this effect persists, at least to some extent, even after reemployment (Clark et al., 2004; Di Tella et al., 2007). These results can be read as indicating an erosion of personal autonomy due to insecurity, because unemployment is evidently an involuntary condition for both income insecurity and identity insecurity in the social context. Economic policy should thus pay particular attention to unemployment even in the short run.

But autonomy can also be eroded in the workplace if social and technological conditions exert a control on workers under the threat of unemployment. A policy that directly influences personnel management is hardly appropriate, but motivational research can do the job by making evident that more autonomous employees

---

[18] A study has even found that the locus of causality measured on the Rotter scale in the USA persists from parents to offspring, and influences earnings in a significant way (Osborne, 2005).

can be both more satisfied and more productive (Pugno & Depedri, 2010). In particular, self-determination theory shows that personal motivation and psychological needs satisfaction are associated with job self-commitment and positive job attitude (Baard, Deci, & Ryan, 2004; Lam & Gurland, 2008; Vansteenkiste et al., 2007). An interesting outcome of self-determination seems to be also creativity (Sheldon, 1995). Therefore, productive organizations may properly design job tasks, compensation system, and interpersonal relations in order to enhance employees' participation and empowerment (Gagné & Forest, 2008).

Insecurity in society generally derives from the scarcity of a key ingredient in social life, namely generalized trust. This can be distinguished from strategic trust, since it is a primary attitude or a preference, usually formed in the family, while strategic trust arises from information about specific others accumulated from past experience (Fehr, 2009; Uslaner, 2002, 2008). The segregation of social minorities and corruption are typical phenomena that reveal a lack of generalized trust vis-à-vis the possible consolidation of strategic trust within groups. Policies against segregation and corruption, and for universality and legality, are obviously to be welcomed. Several economists and international organizations recommend strengthening the role of institutions in the economy precisely to develop trust and relax social constraints, e.g. through coordinating actions (World Bank, 2001). It should be added, however, that a certain amount of generalized trust is necessary for the effective working of institutions, so that once again crucial is the role of the family (Uslaner, 2002).[19]

In conclusion, recognizing the importance of people's autonomy for well-being from the decision-making perspective yields policy implications which shed new light on how to close the gap between economic growth and people's well-being. In particular, it seems more effective for enduring well-being to create the conditions for people to improve their autonomy, rather than directly targeting policy on their happiness, or even simply income. Targeting income growth, in fact, may have negative feedbacks, whereas personal autonomy ensures both well-being and favorable conditions for economic growth, through motivation for personal growth and trust in others.

References

Ainsworth, M. D. S., Blehar, M. C., Waters, E., & Wall, S. (1978). *Patterns of attachments*. Hillsdale, NJ: Erlbaum.
Alesina, A., Glaeser, E. L., & Sacerdote, B. (2005). *Work and leisure in the U.S. and Europe: Why so different?* (NBER Working Papers 11278). Cambridge, MA: National Bureau of Economic Research, Inc.
Alkire, S. (2008). Subjective measures of agency. In L. Bruni, F. Comim, & M. Pugno (Eds.), *Capabilities and happiness* (pp. 254–285). Oxford: Oxford University Press.

---

[19]For example, a study on the introduction of an apparently desirable though intrusive norm in familiar relationship, like mandatory arrest for domestic violence in some states of the USA, have had a perverse effect (Iyengar, 2009).

Amato, P. R., Johnson, D. R., & Booth, A. (2003). Continuity and change in marital quality between 1980 and 2000. *Journal of Marriage & Family*, 65(1), 1–22.
Anderson, C. A., & Bushman, B. J. (2001). Effects of violent video games on aggressive behavior, aggressive cognition, aggressive affect, physiological arousal and prosocial behavior: A meta-analysis. *Psychological Science*, 12, 353–359.
Antoci, A., Sacco, P., & Vanin, P. (2007). Participation, growth and social poverty: Social capital in a homogeneous society. *Open Economics Journal*, 1, 1–13.
Antoci, A., Sacco, P., & Vanin, P. (2008). Social capital accumulation and the evolution of social participation. *Journal of Socio-Economics*, 36, 128–143.
Assor, A., Roth, G., & Deci, E. L. (2004). The emotional costs of perceived parental conditional regard. *Journal of Personality*, 72, 47–87.
Baard, P. P., Deci, E. L., & Ryan, R. M. (2004). Intrinsic need satisfaction: A motivational basis of performance and well-being in two work settings. *Journal of Applied Social Psychology*, 34, 2045–2068.
Barrington-Leight, C. P., & Helliwell, J. F. (2008). *Empathy and emulation* (NBER Working Paper 14593). Cambridge, MA: National Bureau of Economic Research, Inc.
Bartolini, S., Bilancini, E., & Pugno, M. (2008). *Did the decline in social capital depress Americans' happiness?* Quaderni del Dipartimento di Economia Politica, n. 540, University of Siena.
Bartolini, S., & Bonatti, L. (2002). Environmental and social degradation as the engine of economic growth. *Ecological Economics*, 41, 1–16.
Bartolini, S., & Bonatti, L. (2006). The mobilization of human resources as an effect of the depletion of environmental and social assets. *Metroeconomica*, 57, 193–213.
Bartolini, S., & Bonatti, L. (2008). How can the decline in social capital be reconciled with a satisfactory growth performance? *Journal of Socio-Economics*, 37, 1539–1553.
Baumeister, R. F., & Leary, M. R. (1995). The need to belong: Desire for interpersonal attachments as a fundamental human motivation. *Psychological Bulletin*, 117(3), 497–529.
Baumol, W. J. (1967). Macroeconomics of unbalanced growth. *American Economic Review*, 57, 415–426.
Bell, L., & Freeman, R. B. (2001). The incentive for working hard. *Labor Economics*, 8(2), 181–202.
Berlinski, S., Galiani, G., & Gertler, P. (2009). The effect of pre-primary education on primary school performance. *Journal of Public Economics*, 93, 219–234.
Berlinski, S., Galiani, G., & Manacorda, M. (2008). Giving children a better start: Preschool attendance and school-age profiles. *Journal of Public Economics*, 92, 1416–1440.
Bhattacharya, S., & Munasib, A. (2007). *Can too much TV ground you for life?* Television and child outcomes, mimeo (available at http://ssrn.com/abstract=983825)
Björntorp, P. (2001). Do stress reactions cause abdominal obesity and comorbidities? *Obesity Reviews*, 2, 73–86.
Bjørnskov, C. (2008). Social capital and happiness in the United States. *Applied Research Quality Life*, 3, 43–62.
Blanchard, O. (2005). *Macroeconomics*. Upper Saddle River, NJ: Prentice Hall.
Blanchflower, D. G., & Oswald, A. J. (1999). Well-being, insecurity and the decline of American job satisfaction. Darmouth College, Usa, and Warwick University, UK. Mimeo.
Blanchflower, D. G., & Oswald, A. J. (2000). In Blanchflower, D. G., and Freeman R. B. (Eds.) The rising well-being of the young. In *Youth Employment and Joblessness in Advanced Countries* (pp. 289–328). Chicago/London: University of Chicago Press.
Blanchflower, D. G., & Oswald, A. J. (2004). Well-being over time in Britain and the US. *Journal of Public Economics*, 88(7–8), 1359–1386.
Blanchflower, D. G., & Oswald, A. J. (2008). Hypertension and happiness across nations. *Journal of Health Economics*, 27(2), 218–233.
Blanchflower, D. G., Oswald, A. J., & Van Landeghem, B. (2008). Imitative obesity and relative utility. *Journal of the European Economic Association*, 7(2–3), 528–538.

Blomeyer, D., Coneus, K., Laucht, M., & Pfeiffer, F. (2008). *Self-productivity and complementarities in human development* (IZA Discussion Papers No. 3734 available at http://ftp.iza.org/dp3734.pdf).

Borghans, L., Duckworth, A. L., Heckman, J. J., & ter Weel, B. (2008). *The economics and psychology of personality traits* (NBER Working Paper 13810). Cambridge, MA: National Bureau of Economic Research, Inc.

Borghesi, S., & Vercelli, A. (2003). Sustainable globalisation. *Ecological Economics, 44*(1), 77–89.

Bowlby, J. (1969). *Attachment and loss*. New York: Basic Books.

Brickman, P., Coates, D., & Janoff-Bulman, R. (1978). Lottery winners and accidents victims. *Journal of Personality and Social Psychology, 36*, 917–927.

Brown, K. W., & Ryan, R. M. (2003). The benefits of being present: Mindfulness and its role in psychological well-being. *Journal Of Personality and Social Psychology, 84*, 822–848.

Brown, K. W., Kasser, T., Ryan, R. M., Linley, P. A., & Orzech, K. (2009). When what one has is enough. *Journal of Research in Personality, 43*, 727–736.

Brunello, G., Michaud, P. C., & Sanz-de-Galdeano, A. (2009). The rise of obesity in Europe: An economic perspective. *Economic Policy, 24*(59), 551–596.

Bruni, L. (2005). *Hic sunt leones*: Interpersonal relations as unexplored territory in the tradition of economics. In B. Gui & R. Sugden (Eds.), *Economics and social interaction* (pp. 206–228). Cambridge: Cambridge University Press.

Bruni, L., Comim, F., Pugno, M. (Eds.). (2008). *Capabilities and happiness*. Oxford: Oxford University Press.

Bruni, L., & Stanca, L.. (2008). Watching alone: Happiness, relational goods and television. *Journal of Economic Behavior and Organization, 65*(3–4), 506–528.

Buijzen, M., & Valkenburg, P. M. (2003). The unintended effects of television advertising. *Communication Research, 30*(5), 483–503.

Buijzen, M., & Valkenburg, P. M. (2005). Parental mediation of undesired advertising effects. *Journal of Broadcasting & Electronic Media, 49*(2), 153–165.

Buijzen, M., van der Molen, J. H. W., & Sondij, P. (2007). Parental mediation of children's emotional responses to a violent news event. *Communication Research, 34*(2), 212–230.

Carnagey, N. L., Anderson, C. A., & Bushman, B. J. (2007). The effect of video game violence on physiological desensitization to real-life violence. *Journal of Experimental Social Psychology, 43*, 489–496.

Cascio, E. U. (2009). *Do investments in universal early education pay off?* (NBER Working Paper No. 14951 available at http://www.nber.org/papers/w14951).

Cawley, J. (2004). The impact of obesity on wages. *Journal of Human Resources, 39*, 451–474.

Cawley, J., & Spiess, C. K. (2008). *Obesity and developmental functioning among children aged 2–4 years*. (Discussion paper). DIW Berlin 786 http://www.diw.de/documents/publikationen/73/82383/dp786.pdf.

CDC. *Vital statistics*. Available from http://www.cdc.gov/nchs/data/hus/hus09.pdf#026. Accessed 3 October 2010.

Chamberlain, L. J., Wang, Y., & Robinson, T. N. (2006). Does children's screen time predict requests for advertised products? *Stanford University Archives of Pediatrics & Adolescent Medicine, 160*(4), 363–368.

Chishti, P., Stone, D. H., Corcoran, P., Williamson, E., & Petridou, E. (2003). Suicide mortality in the European Union. *European Journal of Public Health, 13*, 108–114.

Clark, A. E., Frijters, P., & Shields, M. (2008). Relative income, happiness and utility: An explanation for the Easterlin paradox and other puzzles. *Journal of Economic Literature, 46*(1), 95–144.

Clark, A. E., Georgellis, Y., Lucas, R. E., & Diener, E. (2004). Unemployment alters the set-point for life satisfaction. *Psychological Science, 15*(1), 8–13.

Clark, A. E., & Oswald, A. J. (1994). Happiness and unemployment. *Economic Journal, 104*(424), 648–659.

Clark, A. E., & Oswald, A. J. (2002). Well-being in panels, available at http://www2.warwick.ac.uk/fac/soc/economics/staff/academic/oswald/revwellbeinginpanelsclarkosdec2002.pdf. mimeo.

Collishaw, S., Maughan, B., & Goodman, R. (2004). Time trend in adolescent mental health. *Journal of Child Psychology and Psychiatry, 45*(8), 1350–1362.

Corneo, G. (2005). Work and television. *European Journal of Political Economy, 21*, 99–113.

Costa, D. L., & Kahn, M. E. (2003). Understanding the decline in social capital, 1952–1998. *Kyklos, 56*, 17–46.

Costa, P. T., & McCrae, R. R. (1980). Influences of extraversion and neuroticism on subjective well-being. *Journal of Personality and Social Psychology, 38*, 668–678.

Crawford, D. W., Houts, R. M., Huston, T. L., & George, L. J. (2002). Compatibility, leisure, and satisfaction in marital relationships. *Journal of Marriage and Family, 64*(2), 433–449.

Cunha, F., & Heckman, J. J. (2009). *The economics and psychology of inequality and human development* (NBER Working Paper No. 14695 available at http://www.nber.org/papers/w14695).

Cunha, F., Heckman, J. J., Lochner, L. J., & Masterov, D. V. (2006). Interpreting the evidence on life cycle skill formation. In E. A. Hanusheck & F. Welch (Eds.), *Handbook of the economics of education* (pp. 697–812). Amsterdam: North-Holland.

Cutler, D. M., Glaeser, E. L., & Norberg, K. E. (2001). *Explaining the rise in youth suicide*. In J. Gruber (Ed.), Risky behavior among youths (pp. 219–270). Chicago: Chicago University Press.

Cutler, D. M., Glaeser, E. L., & Shapiro, J. M. (2003). Why have Americans become more obese? *Journal of Economic Perspectives, 17*(3), 93–118.

Deaton, A. (2002). Health, inequality, and economic development. *Journal of Economic Literature, 41*, 113–158.

Deaton, A. (2008). Income, health and well-being around the world: Evidence from the Gallup World Poll. *Journal of Economic Perspectives, 22*(2), 53–72.

Deci, E. L., & Ryan, R. M.. (1985). *Intrinsic motivation and self-determination in human behavior*. New York: Plenum Press.

Deci, E. L., & Ryan, R. M. (2000). The "what" and "why" of goal pursuits: Human needs and the self-determination of behavior. *Psychological Inquiry, 11*, 227–268.

Di Tella, R., Haisken-De New, J., & McCulloch, R. J. (2007). *Happiness adaptation to income and to status in an individual panel* (NBER Working Paper No. 13159 available at http://www.nber.org/papers/w13159).

Di Tella, R., & McCulloch, R. J. (2008). Gross national happiness as an answer to the Easterlin Paradox? *Journal of Development Economics, 86*, 22–42.

Di Tella, R., McCulloch, R. J., & Oswald, A. J. (2003). The macroeconomics of happiness. *Review of Economics and Statistics, 85*(4), 809–827.

Diener, E., & Lucas, R. E. (1999). Explaining differences in societal levels of happiness. *Journal of Happiness Studies, 1*, 41–78.

Downs, J. S., Loewenstein, G., & Wisdom, J. (2009). Strategies for promoting healthier food choices. *American Economic Review: P&P, 99*(2), 1–10.

Easterlin, R. A. (1974). Does economic growth improve the human lot? Some empirical evidence. In P. A. David, W. R. Melvin (Eds.), *Nations and households in economic growth* (pp. 89–125). New York: Academic Press.

Easterlin, R. A. (1995). Will raising the incomes of all increase the happiness of all? *Journal of Economic Behavior & Organization, 27*(1), 35–47.

Easterlin, R. A. (2001). Income and happiness: Towards a unified theory. *The Economic Journal, 111*(473), 465–484.

Easterlin, R. A. (2005a). Diminishing marginal utility of income? Caveat Emptor. *Social Indicators Research, 70*, 243–255.

Easterlin, R. A. (2005b). Building a better theory of well-being. In L. Bruni & P. Porta (Eds.), *Economics and happiness* (pp. 29–64). Oxford: Oxford University Press.

Easterlin, R. A., & Angelescu, L. (2009, March). *Happiness and growth the world over: Time series evidence on the happiness-income paradox* (IZA Discussion Paper No. 4060).

Easterlin, R. A., & Crimmins, E. M. (1991). Private materialism, personal self-fulfillment, family life, and public interest. *Public Opinion Quarterly, 55*(4), 499–533.

Eckersley, R., & Dear, K. (2002). Cultural correlates of youth suicide. *Social Science & Medicine, 55,* 1891–1904.

Ekman, P., Davidson, R., & Friesen, W. (1990). The Duchenne smile: Emotional expression and brain physiology II. *Journal of Personality and Social Psychology, 58,* 342–353.

Fajnzylber, P., Lederman, D., & Loayza, N. (2000). Crime and victimization: An economic perspective. *Economía, 1,* 219–278.

Fehr, E. (2009). *On the economics and biology of trust. Journal of the European Economic Association, 7*(2–3), 235–266.

Ferguson, C. J. (2007). Evidence for publication bias in video game violence effects literature: A meta-analytic review. *Aggression and Violent Behavior, 12,* 470–482.

Ferrer-i-Carbonell, A. (2005). Income and well-being: An empirical analysis of the comparison income effect. *Journal of Public Economics, 89,* 997–1019.

Ferrer-i-Carbonell, A., & Van Praag, B. M. S. (2008). *Do people adapt to changes in income and other circumstances*? mimeo available at http://ferrer.iae-csic.org/Adaptation&IncomeChanges.pdf

Fombonne, E., Simmons, H., Meltzer, H., & Goodman, R. (2003). Prevalence of pervasive developmental disorders in the British national wide survey of child mental heath. *International Review of Psychiatry, 15*(1–2), 158–165.

Ford, M. T., Heinen, B. E., & Langkamer, K. L. (2007). Work and family satisfaction and conflict: A meta-analysis of cross-domain relations. *Journal of Applied Psychology, 92*(1), 57–80.

Frank, R. H. (1999). *Luxury fever*. New York: The Free Press.

Frank, R. G., & Meara, E. (2009). *The effect of maternal depression and substance abuse on child human capital development* (NBER Working Paper No. 15314).

Frederick, S., & Loewenstein, G. (1999). Hedonic adaptation. In D. Kahneman, E. Diener, N. Schwarz (Eds.), *Well-being: The foundations of hedonic Psychology* (pp. 302–329). New York: Russell Sage Foundation.

Frey, B., & Stutzer, A.. (2001). Maximizing happiness? *German Economic Review, 1*(2), S. 145–167.

Frey, B., & Stutzer, A. (2006). Does marriage make people happy, or do happy people get married? *Journal of Socio-Economics, 35,* 326–347.

Gagné, M., & Forest, J.. (2008). The study of compensation systems through the lens of self-determination theory. *Canadian Psychology, 49*(3), 225–232.

Gardner, J., & Oswald, A. J. (2007). Money and mental wellbeing. *Journal of Health Economics, 26*(1), 49–60.

Gentile, D. A., Saleem, M., & Anderson, C. A. (2007). Public policy and the effects of media violence on children. *Social Issues and Policy Review, 1,* 15–61.

Glenn, N., & Weaver, C. N. (1998). The changing relationship of marital status to reported happiness. *Journal of Marriage and the Family, 50*(2), 317–324.

Gopnik, A., Meltzoff, A. N., & Kuhl, P. K. (2000). *The scientist in the crib: What early learning tells us about the mind*. New York: HarperCollins.

Graham, C., & Pettinato, S. (2002). *Happiness and hardship*. Washington, DC: The Brookings Institution.

Green, F. (2007). *Demanding work. The paradox of job quality in the affluent economy*. Princeton, NJ: Princeton University Press.

Green, F., & Gallie, D. (2002), *High skills and high anxiety: Skills, hard work and mental well-being*, Oxford & Warwick Universities, SKOPE research paper no. 27. Available at http://www.skope.ox.ac.uk/sites/default/files/SKOPEWP27.pdf

Green, F., & Tsitsianis, N. (2005). An investigation of national trends in job satisfaction in Britain and Germany. *British Journal of Industrial Relations, 43*(3), 401–430.

Gronlick, W. S. (2003). *The psychology of parental control*. Mahwah, NJ: Taylor & Francis.

Grönlund, A. (2007). More control, less conflict? Job demand-control, gender and work-family conflict gender. *Work and Organization, 14*(5), 476–497.

Guay, F., Chanal, J., & Ratelle, C. F. (2008). Optimal learning in optimal contexts: The role of self-determination in education. *Canadian Psychology, 49*(3), 233–240.

Gui, B. (2005). From transactions to encounters. In B. Gui & R. Sugden (Eds.), *Economics and social interaction* (pp. 23–50). Cambridge: Cambridge University Press.

Guryan, J., Hurst, E., & Kearney, M. (2008). Parental education and parental time with children. *Journal of Economic Perspectives, 22*(3), 23–46.

Hacker, J. S. (2006). *The great risk shift.* New York: Oxford University Press.

Heckman, J. J. (2008). School, skills, and synapses. Economic Inquiry, *46*(3), 289–492.

Helliwell, J. F. (2006). Well-being, social capital and public policy: What's new? *The Economic Journal, 116*(510), C34–C45.

Helliwell, J. F. (2007). Well-being and social capital: Does suicide pose a puzzle? *Social Indicators Research, 81*, 455–496.

Helliwell, J. F., Barringon-Leigh, C. P., Harris, A., & Huang, H. (2009). *International evidence on the social context of well-being* (NBER Working Paper No. 14720 available at http://www.nber.org/papers/w14720).

Hertzenberg, S. A., Alic, J. A., & Wial, H.. (1998). *New rules for a new economy: Employment and opportunity in postindustrial America.* Ithaca, NY: Cornell University Press.

Hirsch, F. (1976). *Social limits to growth.* Cambridge, MA: Harvard University Press.

Hodiamont, P. P. G., Rijnders, C. A. T., Mulder, J., & Furer, J. W. (2005). Psychiatric disorders in a Dutch health area: A repeated cross-sectional survey. *Journal of Affective Disorders, 84*(1), 77–83.

Huang, W. C. (1996). Religion, culture, economic and sociological correlates of suicide rates. *Applied Economics Letters, 3*, 779–782.

Huang, F. (2006, February 28). *Child development production functions.* Singapore: Singapore Management University.

Huppert, F. A. (2005). Positive mental health in individuals and populations. In F. A. Huppert, B. Keverne, N. Baylis (Eds.), *The science of well-being* (pp. 306–340). Oxford: Oxford University Press.

Iyengar, R. (2009). Does the certainty of arrest reduce domestic violence? *Journal of Public Economics, 93*, 85–98.

Jagannathan, R., Kapoor, M., & Schaumburg, E. (2009). *Why are we in a recession?* (NBER Working Papers No. 15404). Cambridge, MA: National Bureau of Economic Research, Inc.

Jungeilges, J., & Kirchgaessner, G. (2002). Economic welfare, civil liberty, and suicide. *Journal of Socio-economics, 31*, 215–231.

Jäntti, M., Røed, K., Naylor, R., Björklund, A., Bratsberg, B., Raaum, O., et al. (2006). *American exceptionalism in a new light: A comparison of intergenerational earnings mobility in the Nordic countries, the UK and the US* (ZA Discussion Paper No. 1938).

Kahneman, D., Wakker, P. P., & Sarin, R. (1997). Back to Bentham? Explorations of experienced utility. *Quarterly Journal of Economics, 112*, 375–405.

Kamp Dush, C. M., Cohan, C. L., & Amato, P. R. (2003). The relationship between cohabitation and marital quality and stability: Change across cohorts? *Journal of Marriage and Family, 65*(3), 539–549.

Karoly, L. A., Kilburn, M. R., & Cannon, J. S. (2003). Early childhood interventions: Proven results, future promises. *Rand labor and population* (Available at http://www.rand.org/pubs/monographs/MG341/)

Kashdan, T. B., & Breen, W. E.. (2007). Materialism and diminished well-being: Experiential avoidance as a mediating mechanism. *Journal of Social & Clinical Psychology, 26*(5), 521–539.

Kasser, T. (2002). *The high price of materialism.* Cambridge, MA: MIT Press.

Kasser, T., Cohn, S., Kanner, A. D., & Ryan, R. M. (2007). Some costs of American Corporate Capitalism: A psychological exploration of value and goal conflicts. *Psychological Inquiry, 18*, 1–22.

Kasser, T., Ryan, R. M., Couchman, C. E., & Sheldon, K. M. (2004). Materialistic values. In T. Kasser & A. D. Kanner (Eds.), *Psychology and consumer culture* (pp. 11–28). Washington, DC: American Psychological Association.

Kasser, T., Ryan, R. M., Zax, M., & Sameroff, A. J. (1995). The relations of maternal and social environment to adolescents' materialistic and prosocial values. *Developmental Psychology, 31*, 907–914.

Katsaiti, M.-S. (2009). *Obesity and happiness* (Working papers 2009-44). Connecticut: University of Connecticut, Department of Economics.

Kawachi, I., Kennedy, B. P., Lochner, K., & Prothrow-Stith, D. (1997). Social capital, income inequality and mortality. *American Journal of Public Health, 87*, 1491–1498.

Kessler, R. C., Berglund, P., Borges, G., Nock, M., & Wang, P. S. (2005). Trends in suicide ideation, plans, gestures, and attempts in the US, 1990–1992 to 2001–2003. *Journal of the American Medical Association, 293*(20), 2487–2495.

Klerman, G. L. (1988). The current age of youthful melancholia. *British Journal of Psychiatry, 152*, 4–14.

Klerman, G. L. (1993). The postwar generation and depression. In M. A. Ghadirian Abdu'l & H. E. Lehmann (Eds.), *Environment and psychopathology* (pp. 73–86). New York: Springer.

Knight, J., & Gunatilaka, R. (2009). *Income, aspirations and the hedonic Treadmill in a poor society* (Economics Series Working Papers 468). Oxford: University of Oxford, Department of Economics.

Knight, J., Song, L., & Gunatilaka, R. (2009). Subjective well-being and its determinants in rural China. *China Economic Review, 20*(4), 635–649.

Koestner, R., & Losier, G. F. (2006). Distinguishing reactive versus reflective autonomy. *Journal of Personality, 64*(2), 465–494.

Kuhn, P., & Lozano, F.. (2008). The expanding workweek? Understanding trends in long work hours among U.S. men, 1979–2006. *Journal of Labor Economics, 26*(2), 311–343.

Kyrou, I., Chrousos, G. P., & Tsigos, C. (2006). Stress, visceral obesity, and metabolic complications. *New York Academy of Sciences, 1083*(1), 77–110.

Lam, C. F., & Gurland, S. T. (2008). Self-determined work motivation predicts job outcomes, but what predicts self-determined work motivation. *Journal of Research in Personality, 42*, 1109–1115.

Lavori, P. W., Warshaw, M., Klerman, G. L., & Mueller, T. I. (1993). Secular trends in lifetime onset of MDD stratified by selected sociodemographic risk factors. *Journal of Psychiatric Research, 27*(1), 95–109.

Layard, R. (2005). *Happiness: Lessons from a new science*. New York: Penguin Press (on-line Annex available at http://cep.lse.ac.uk/layard/annex.pdf).

Layard, R., & Dunn, J. (2009). *A good childhood*. London: Penguin.

Layard, R., Mayraz, G., & Nickell, S. (2009, March). Does relative income matter? Are the critics right? (CEP Discussion Paper No. 918 available at http://cep.lse.ac.uk/pubs/download/dp0918.pdf).

Layzer, J. I., Goodson, B. D., Bernstein, L., & Price, C. (2001). *National evaluation of family support programs*. Cambridge, MA: Abt Associates Inc.

Lester, D., & Yang, B. (1997). *The economy and suicide*. Commack, NY: Nova Science.

Levi, F., La Vecchia, C., & Saraceno, B. (2003). Global suicide rates. *European Journal of Public Health, 13*, 97–98.

Lucas, R. E., Clark, A. E., Georgellis, Y., & Diener, E. (2003). Reexamining adaptation and the set point model of happiness. *Journal of Personality and Social Psychology, 84*(3), 527–539.

Luthar, S. S. (2003). The culture of affluence. *Child Development, 74*(6), 1581–1593.

Luttmer, E. F. P. (2005). Neighbors as negatives; relative earnings and well-being. *Quarterly Journal of Economics, August, 120*(3), 923–1002.

Maughan, B., Iervolino, A. C., & Collishaw, S. (2005). Time trends in child and adolescent mental disorders. *Current Opinion in Psychiatry, 18*(4), 381–385.

McEwen, B. S. (1998). Protective and damaging effects of stress mediators. *New England Journal of Medicine, 338*, 171–179.

McFadden, D. (1999). Rationality for economists? *Journal of risks and uncertainty, 19*, 73–105.
McKeown, R. E., Cuffe, S. P., & Schulz, R. M. (2006). US suicide rates by age group, 1970–2002: An examination of recent trends. *American Journal of Public Health, 96*, 1744–1751.
McPherson, M., Smith-Lovin, L., & Brashears, M. E. (2006, June). Social isolation in America: Changes in core discussion networks over two decades. *American Sociological Review, 71*, 353–375.
Mellor, J. M., & Milyo, J. (2001). Reexamining the evidence of an ecological association between income inequality and health. *Journal of Health, Politics, Policy, Law, 26*, 487–522.
Merrick, J., Kandel, I., & Vardi, G. (2003). Trends in adolescent violence. *International Journal of Adolescent Medicine and Health, 15*(3), 285–287.
Michalos, A. C. (1985). Multiple discrepancies theory. *Social Indicator Research, 16*, 347–413.
Mihalopoulos, C., Sanders, M. R., Turner, K. M. T., Murphy-Brennan, M., & Carter, R. (2007). Does the triple P-Positive Parenting Program provide value for money? *Australian and New Zealand Journal of Psychiatry, 41*(3), 239–246.
Miringoff, M., & Opdyke, S. (2008). *America's social health*. Armonk, NY: M.E. Sharpe.
Mishel, L., Bernstein, J., & Schmitt, J. (1999). *The state of working America 1998–1999*. Ithaca, NY: Cornell University Press.
Mojon-Azzi, S., & Sousa-Poza, A. (2007). *Hypertension and life satisfaction: A comment and replication of Blanchflower and Oswald* (Working Paper Series, 44). Switzerland: University of St. Gallen, Department of Economics.
Moran, P., Ghate, D., & van der Merwe, A. (2004). *What works in parenting support? A review of the international evidence* (Research Report RR574). London: Department for Education and Skills, Policy Research Bureau.
Nussbaum, M. (2000). *Women and human development*. Cambridge: Cambridge University Press.
Nussbaum, M. (2003). Capabilities as fundamental entitlements: Sen and social justice. *Feminist Economics, 9*(2–3), 33–59.
OECD. (2008). *Growing unequal? Income distribution and poverty in OECD countries*. Paris: Author.
Offer, A. (2006). *The challenge of affluence*. Oxford: Oxford University Press.
Olfson, M., Marcus, S. C., Weissman, M. M., Jensen, P. S., & Peter, S. (2002). National trends in the use of psychotropic medications by children. *Journal of the American Academy of Child and Adolescent Psychiatry, 41*(5), 514–521.
Osborne. (2005). Personality and the intergenerational transmission of economic status. In S. Bowles, H. Gintis, M. Osborne Groves (Eds.), *Unequal chances* (pp. 208–230). Princeton, NJ: Princeton University Press.
Ostchega, Y., Dillon, C. F., Hughes, J. P., Carroll, M., & Yoon, S. (2007). Trends in hypertension prevalence, awareness, treatment, and control in older U.S. adults: Data from the National Health and Nutrition Examination Survey 1988 to 2004. *Journal of the American Geriatrics Society, 55*(7), 1056–1065.
Oswald, A. J., & Powdthavee, N. (2007). Obesity, unhappiness, and the challenge of affluence: Theory and evidence. *Economic Journal, 117*(521), 441–454.
Paxton, P. (1999). Is social capital declining in the US? *American Journal of Sociology, 105*(1), 88–127.
Pichler, F. (2006). Subjective quality of life of young Europeans. Feeling happy but who knows why? *Social Indicators Research, 75*, 419–444.
Polanyi, K. (1968). *The great transformation*. Boston: Beacon.
Pritchard, C., & Butler, A. (2003). A comparative study of children and adult homicide rates in the US and the major Western countries 1974–1999. *Journal of Family Violence, 18*(6), 341–350.
Pryor, J. H., Hurtado, S., Sharkness, J., & Korn, W. S. (2007). *The American freshmen: National norms*. Los Angeles: HERI.
Pugno, M. (2008a). Capabilities, the self, and well-being. In L. Bruni, F. Comim, M. Pugno (Eds.), *Capabilities and happiness* (pp. 224–253). Oxford: Oxford University Press.

Pugno, M. (2008b). Economics and the self. A formalisation of self-determination theory. *Journal of Socio-Economics, 37*, 1328–1346.

Pugno, M.. (2009). The Easterlin paradox and the decline of social capital: An integrated explanation. *Journal of Socio-Economics, 38*(4), 590–600.

Pugno, M., & Depedri, S.. (2010). Job performance and job satisfaction: An integrated survey. *Economia Politica-Journal of Analytical and Institutional Economics, 26*(1), 139–174.

Putnam, R. D.. (2000). *Bowling alone*. New York: Simon & Schuster.

Reeve, J.. (2006). Teachers as facilitators. *The Elementary School Journal, 106*(3), 225–236.

Robinson, R. V., & Jackson, E. F.. (2001). Is trust in others declining in America? *Social Science Research, 30*, 117–145.

Robinson, T. N., Saphir, M. N., Kraemer, H. C., Varady, A., & Haydel, K. F.. (2001). Effects of reducing television viewing on children's requests for toys. *Journal of Developmental and Behavioral Pediatrics, 3*(22), 179–184.

Rogers, S. J., & Amato, P. R.. (1997). Is marital quality declining? *Social Forces, 75*, 1089–1100.

Roth, G., Assor, A., Niemiec, C. P., Ryan, R. M., & Deci, E. L.. (2009). The emotional and academic consequences of parental conditional regard. *Developmental Psychology, 45*, 1119–1142.

Routledge, B., & von Amsberg, J.. (2003). Social capital and growth. *Journal of Monetary Economics, 50*(1), 167–193.

Rutter, M., & Smith, D. J. (Eds.). (1995). *Psychosocial disorders in young people*. Chichester: Wiley.

Ryan, R. M., & Brown, K. W.. (2003). Why we don't need self-esteem. *Psychological Inquiry, 14*(1), 71–82.

Ryan, R. M., & Deci, E. L.. (2001). On happiness and human potentials. *Annual Review of Psychology, 52*, 141–166.

Ryan, R. M., & Deci, E. L.. (2006). Self-regulation and the problem of human autonomy? *Journal of Personality, 74*(6), 1557–1585.

Ryan, R. M., Huta, V., & Deci, E. L.. (2008). Living well: A self-determination theory perspective on eudaimonia. *Journal of Happiness Studies, 9*, 139–170.

Ryff, C. D., & Singer, B. H.. (1998). The contours of positive human health. *Psychological Inquiry, 9*(1), 1–28.

Sacker, A., & Wiggins, R. D.. (2002). Age-period-cohort effects on inequalities in psychological distress. *Psychological Medicine, 32*, 977–990.

Saffer, H., & Lamiraud, K. (2008). *The effects of hours of work on social interaction* (NBER working paper No. 13743 available at http://www.nber.org/papers/w13743).

Sandvik, E., Diener, E., & Seidlitz, L.. (1993). Subjective well-being: The convergence and stability of self and non self report measures. *Journal of Personality, 61*, 317–342.

Sansone, C., & Harackiewicz, J. M. (Eds.). (2000). *Intrinsic and extrinsic motivation*. San Diego, CA: Academic Press.

Sapolsky, R. M. (1993). Endocrinology alfresco. *Recent Progress in Hormone Research, 48*, 437–468.

Sarracino, F. (2009). *Social capital and subjective well-being trends: Evidence from 11 European countries* (Quaderni del Dipartimento di Economia Politica No. 558). Siena: University of Siena, Department of Economics.

Savage, J.. (2004). Does viewing violent media really cause criminal violence? A methodological review. *Aggression and Violent Behavior, 10*, 99–128.

Schmitt, N. M., Wagner, N., & Kirch, W. (2007). Consumers' freedom of choice. *Journal of Public Health, 15*(1), 943–1853.

Schor, J.. (1998). *The overspent American*. New York: Basic Books.

Schor, J. (2004). *Born to buy*. New York: Scribner.

Scitovsky, T. (1976). *The joyless economy*. New York: Oxford University Press.

Sen, A. (1985). *Commodities and capabilities*. Oxford: Oxford University Press.

Sen, A. (1999a). *Development as freedom*. New York: Knopf.
Sen, A. (1999b). *Reason before identity*. New Delhi: Oxford University Press.
Senik, C. (2008). Is man doomed to progress? *Journal of Economic Behavior & Organization*, 68(1), 140–152.
Senik, C. (2009). *Income distribution and subjective happiness. A survey* (OECD Social Employment and Migration Working Papers No. 96 OECD Publishing. doi: 10.1787/218860720683).
Shedler, J., Mayman, M., & Manis, M. (1993). The illusion of mental health. *American Psychologist*, 48(11), 1117–1131.
Sheldon, K. M.. (1995). Creativity and self-determination in personality. *Creativity Research Journal*, 8(1), 25–36.
Sheldon, K. M., & Lyubomirsky, S.. (2009). Change your actions, not your circumstances: An experimental test of the Sustainable Happiness model. In A. K. Dutt & B. Radcliff (Eds.), *Happiness, economics, and politics: Towards a multi-disciplinary approach* (pp. 324–342). Cheltenham: Elgar.
Siegel, D. J.. (2001). Toward an interpersonal neurobiology of the developing mind. *Infant Mental Health Journal*, 22(1–2), 67–94.
Soenens, B., Vansteenkiste, M., Duriez, B., & Goossens, L.. (2006). In search of the sources of psychologically controlling parenting. *Journal of Research on Adolescence*, 16(4), 539–559.
Stevenson, B., & Wolfers, J. (2008, May). Economic growth and happiness. *Brookings Papers on Economic Activity*.
Stiglitz, S., Sen, A., & Fitoussi, J. P. (2009). *Report by the Commission on the Measurement of Economic Performance and Social Progress*, www.stiglitz-sen-fitoussi.fr/documents/rapport_anglais.pdf
Stutzer, A.. (2004). The role of income aspirations in individual happiness. *Journal of Economic Behaviour and Organization*, 54(1), 89–109.
Stutzer, A. (2007). *Limited self-control, obesity and the loss of happiness* (IZA Discussion Paper No. 2925 available at http://ftp.iza.org/dp2925.pdf).
Sugden, R. (2007, June 14–17). *Is happiness a matter for governments? A comparison of the utilitarianisms of Richard Layard and John Stuart Mill*. Paper presented at the Conference on Policies for Happiness, Siena.
Sutton, S. K., & Davidson, R. J.. (1997). Prefrontal brain asymmetry: A biological substrate of the behavioral approach and inhibition systems. *Psychological Science*, 8(3), 204–210.
Sweeting, H., Young, R., & West, P.. (2009). GHQ increases among Scottish 15 year olds 1987–2006. *Social Psychiatry & Psychiatric Epidemiology*, 44(7), 579–586.
Sylva, K., Melhuish, E., Sammons, P., Siraj-Blatchford, I., & Taggart., B.. (2010). *Early childhood matters*. London: Routledge.
Twenge, J. M. (2000). The age of anxiety? The birth cohort change in anxiety and neuroticism, 1952–1993. *Journal of Personality and Social Psychology*, 79(6), 1007–1021.
Twenge, J. M., Zhang, L., & Im, C. (2004). Beyond my control: A cross-temporal meta-analysis of increasing externality in locus of control, 1960–2002. *Personality and Social Psychology Review*, 8(3), 308–319.
Uslaner, E. M.. (2002). *The moral foundations of trust*. Cambridge: Cambridge University Press.
Uslaner, E. M.. (2008). Where you stand depends upon where your grandparents sat: The inheritability of generalized trust. *Public Opinion Quarterly*, 72(4), 725–740.
Van de Stadt, H., Kapteyn, A., & de Geer, V.. (1985). The relativity of utility. *Review of Economics and Statistics*, 67, 179–187.
van Hemert, D. A., van de Vijver, F. J. R., & Poortinga, Y. H.. (2002). The beck depression inventory as a measure of subjective well-being: A cross national study. *Journal of Happiness Studies*, 3, 257–286.
Vansteenkiste, M., Neyrinck, B., Niemiec, C. P., Soenens, B., De Witte, H., & Van Den Broeck, A.. (2007). On the relations among work value orientations, psychological need satisfaction,

and job outcomes: A self-determination theory approach. *Journal of Occupational and Organizational Psychology, 80*, 251–277.

Verhaak, P. F. M., Hoeymans, N., & Westert, G. P.. (2005). Mental health in the Dutch population and in general practice: 1987–2001. *British Journal of General Practice, 55*(519), 770–775.

Verme, P.. (2009). Happiness, freedom and control. *Journal of Economic Behavior & Organization, 71*(2), 146–161.

Weintraub, A. E.. (2000). The role of interpretation processes and parental discussion in the media's effects on adolescents' use of alcohol. *Pediatrics, 105*(2), 343–349.

Wilkinson, R. G.. (2005). *The impact of inequality*. New York: Routledge.

Williams, G. C., Cox, E. M., Hedberg, V. A., & Deci, E. L.. (2000). Extrinsic life goals and health risk behaviors in adolescents. *Journal of Applied Social Psychology, 30*, 1756–1771.

Wisman, J. D., & Capehart, K. (2010). *Creative destruction, economic insecurity, stress and epidemic obesity*. American Journal of Economics and Sociology, *69*, 936–982.

Wooten, M. G.. (2003). Pestering parents. *Social Policy Report, 20*(2), 3–17.

World Bank. (2001). *Understanding and measuring social capital* (Working Paper No. 24). World Bank: Washington.

Zimmermann, A. C., & Easterlin, R. A.. (2006). Happily ever after? Cohabitation, marriage, divorce, and happiness in Germany. *Population and Development Review, 32*(3), 511–528.

Chapter 11
The Development of Conceptions of Personal Autonomy, Rights, and Democracy, and Their Relation to Psychological Well-Being

Charles C. Helwig and Justin McNeil

Self-determination theory holds that people are rational, meaning-making agents who are self-governing (autonomous) and who exercise their autonomy and develop their competencies in relations with others. Because all individuals as seen as possessing autonomy as a universal psychological need, optimal social relations can be conceived as those which are characterized by a respect for personal autonomy, mutuality, and rationality (Ryan & Deci, 2001). This assumption of a self-governing or autonomous agent as psychologically normative has much in common with the view of the person inherent within modern philosophical theorizing about democracy, freedoms, and rights (e.g., Dworkin, 1977; Gewirth, 1978; Larmore, 2008; Rawls, 1971; Sen, 1999). Each of these contemporary moral philosophical perspectives, in different ways, postulates that human beings are agents who act in the world and pursue personal interests, and as such are the moral bearers of rights and freedoms. At the same time, as social beings, people are entitled to equal respect in their mutual relations with one another and with the social institutions in which they participate. Social relationships of mutual respect and reciprocity are thus seen as fostering the development of autonomy, and individual needs for autonomy correspondingly place limits on the forms of social organization that are seen as just (Nussbaum, 2000). Democratic social forms that are non-coercive and that permit individuals to develop their own spheres of personal choice and to have a say in how things are run are argued to be both more just and more promoting of psychological well-being than are social forms that are coercive, that intrude on spheres of personal choice and autonomy, or that fail to provide individuals with a voice in decisions that affect them (Sen, 1999).

Perhaps partly as a result of these shared assumptions with contemporary democratic perspectives and theorizing, self-determination theory recently has been criticized for holding an allegedly "Western" or ethnocentric view of the self, and thus for failing to account for the psychology and moral perspectives of individuals throughout much of the non-Western world. For example, it has been argued

---

C.C. Helwig (✉)
Department of Psychology, University of Toronto, Toronto, ON, Canada, M5S 3G3
e-mail: helwig@psych.utoronto.ca

by some cultural psychologists that the psychology of non-Western peoples is best characterized in terms of an "interdependent self" for whom autonomy or personal choice has little or no significance (Heinrich, Heine, & Norenzayan, 2010; Markus & Kitayama, 1991). Correspondingly, in contrast to the emphasis on autonomy and rights found in the West, the thinking of non-Western peoples about social relations and morality has been characterized as "duty-based" rather than "rights-based" (Miller, 1994; Shweder, Mahapatra, & Miller, 1987), and thus focused on obedience to authority, the maintenance of social harmony, and following the group (Greenfield, Keller, Fuligni, & Maynard, 2003; Markus, 2008; Triandis, 1989).

Self-determination theory has typically approached this debate through an emphasis on the consequences for psychological functioning associated with the satisfaction or thwarting of basic needs such as autonomy in different cultural settings (e.g., Ryan & Deci, 2001). However, as Roth and Deci (2009) point out, cognition is an important foundation for autonomy as it provides the organizational structure within which basic psychological needs are experienced. Recent research within developmental psychology has examined directly the development of conceptions of personal autonomy and rights and democratic understandings in both Western and non-Western cultures, and has contributed some important findings that bear directly on these issues. In this chapter, we will examine this new and emerging research and illustrate how its findings are compatible with many of the core propositions of self-determination theory. It is hoped that, in bringing this body of recent work in developmental psychology to light to self-determination theorists, this discussion may provide the basis for a fruitful synthesis of social cognitive developmental perspectives and self-determination theory. Such a synthesis may provide a more comprehensive understanding of how psychological needs functioning and social cognition may interact in development and in different cultural settings.

Conceptions of Personal Autonomy, Freedoms, and Rights

The notion of personal freedom is one of the cornerstones of modern democratic societies (Dworkin, 1977). Personal freedom implies the demarcation of a private sphere, in which individuals may pursue their own projects or interests free from interference by others, including societal agents such as religion or the state. This private sphere is believed to assist individuals to develop as free and autonomous agents who have control of key aspects of their lives, and help them to develop their capacities as human beings (Nussbaum, 2000; Sen, 1999). Formally, within modern liberal democratic societies, personal freedom takes the form of guarantees of civil liberties and freedoms, such as free access to information, freedom of religion and belief, and rights to basic privacy and freedom of association. In addition to serving individual ends of self-development, personal autonomy is also viewed as essential for the development of civic commitment (Hart, Atkins, & Donnelly, 2006; Youniss & Yates, 1997). Democratic societies need citizens who will actively participate in society's institutions, including its political and civic organizations. Individuals who have the freedom of action to pursue their interests, to belong to diverse social organizations and groups, and who are guaranteed access to information and opportunities to discuss public policy with like-minded others are more likely to develop a sense of political agency and thereby to participate effectively in democratic social institutions as citizens.

These features of democratic theorizing and practice bear important relations to self-determination theory's core propositions about universal psychological needs. Most obvious in this context is the need for autonomy, conceptualized as individuals' need to regulate their own behavior (to be "self-determining") in accordance with their deeply held interests and values (Ryan & Deci, 2001). Autonomy, thus, is different from "independence" or self-sufficiency, and is not the opposite of relatedness, as it is often mistakenly conceived, since individuals may be either autonomously independent or autonomously related (see Kagitcibasi, 2005, for a discussion). Rather, autonomy in this perspective is conceived of as the opposite of heteronomy, or being under the authority or rule of another (Piaget, 1932). To the extent that democratic forms of social organization afford individuals the freedom to regulate their own behavior in accordance with their interests, and protect this autonomy by formal guarantees of freedoms or rights, they are more likely to be autonomy supportive than other forms of social organization that fail to protect individual autonomy and personal choice (Chirkov, 2007). Thus, when social institutions are seen as limiting individuals' autonomy, or compelling them to act in ways that they would not endorse, such restrictions or dictates would be expected to be experienced as coercive and therefore not fully internalized or endorsed.

Over the last few decades, developmental psychologists working within a perspective known as social domain theory (Turiel, 2006) have examined children's conceptions of different types of issues or "domains." One of these domains involves conceptions of "personal issues" or those issues over which people believe that they should have personal jurisdiction and control. The personal domain is theorized to be an important source of children's emerging conceptions of autonomy and is believed to aide in the construction of a unique self and identity (Nucci, 2001). Children's own conceptions of personal issues have been examined in research that asks children to consider whether a variety of different types of acts should be regulated by authorities, and to provide justifications or reasons for these judgments (Nucci & Weber, 1995; Nucci, 1981). This research has shown that even young children consider some actions (e.g., recreational pursuits, choice of friends, what they wear) as not legitimately regulated by authorities and as up to the individual to decide. In their reasoning, children appeal to personal choice, the desires or needs of individuals, and explicit references to freedoms in explaining why it would be wrong for authorities to regulate these acts (e.g., "it's your choice"; "it's personal freedom"). Children also consider issues of identity and self-expression when reasoning about the personal. For example, Lagatutta, Nucci, & Bosacki (2010) presented 4–8 year old children with hypothetical examples in which an authority prohibits children from acting in various ways, including issues falling within the personal domain (e.g., clothing, activity, friendship choice). Children of all ages predicted that agents would be less likely to comply and feel good if the prohibited personal issue was strongly associated with the agent's identity then if it was not. These findings illustrate children's emerging awareness of the psychological significance of basic needs for autonomy and the consequences associated with heteronomous control of the personal.

Importantly, children's conceptions of personal autonomy do not reflect an unbridled individualism or egoism, as children do acknowledge the legitimacy of social control and authority commands for other kinds of social rules and issues. For example, children accept the legitimacy of authorities such as parents or teachers over moral issues involving harm to others, injustice, or violation of their rights, or social conventional issues such as culturally relative customs or practices (e.g., forms of address, etiquette). Authorities may legitimately make rules governing moral and social conventional issues, and violations of these rules by children are judged to be wrong (Turiel, 2006). In their reasoning about moral and social conventional issues, children themselves appeal to concepts of harm, rights, or justice for moral issues, and to the disruption of social organization or the presence of shared norms or customs or explicit social rules in the case of social conventions (Smetana, 2006). These findings show how the development and demarcation of a domain of personal autonomy occurs alongside the development of simultaneous commitments to both moral conceptions of justice or concern for others along with the construction of concepts of shared social conventional rule systems to which children are also committed. Autonomy needs are therefore regulated and integrated with considerations emerging out of children's relatedness with others, such as reciprocity and justice or commitment to cultural traditions and conventions.

The idea of a personal domain defining areas of autonomy that authorities may not legitimately interfere with is not restricted to Western cultural settings but has been found among children from a wide variety of cultures often characterized as "collectivistic" or holding an interdependent view of the self, such as Colombia (Ardilla-Rey & Killen, 2001), Brazil (Nucci & Camino-Sapiro, 1996), Hong Kong (Yau & Smetana, 2003a), Korea (Kim & Turiel, 1996), and Japan (Yamada, 2009). In each of these societies, children identify similar sorts of issues (e.g., recreational pursuits, choice of friends) as beyond the boundaries of legitimate authority regulation, and violations of authority restrictions on these activities are judged by children as acceptable. Although the boundaries of the personal may, of course, vary in ways that show influences of culture (e.g., certain aspects of how one dresses may not be up to personal choice in some cultures), children in a variety of cultural contexts do believe that individuals should be given a space to enact their needs for self-expression, personal choice, and identity formation that may not be arbitrarily infringed upon by authorities. These findings are not compatible with the view that people in non-Western cultures generally value obedience over autonomy or do not recognize autonomy as an important human need or good, as critics of self-determination theory sometimes claim.

The particular issues that children see as part of their personal domain undergo transformation throughout childhood and adolescence, as children's competencies develop and they increasingly assert their autonomy over expanding areas of personal jurisdiction and control. In early childhood, children's conceptions of personal autonomy are generally tied to concrete issues of control over their bodies and basic recreational pursuits such as play, choice of friends, or food preferences. Beginning in middle childhood, areas of personal autonomy expand to include issues of privacy and freedom of thought or other basic freedoms related to children's exercise of self-determination (Ruck, Abramovitch, & Keating, 1998). Research on children's developing conceptions of civil liberties such as freedom of speech and religion conducted in North America indicates that by middle-childhood, children define these areas as important to people's needs for self-expression, and they judge arbitrary or restrictive government laws restricting these civil liberties as wrong in all countries, regardless of variations in local practices or laws (Helwig, 1995, 1998).

Although freedom of speech and religion are often thought of as uniquely "Western" notions, endorsement of these rights as universal human rights by adolescents has been found in several non-Western cultural settings, including among the Druze of Israel (Turiel & Wainryb, 1998), among Muslim immigrants in the Netherlands (Verkuyten & Slooter, 2008, in Malaysia (Cherney & Shing, 2008), and even in Mainland China (Lahat, Helwig, Yang, Tan, & Liu, 2009). For example, Lahat et al. (2009) examined urban and rural Chinese adolescents' judgments about issues such as whether a school principal could prohibit a high school student from publishing an article critical of the school's rules in the school newspaper, or whether parents who are atheists could prohibit their child from belonging to a religion of the child's choice. In both urban and rural settings, the majority of Chinese adolescents supported these rights and judged restrictions of children's rights by authorities as wrong, although rural adolescents supported freedoms in somewhat less proportions than urban adolescents. In their reasoning, Chinese adolescents appealed to needs for self-determination, autonomy, and personal choice in supporting children's freedom to make these choices. Interestingly, the same developmental pattern was found across both urban and rural contexts within China, with older adolescents supporting freedoms and rights more strongly than younger adolescents. These findings illustrate how the developmental tendency of children to assert greater autonomy as they get older is found in a non-Western cultural environment, even for issues such as civil liberties that may not have strong support in certain cultural settings.

Studies of direct observations of children's interactions around violations of social rules or other conflicts with authorities have provided insights into the complex interactional processes involved in children's construction of a domain of personal autonomy (e.g., Nucci & Weber, 1995). Nucci and Weber (1995) examined the types of social interactions that surrounded 3- and 4-year-old children's violations of social rules or their attempts to assert their own autonomy, and how their mothers responded. They found, first, that children tended to assert their own personal autonomy or prerogative around personal issues (e.g., dress or recreational pursuits), or those that combined a strong element of personal choice with other issues, such as social-convention or prudence (i.e., acts with the potential for harm to the self). Interestingly, children rarely asserted their personal prerogative around moral issues (e.g., hurting or treating others unfairly) or in the context of straightforward social conventional violations. Children's assertions of their own autonomy and personal choice in real-life interactions thus paralleled the types of distinctions found in their judgments of hypothetical rules and situations discussed earlier.

Moreover, closer examination of children's interactions with their mothers around personal issues revealed several features associated with the process of autonomy formation in early childhood. First, as might be expected, mothers do grant children autonomy and provide them with opportunities for personal choice. Importantly, however, autonomy development does not represent merely that which is granted by adults or authorities. Rather, children themselves also actively claim areas of personal jurisdiction in ways that frequently bring them into conflict with adults. In these conflicts, parents themselves often acknowledge children's emerging autonomy needs, and parents (and also children) sometimes compromise so as to enable children to exercise their autonomy within the context of adult structure or guidance (e.g., by permitting the expression of children's personal desires or choice but in a way that is safe for them). Thus, processes of autonomy granting (by parents) and autonomy claiming (by children) both contribute to the formation of children's early notions of personal autonomy, and this process is often characterized by moderate levels of conflict as children and parents mutually negotiate the expression of children's autonomy needs (Smetana, 2005).

Subsequent research with adolescents has shown that these sorts of processes continue throughout development (Smetana, 1988, 1989). Conflicts between parents and adolescents tend to be over issues that combine aspects of personal choice and other domains, especially social convention or prudential issues, and not over moral issues. Often, adolescents and parents would tend to define these issues differently, leading to conflicts. For example, adolescents might see issues such as the state of cleanliness of the child's room as a personal issue and therefore adolescents' own business, whereas parents might assert their social conventional authority to determine matters "under their roof." Similarly, parents may have concerns over safety in regard to many issues that adolescents see as part of their personal jurisdiction (e.g., how late they stay out with friends or whom they may date). In general, research indicates that moderate amounts of conflict are normal in adolescence, and that these conflicts tend to subside beyond early or middle adolescence as adolescents' competences develop and as they claim and are given increasing autonomy by parents (Smetana, 2005).

Research with adolescents from a variety of cultures, including Mainland China, Chile, and the Philippines, has shown that relations between adolescents and parents in these cultures are characterized by similar disputes about the legitimate boundaries of parental authority and its perceived implications for adolescents' autonomy (Darling, Cumsille, & Pena-Alampay, 2005; Yau & Smetana, 2003b). Typically, such conflicts arose over issues that combined elements of personal issues and concerns over prudence or social convention, as in the research conducted in the United States. Furthermore, adolescents in all cultural contexts tended to assert or desire greater autonomy at earlier ages than parents were willing (initially) to give them. Cultures also tend to vary in the ages at which autonomy is granted, with some cultures granting autonomy over many issues fairly early and other cultures granting it fairly late in adolescence. The context of the Philippines is especially interesting, as parents in this culture tended to impose rules in a fairly constant fashion across adolescence, whereas adolescents in this culture tended, with increasing age, to see parentally imposed rules as illegitimate (Darling et al., 2005). Interestingly, the greatest frequency of conflict in this culture occurred over those rules that adolescents thought were illegitimate but that they felt they had to obey anyway. Thus, it can be inferred that the motivation of these adolescents to obey these rules was either heteronomous or introjected (Deci & Ryan, 2008). This motivational basis, however, did not lead to obedience, as might be expected according to a culturally defined developmental pathway of interdependence and increasing harmony between children and adults often claimed to hold in a strongly collectivist culture such as the Philippines (Greenfield et al., 2003), but rather to higher levels of conflict with authority as adolescents resisted the internalization of adult expectations. Taken together, the findings of this research, conducted within different kinds of cultures, indicates that the leading edge of autonomy development is driven by adolescents' increasing claims for more autonomy—and by parents ultimately giving in—and not simply by parental granting of autonomy at certain culturally defined ages. These findings provide strong support for self-determination theory's claim that autonomy is a universal human need that underlies and drives the development of a personal sphere of decision making, within the context of the child's emerging capacities and capabilities and interactions with adults. Clearly, these findings are not consistent with the idea that autonomy is an aspect of the self that may or may not be constructed and transmitted at the cultural level by authorities or other agents of socialization, in accordance with general cultural orientations or ideologies (Shweder, 2003).

Research from the social domain perspective also has uncovered how conflicts about autonomy may occur within cultures and may stem from variations in the scope of the personal domain accorded to different classes of persons, including among adults. Many of these variations revolve around different norms regarding the rights and entitlements of men and women. For example, in many traditional societies, males are conventionally accorded far greater entitlements to personal choice and the freedom to pursue their desires and wishes than are females. Research conducted in a several cultures, including among the Druze, a traditional Arab society in Israel (Wainryb & Turiel, 1994), in India (Neff, 2001), and in Benin, Africa (Conry-Murray, 2009), has shown that females in these societies are generally more likely to perceive these practices as a restriction of women's personal autonomy, and therefore as unfair, than are males. Nevertheless, in many circumstances, females within these societies do endorse obedience to gender-related restrictions on personal choice, largely out of concern with punishment or the negative social consequences associated with their violation (Wainryb & Turiel, 1994). These findings of diversity within cultures in judgments of freedoms and rights are difficult to reconcile with global characterizations of traditional or non-Western societies in terms of duty-based moralities and the acceptance of inequality by those in subordinate positions (Shweder et al., 1987). Further, they show how certain cultural practices relating to issues of personal choice and autonomy may be critically evaluated by people within a culture, especially by those whose needs for autonomy are perceived as significantly restricted by certain cultural norms. These findings also parallel research from self-determination theory showing that individuals from diverse cultures (e.g., Korea, Turkey, Russia, and the United States) are much less likely to internalize vertical cultural norms (or those emphasizing authority, power, and obedience), when compared to more horizontal cultural norms characterized by equality, autonomy, and mutual respect (Chirkov, Ryan, Kim, & Kaplan, 2003).

Democratic Participation and Voice

The preceding review of the development of autonomy and its relation to other moral norms such as justice and fairness illustrates an important feature of autonomy that is often misunderstood when autonomy is caricatured or reduced to simple individualism or egoism (see Kacitcibasi, 2005, for a discussion of this issue). Psychological needs for autonomy must be situated within a moral context that includes mutual respect and regard for the situation of others, including the autonomy needs of everyone. This idea corresponds to one of the defining features of morality—i.e., generalizability (Gewirth, 1978; Rawls, 1971)—or the idea that moral norms are "impersonal" and hold for all individuals, regardless of one's own purely personal perspective. Within a democratic social organization, individuals are involved in making the rules or otherwise participating with others in the creation and maintenance of the social order, sometimes through processes of deliberation, discussion, and even debate or disagreement. Because democratic social organization treats people as equals who may all contribute to decision making, it can provide the mutual respect on which true (moral) autonomy is based (Piaget, 1932). This point corresponds to a key proposition within self-determination theory, essential for understanding its relation to democratic social organization, and this is that autonomy and relatedness needs are intertwined and mutually supportive of one another (Ryan & Deci, 2001). Social relationships of mutual respect and reciprocity foster the experience of autonomy, and individual needs for autonomy correspondingly place limits on the forms of social organization that can be rationally justified. Seen in this way, autonomy is not a form of self-interest that is necessarily opposed to the common good, but must include a wider perspective, based on reciprocity, that transcends unbridled egoism. As many theorists of democracy have long argued (e.g., Dewey, 1916), personal autonomy and the common good are two related poles of democratic consciousness that, although always in a delicate balance, should not be seen as mutually exclusive.

This point may be illustrated by the findings of a study of a large-scale, real world implementation of an educational program designed to foster children's understanding of their own rights. Covell, McNeil, and Howe (2009) assessed the effects of a rights-consistent educational curriculum, entitled "Rights, Respect, & Responsibility" (RRR) program, in Hampshire, England, over a 3-year period. Whereas civic education in England was recommended for children from the age of 5 onward, it only became mandatory for children 11 years and older, and thus many children between the ages of 5–11 were not adequately educated about civic issues such as rights and responsibilities. The RRR program was designed to implement a rights-consistent curriculum in schools with students in this age range, and incorporated a broad change in the school ethos to give children at even these young ages the ability to have meaningful input into how the schools were run, including over issues such as hiring practices, school activities, and academic programs. Interviews conducted with children from these schools indicated that children from schools in which the program was fully implemented, i.e. in which children's rights were embedded within the school's overall ethos, had more advanced reasoning regarding rights, particularly their rights to education. However, the students also tended to display more advanced understandings of their responsibilities as well, especially with regard to respecting the rights of other students. Thus, children who were educated about their rights were not only more cognizant of the rights afforded to them, but also of their responsibilities to others.

Other research has directly examined children's developing understandings of democratic decision-making processes themselves in a variety of social contexts, such as the peer group, school, family, and government (Helwig & Kim, 1999; Helwig, 1998; Helwig, Arnold, Tan, & Boyd, 2003, 2007; Kinoshita, 2006; Moessinger, 1981). This research has shown that children from a variety of cultures (including Canada, Mainland China, Switzerland, and Japan) often endorse and understand basic principles of democratic participation. For example, democratic decision-making procedures that give children full input into making decisions, such as majority rule or consensus, are endorsed for decisions over recreational pursuits or for matters involving the coordination of conflicting personal preferences in a group (Helwig & Kim, 1999). Specifically, children believe that they should decide democratically what game a group of children would play or what television show they would watch, or have input into family decisions such as where a family goes on vacation, and they critically evaluate unilateral adult decision making that does not take into account children's own perspectives in these instances (Helwig & Kim, 1999). In justifying their judgments, children appeal directly to their need to have a voice in decisions and to fairness principles based on majority rule. Moreover, children sometimes extended this support for democratic decision making into social contexts in which adults traditionally have decision-making authority, such as decisions made by teachers within classrooms. For instance, when the decision to be made was perceived as largely recreational in nature or as involving children's own personal interests, such as where a school class should go on a field trip, children saw democratic decision making by children themselves as more fair than unilateral decision making by teachers alone. However, at the same time, children ceded decision-making autonomy to adults when the decision was seen as impacting children's welfare or when adults were perceived to be more competent to make better decisions, as in decisions over school curriculum (Helwig & Kim, 1999). These findings indicate that children are sensitive to issues of children's competence and developmental level in deciding the types of matters over which they should be given decision-making autonomy.

Cross-cultural studies of evaluations of democratic versus authority-oriented decision making in non-Western societies such as Mainland China have suggested that endorsements of democratic decision making do not always follow a simple cultural pattern (e.g., Helwig et al., 2003, 2007). For instance, although the educational system in China is more hierarchical than in the West, with a standardized curriculum in effect across the country and highly competitive nation-wide entrance examinations at each level beginning with Junior High school, Chinese adolescents tended not to endorse adult decision making over the curriculum and were more positive about children's own democratic involvement in curriculum decisions than were Western adolescents, who presumably have more autonomy in general over academic matters (Helwig et al., 2003). In their justifications, Chinese adolescents often criticized adult decision making over the curriculum as leading to unfair outcomes and as counterproductive because it may stifle children's autonomy needs, freedom, and initiative (see Helwig, 2005, for extended examples of justifications given by Chinese adolescents).

In a subsequent study examining Chinese and Canadian adolescents' reasoning about various hypothetical forms of democratic and non-democratic government (Helwig et al., 2007), both Chinese adolescents from rural and urban settings and urban Canadian adolescents were found to prefer democratic forms of government, such as a representative democracy (in which the people elect representatives to govern for them), or a direct democracy (in which the people themselves directly vote on policy decisions), over various forms of non-democratic government such as a meritocracy or oligarchy. In justifying their responses, both Chinese and Canadian adolescents appealed to the principle of voice or the people having a say, and to the accountability afforded by elections that would allow for the removal of officials who do not govern in the people's interest, despite the fact that such opportunities for citizen's involvement in political decision making are highly limited or non-existent within China's current political system. Taken together, these findings indicate that democratic principles are not restricted to Western, liberal democracies, and are applied by adolescents in a variety of cultures to critically evaluate existing forms of nondemocratic social organization that are perceived to be lacking in provision for individuals' autonomy needs.

Recent research in Western and non-Western cultures has shown that democratic principles of group decision making, such as majority rule, are applied in ways that also take into account individual freedom and autonomy (e.g., Helwig, Yang, Tan, Liu, & Shao, in press; Kinoshita, 2006). This research, conducted with children and adolescents in Canada, England, Mainland China, and Japan, examined the issues over which democratic group decision making by majority rule (in a school classroom) was judged as acceptable. Across all cultures, majority rule was judged acceptable for deciding social-conventional or social-organizational issues, such as how to organize a class party or what to paint on a class mural, but it was not seen as acceptable for deciding personal issues such as what a class would eat for lunch or with whom they would be friends. These findings reveal that, even in cultures such as China and Japan that are often characterized as "group-oriented" and collectivistic (Triandis, 1989), conceptions of areas of personal autonomy and freedom constrain and define areas over which the group should not interfere in people's lives.

Autonomy, Democratic Participation, and Well-Being

The findings of this emerging body of research indicate that notions of autonomy, personal freedoms, and democratic decision making are not uniquely Western concepts but have general appeal across a wide variety of cultural contexts and settings. One of the important questions raised by self-determination theory is whether or not these aspects of democratic social organization themselves are positively related to human well-being. In the this section, we will examine some recent cross-cultural research findings tracing the unique relations between democratic features of social organization, such as support for autonomy, personal choice, and democratic involvement in decision making, and psychological outcomes related to individual's psychological health and well-being. Our aim is to illustrate how children's and adolescents' autonomy needs are construed and constructed in accordance with children's emerging notions of freedoms and democratic conceptions. Accordingly, we will show how the thwarting of children's needs to exercise autonomy over *democratic* issues of freedom and participation has been found to be associated with negative psychological outcomes across diverse cultural settings.

As noted earlier, one of the important features of autonomy pertains to areas of personal freedom over which individuals may exercise autonomous control, free from unwanted intrusion. Recent research (Hasebe, Nucci, & Nucci, 2004; Helwig, Yang, Nucci, & To, 2009; Qin, Pomerantz, & Wang, 2009) has examined the effects on psychological well-being of adolescents' (from the United States, Japan, and China) perceptions of parental control over a variety of issues falling within different social domains. This research has found that adolescents from all of these cultural settings tend to accept parental control over social conventional or prudential issues, but not over personal issues (or over issues in which adolescents' personal autonomy was perceived to overlap with other domains). When adolescents perceived their parents as being overcontrolling with regard to personal issues (or those overlapping with their autonomy), they tended to report internalizing symptoms of psychopathology, such as anxiety and depression. However, adolescents did not tend to report symptoms of psychopathology in relation to perceived parental control over social conventional or prudential issues, where parental control was generally accepted as legitimate. These findings suggest that behavioral or psychological control (Barber, Stolz, & Olsen, 2005), and its potential for negative psychological effects, is mediated by adolescents' emerging constructions of spheres of personal autonomy and freedom. Thus, the harmful effects of parental control, when found, appear not to be due to control *per se*, but to the mismatch between parental attempts to intrude on or regulate areas over which adolescents perceive and claim personal freedom and autonomy.

These similarities across cultures in the psychological outcomes of parental intrusion on the exercise of adolescents' emerging freedoms and autonomy should not be taken to suggest that this process may not also be culturally inflected or patterned. Cultural differences have been found in the timetable and patterning of the development of autonomy and associated outcomes for psychological well-being.

For example, Qin et al. (2009), in a short-term cross-cultural longitudinal study conducted over the 7th and 8th grades, found that American adolescents reported greater gains in autonomy (mainly in the form of unilateral child decision making) during this time than did Chinese children, who reported more joint decision making between children and parents. American adolescents' gains in autonomy were associated with positive emotional outcomes, but the correspondingly more modest gains in autonomy that Chinese adolescents experienced over this time period did not similarly lead to more positive emotional functioning. However, in families where unilateral parental decision making was predominant or continued over time, there were negative effects on adolescents' emotional functioning (e.g., depressive symptoms, anxiety, lower self-esteem) in both cultures, although these effects were somewhat stronger in the United States than in China. Thus, although Chinese and American adolescents may claim autonomy in somewhat different ways and at different ages, overly restrictive parental control was detrimental to well-being in both cultural settings.

Other research has begun to examine how aspects of the school environment (termed "school climate") affect children's well-being and adjustment. A recent, large-scale longitudinal study (Way, Reddy, & Rhodes, 2007) of over 1,400 American adolescents in 6th–8th grades examined relations between a variety of features of school climate, one of which was student perceptions of opportunities for autonomy (measured, for example, as having a say in how things worked in school or having input into decisions and curriculum), and various health outcomes such as depression, self-esteem, and behavioral problems. It was found that perceptions of student autonomy became more negative over the 3-year period of middle school, and that as students perceived fewer opportunities for involvement in decision making, there were increases in depressive symptoms and behavioral problems and decreases in reported self-esteem. Moreover, the researchers were able to use path analyses to determine the direction of these effects; the direction was found to be unidirectional and went from changes in perceptions of autonomy to well-being, rather than in the opposite direction (students' adjustment predicting their perceptions of the school climate). It is probably unlikely that these declines in student autonomy reported by adolescents represent actual declines in the decision-making opportunities offered to them. More plausibly, adolescents' increasing dissatisfaction with what the school provides may be driven by expansions in their expectations for autonomy, as documented by the social cognitive developmental research reviewed earlier (Helwig, 2006; Smetana, 2006). These findings thus are fully consistent with the proposition that children and adolescents increasingly internalize and define autonomy in democratic terms (e.g., as necessitating an increasing say in decisions). These associations between the level of decision-making autonomy granted to children in school settings and important aspects of well-being (e.g., self-esteem and depression and anxiety) have been replicated in a recent study of adolescents in the mainland Chinese city of Nanjing (Jia et al., 2009), indicating that adolescents in a collectivistic culture also benefit from enhanced decision-making opportunities in schools. Overall, these new lines of research suggest that children's emerging perceptions of autonomy, rights, and democratic decision making are essential pathways through which autonomy needs may be satisfied in different cultural settings. Accordingly, understanding these pathways is essential for illuminating the ways in which social institutions may act to enhance or diminish children's well-being.

Conclusions

Children in a variety of cultural contexts have been shown to develop concerns with personal autonomy and rights, and these conceptions not only place limits on the forms of social organization seen as legitimate but also have relevance for children's psychological well-being, consistent with self-determination theory. Although many current psychological theories relegate freedoms, rights, and democracy to products of Western intellectual traditions or cultural settings, a body of new and emerging psychological evidence, conducted in a variety of cultural settings, both Eastern and Western, and from a variety of theoretical perspectives, including self-determination theory, suggests otherwise. Individuals in diverse cultural environments have been found to define areas of personal jurisdiction or freedom that limit the forms of social control that are perceived to be legitimately imposed on individuals. These areas of personal jurisdiction are justified in terms of appeals to personal agency, choice, and freedom, and are relevant to both children and to adults. Rather than reflecting an unbridled egoism or individualism, as sometimes claimed, areas of personal jurisdiction are connected to beliefs about autonomy and personal choice and exist alongside and in relation to equally important and equally internalized commitments to social norms, traditions, and moral conceptions of justice and the avoidance of harm to others. Individuals in diverse cultural settings sometimes extend their needs for autonomy to embrace democratic social organization grounded on the principle of voice and the need for individuals to participate in decision making, in ways that may go beyond what is granted to them by their cultural environment or by powerful authorities. These democratic concepts are comprehended and often claimed by children and adolescents themselves as they develop explicit conceptions of their own autonomy and reflect on the different types of social rules and structures that they experience in their daily lives. More than mere intellectual constructions, conceptions of autonomy and democracy have been shown to have functional psychological significance for the realization of individuals' psychological well-being. Social scientists need to pay attention to these emerging findings as they have important implications for how conceptions of self, morality, and society are defined and studied. Beyond this, policy makers, governments, and citizens alike need to ensure that the institutions in which children and adults participate are structured to suitably respect individuals' universal needs for personal autonomy, in order to foster human happiness and full participation in shared social life.

References

Ardilla-Rey, A., & Killen, M. (2001). Middle-class Colombian children's evaluations of personal, moral, and social conventional interactions in the classroom. *International Journal of Behavioral Development, 25,* 246–255.

Barber, B. K., Stolz, H. E., & Olsen, J. A. (2005). Parental support, psychological control, and behavioral control: Assessing relevance across time, culture, and method. *Monographs of the Society of Research in Child Development, 70,* 1–137.

Cherney, I. D., & Shing, Y. L. (2008). Children's nurturance and self-determination rights: A cross-cultural perspective. *Journal of Social Issues, 64,* 835–856.

Chirkov, V. I. (2007). Culture, personal autonomy, and individualism: Their relationships and implications for personal growth and well-being. In G. Zheng, K. Leung, & J. G. Adair (Eds.), *Perspectives and progress in contemporary cross-cultural psychology* (pp. 247–263). Beijing: China Light Industry Press.

Chirkov, V., Ryan, R. M., Kim, Y., & Kaplan, U. (2003). Differentiating autonomy from individualism and independence: A self-determination theory perspective on internalization of cultural orientations and well-being. *Journal of Personality and Social Psychology, 84,* 97–109.

Conry-Murray, C. (2009). Adolescent and adult reasoning about gender and fairness in traditional practices in Benin, West Africa. *Social Development, 18,* 427–446.

Covell, K., McNeil, J., & Howe, B. R. (2009). Reducing teacher burnout by increasing student engagement: A children's rights approach. *School Psychology International, 30,* 282–290.

Darling, N., Cumsille, P., & Pena-Alampay, L. (2005). Rules, legitimacy of parental authority, and obligation to obey in Chile, the Philippines, and the United States. In J. G. Smetana (Ed.), *Changing boundaries of parental authority during adolescence: New directions for child and adolescent development* (Vol. 108, pp. 47–60). San Francisco, CA: Jossey-Bass.

Deci, E. L., & Ryan, R. M. (2008). Self-determination theory: A macrotheory of human motivation, development, and health. *Canadian Psychology, 49,* 182–185.

Dewey, J. (1916). *Democracy and education: An introduction to the philosophy of education.* New York: Free Press.

Dworkin, R. A. (1977). *Taking rights seriously.* Cambridge, MA: Harvard University Press.

Gewirth, A. (1978). *Reason and morality.* Chicago, IL: University of Chicago Press.

Greenfield, P. M., Keller, H., Fuligni, A., & Maynard, A. (2003). Cultural pathways through universal development. *Annual Review of Psychology, 54,* 461–490.

Hart, D., Atkins, R., & Donnelly, T. M. (2006). Community service and moral development. In M. Killen, & J. Smetana (Eds.), *Handbook of moral development.* Hillsdale, NJ: Lawrence Erlbaum Associates.

Hasebe, Y., Nucci, L., & Nucci, M. S. (2004). Parental control of the personal domain and adolescent symptoms of psychopathology: A cross-national study in the United States and Japan. *Child Development, 75,* 815–828.

Heinrich, J., Heine, S. J., & Norenzayan, A. (2010). The weirdest people in the world? *Behavioral and Brain Sciences, 33*(2–3), 61–83.

Helwig, C. C. (1995). Adolescents' and young adults' conceptions of civil liberties: Freedom of speech and religion. *Child Development, 66,* 152–166.

Helwig, C. C. (1998). Children's conceptions of fair government and freedom of speech. *Child Development, 69,* 518–531.

Helwig, C. C. (2005). Culture and the construction of concepts of personal autonomy and democratic decision making. In J. E. Jacobs & P. A. Klazynski (Eds.), *The development of judgement and decision making in children and adolescents.* Mahwah, NJ: Lawrence Erlbaum Associates.

Helwig, C. (2006). The development of personal autonomy throughout cultures. *Cognitive Development, 21,* 458–473.

Helwig, C. C., Arnold, M. L., Tan, D., & Boyd, D. (2003). Chinese adolescents' reasoning about democratic and authority-based decision making in peer, family, and school contexts. *Child Development, 74,* 783–800.

Helwig, C. C., Arnold, M. L., Tan, D., & Boyd, D. (2007). Mainland Chinese and Canadian adolescents' judgments and reasoning about the fairness of democratic and other forms of government. *Cognitive Development, 22*, 96–109.

Helwig, C. C., & Kim, S. (1999). Children's evaluations of decision-making procedures in peer, family, and school contexts. *Child Development, 70*, 502–512.

Helwig, C. C., Yang, S., Nucci, L. P., & To, S. (2009, April). *Parental control of the personal domain and adolescent symptoms of psychopathology in urban and rural China*. Poster presented at the biennial meeting of the Society for Research in Child Development, Denver.

Helwig, C. C., Yang, S., Tan, D., Liu, C., & Shao, T. (in press). Urban and rural Chinese adolescents' judgments and reasoning about personal and group jurisdiction. *Child Development*.

Jia, Y., Way, N., Ling, G., Yoshikawa, H., Chen, X., Hughes, D., et al. (2009). The influence of student perceptions of school climate on socioemotional and academic adjustment: A comparison of Chinese and American adolescents. *Child Development, 80*, 1514–1530.

Kagitcibasi, C. (2005). Autonomy and relatedness in cultural context: Implications for self and family. *Journal of Cross-Cultural Psychology, 36*, 403–422.

Kim, J. M., & Turiel, E. (1996). Korean and American children's concepts of adult and peer authority. *Social Development, 5*, 310–329.

Kinoshita, Y. (2006). Children's judgment of the legitimacy of group decision making about individual concerns: A comparative study between England and Japan. *International Journal of Behavioral Development, 30*, 117–126.

Lagatutta, K. H., Nucci, L., & Bosacki, S. L. (2010). Bridging theory of mind and the personal domain: Children's reasoning about resistance to parental control. *Child Development, 81*, 616–635.

Lahat, A., Helwig, C. C., Yang, S., Tan, D., & Liu, C. (2009). Mainland Chinese adolescents' judgements and reasoning about self-determination and nurturance rights. *Social Development, 18*, 690–710.

Larmore, C. (2008). *The autonomy of morality*. Cambridge: Cambridge University Press.

Markus, H. R. (2008). Pride, prejudice and ambivalence: Toward a unified theory of race and ethnicity. *American Psychologist, 63*, 651–670.

Markus, H., & Kitayama, S. (1991). Culture and self: Implications for cognition, emotion and motivation. *Psychological Review, 98*, 224–253.

Miller, J. G. (1994). Cultural diversity in the morality of caring: Individually oriented versus duty-based interpersonal moral codes. *Cross-Cultural Research: The Journal of Comparative Social Science, 28*(1), 3–39.

Moessinger, P. (1981). The development of the concept of majority decision: A pilot study. *Canadian Journal of Behavioral Science, 13*, 359–362.

Neff, K. D. (2001). Judgments of personal autonomy and interpersonal responsibility in the context of Indian spousal relationships: An examination of young people's reasoning in Mysore, India. *British Journal of Developmental Psychology, 19*, 233–257.

Nucci, L. P. (1981). The development of personal concepts: A domain distinct from moral and social concepts. *Child Development, 52*, 114–121.

Nucci, L. P. (2001). *Education in the moral domain*. Cambridge: Cambridge University Press.

Nucci, L. P., Camino, C., & Sapiro, C. (1996). Social class effects on northeastern Brazilian children's conceptions of areas of personal choice and social regulation. *Child Development, 67*, 1223–1242.

Nucci, L. P., & Weber, E. (1995). Social interactions in the home and the development of young children's conceptions within the personal domain. *Child Development, 66*, 1438–1452.

Nussbaum, L. C. (2000). *Women and human development: The capabilities approach*. Cambridge: Cambridge University Press.

Piaget, J. (1932). *The moral judgment of the child*. New York: Free Press.

Qin, L., Pomerantz, E. M., & Wang, Q. (2009). Are gains in decision-making autonomy during early adolescence beneficial for emotional functioning? The case of the United States and China. *Child Development, 80*, 1705–1721.

Rawls, J. (1971). *A theory of justice*. Cambridge, MA: Harvard University Press.
Roth, G., & Deci, E. L. (2009). Autonomy. In S. J. Lopez (Ed.), *Encyclopedia of positive psychology* (Vol. 1, pp. 78–82). Hoboken, NJ: Wiley.
Ruck, M. D., Abramovitch, R., & Keating, D. P. (1998). Children's and adolescents' understanding of rights: Balancing nurturance and self-determination. *Child Development, 69*, 404–417.
Ryan, R. M., & Deci, E. L. (2001). On happiness and human potential: A review of research on hedonic and eudaimonic well-being. *Annual Review of Psychology, 52*, 141–166.
Sen, A. (1999). *Development as freedom*. Oxford: Oxford University Press.
Shweder, R. A. (2003). *Why do men barbecue? Recipes for cultural psychology*. Cambridge, MA: Harvard University Press.
Shweder, R. A., Mahapatra, M., & Miller, J. G. (1987). Culture and moral development. In J. Kagan & S. Lamb (Eds.), *The emergence of morality in young children* (pp. 1–82). Chicago: University of Chicago Press.
Smetana, J. G. (1988). Adolescents' and parents' conceptions of parental authority. *Child Development, 59*, 321–335.
Smetana, J. G. (1989). Adolescents' and parents' reasoning about actual family conflict. *Child Development, 60*, 1052–1067.
Smetana, J. G. (2005). Adolescent-parent conflict: Resistance and subversion as developmental process. In L. Nucci (Ed.), *Conflict, contradiction, and contrarian elements in moral development and education* (pp. 69–91). Mahwah, NJ: Erlbaum.
Smetana, J. G. (2006). Social-cognitive domain theory. In M. Killen & J. G. Smetana (Eds.), *Handbook of moral development* (pp. 119–153). Mahwah, NJ: Erlbaum.
Triandis, H. C. (1989). The self and social behavior in differing cultural contexts. *Psychological Review, 96*, 506–520.
Turiel, E. (2006). The development of morality. In W. Damon, R. M. Lerner, & N. Eisenberg (Eds.), *Handbook of child psychology: Vol. 3. Social, emotional, and personality development* (6th ed., pp. 789–857). Hoboken, NJ: Wiley.
Turiel, E., & Wainryb, C. (1998). Concepts of freedoms and rights in a traditional, hierarchically organized society. *British Journal of Developmental Psychology, 16*, 375–394.
Verkuyten, M., & Slooter, L. (2008). Muslim and non-Muslim adolescents' reasoning about freedom of speech and minority rights. *Child Development, 79*, 514–528.
Wainryb, C., & Turiel, E. (1994). Dominance, subordination, and concepts of personal entitlements in cultural contexts. *Child Development, 65*, 1701–1722.
Way, N., Reddy, R., & Rhodes, J. (2007). Students' perceptions of school climate during the middle school years: Associations with trajectories of psychological and behavioral adjustment. *American Journal of Community Psychology, 40*, 194–213.
Yamada, H. (2009). Japanese children's reasoning about conflicts with parents. *Social Development, 18*, 962–977.
Yau, J., & Smetana, J. G. (2003a). Conceptions of moral, social-conventional, and personal events among Chinese preschoolers in Hong Kong. *Child Development, 74*, 1–12.
Yau, J., & Smetana, J. G. (2003b). Adolescent-parent conflict in Hong Kong and Shenzhen: A comparison of youth in two cultural contexts. *International Journal of Behavioral Development, 27*, 201–211.
Youniss, J., & Yates, M. (1997). *Community service and social responsibility in youth*. Chicago: University of Chicago Press.

Chapter 12
Personal Autonomy and Environmental Sustainability

Luc G. Pelletier, Daniel Baxter, and Veronika Huta

The Concept of Environmental Sustainability

The widespread rise of interest in the concept of environmental sustainability represents a significant shift in how people view the relationships between mounting environmental problems, socio-economic growth, and humanity's well-being. The most recent major international scientific consensus is that human activities are changing the climate at a planetary level, that many impacts of this climate change are already evident, and that further effects are inevitable because both socio-economic growth in developing countries and population growth are inevitable (IPCC, 2007). Although predicting population and socio-economic growth is not an exact science, the United Nation Population Fund (2009) reported that, after growing very slowly for most of human history, the world's population has more than doubled in the last half century to reach 6 billion in late 1999. In 2006, the world population reached 6.7 billion, and it is expected to rise by 2.53 billion people to reach a total of 9.1 billion in 2050. This increase alone is close to the total world population in 1950. This dramatic growth in population will increase the number of inhabitants competing for the world's limited resources. In addition, the human activities needed to reach a high quality of life in both developed and developing countries will inevitably lead to an increase in global warming.

This serves to illustrate how complex the problem of sustainable development is, and how closely tied it is to human activity. In fact, many other environmental problems—such as the rise of air pollution, the reduction of clean water supplies, the depletion of the Earth's ozone layer, and the clearing of tropical rain forests—are also the direct result of human activities that were initially designed to improve humanity's well-being, generate economic growth, and correct socio-economic disparities like poverty and low quality of life (Gardner & Stern, 1996; Hopwood, Mellor, & O'Brien, 2005).

L.G. Pelletier (✉)
School of Psychology, University of Ottawa, Ottawa, ON, Canada K1N 6N5
e-mail: Luc.Pelletier@uOttawa.ca

The process of bringing together environmental issues, socio-economic concerns, and humanity's well-being is the central idea encapsulated in the Brundtland Report's definition of environmental sustainability as meeting the needs of the present without compromising the ability of future generation to meet their needs (World Commission on Economic Development, 1987). So far, the proposed model for sustainable development is composed of three connected, interdependent domains: the environment, society, and the economy. Although it is increasingly clear that human activities cause climate change, the solutions that have thus far been proposed simply involve trade-offs between environmental, economical, and social concerns, such as whether it is acceptable to cause large scale pollution when one's country is using tar sands in order to produce energy, stimulate the economy and increase growth, or whether the loss of jobs in the car industry is acceptable for cleaner air. In other words, existing strategies ignore the fact that a sustainable future can only be achieved through a substantial shift in the values, attitudes, and behaviors of the individuals and institutions that caused the harm to the environment (McKenzie-Mohr & Oskamp, 1995). The field of psychology and the subfield of motivation in particular provide crucial understanding of how such a shift could take place. We have learned much about the psychological processes that would be needed for individuals to learn new environmentally responsible behaviors, adopt these behaviors, and more importantly, maintain them and integrate them into their lifestyles.

The current environmental situation has made many people realize that sustainable development needs to be a central goal of society, even though the achievement of this goal is extremely difficult and complex, as it is intertwined with competing socio-economic and well-being goals. In order to make progress toward sustainable development, in this chapter we argue that a central target is the motivation of individual people, whether they are private citizens, heads of industries, or leaders of governments. Also, we propose that self-determination theory provides a useful framework for organizing and understanding psychological science's response to environmental sustainability, and most importantly promoting pro-environmental motivation and behavior. When a person is well integrated, pro-environmental, socio-economic, and well-being goals work in harmony rather than competing with each other.

Psychological Science's Response to a Sustainable Environment

In the 20 or so attempts to synthesize the many studies on pro-environmental behaviors (PEBs) done so far (more than 400), it is repeatedly emphasized that psychological science should play a major role in addressing these problems (Kazdin, 2009; Swim et al., 2009). Some reviews focus on very specific potential theoretical accounts or psychological processes that could predict or lead to change of PEB (Eagly & Kulesa, 1997; Kollmuss & Agyeman, 2002; Oskamp, 2000), while other reviews include meta-analyses (Bamberg & Möser, 2007; Hines, Hungerford,

& Tomera, 1987; Osbaldiston, 2004; Zelesny, 1999) or more traditional narrative descriptions (Dwyer, Leeming, Cobern, Porter, & Jackson, 1993; Gifford, 2007; Stern, 2000) of the effects that different strategies or interventions have on a variety of PEBs. In some of these reviews, the authors go a step further and propose models that combine the diversity of topics, the multiple influences that have been proposed, and the different types of interventions coming from different areas of psychology (Gardner & Stern, 2002; Gifford, 2007; Hines et al., 1987). However, at best, these models provide lists of correlates that one could take into account when designing an intervention. Nevertheless, let us review what we have learned from this research. We will then examine how self-determination theory could provide a more coherent framework for understanding and promoting PEB.

Given the complexity of sustainable development, most of the research in this field (Gardner & Stern, 2008; McKenzie-Morh, 2008) has focused on specific, concrete behaviors like the consumption of bottled water, reusing hotel towels, using special light bulbs, recycling, energy conservation, auto emissions inspection, residential water conservation, or living more modestly. This has been combined with interventions that focus on education and information strategies which provide information about specific environmental conditions (Gardner & Stern, 2002), use social norms in message framing (Goldstein, Cialdini, & Griskevicius, 2008), provide feedback or information on results (Darby, 2006), and/or employ motivational strategies that focus on incentives and disincentives (Clayton, 2009; Gardner & Stern, 2002), social marketing, and the facilitation of behavior (McKenzie-Mohr & Smith, 1999).

With regard to education and information strategies, research on PEB has typically examined the effects of providing information regarding specific topics (e.g., specific environmental problems, health risks, environmental effects of certain behaviors), sometimes combined with information about the extent to which people agree with these perceptions (i.e., social norms), or provision of feedback (e.g., exact amount of electricity consumption). The outcome generally studied has been environmental concern or dissatisfaction. A major limitation of using this outcome, however, is that dissatisfaction and concern are rarely sufficient for action. For one thing, individuals must know what to do and must believe that their actions can change the situation; and even when these requirements are present, people mainly make only specific, simple, and easy changes in their behavior. When behaviors become more difficult or costly, the association between environmental attitudes, knowledge, and pro-environmental behaviors is considerably reduced.

Indeed, several studies and surveys have shown that there is generally a gap between the extent to which people are aware of environmental conditions and the PEB they display (Kollmuss & Agyeman, 2002; Wood, Tam, & Guerrero-Witt, 2005). Several surveys indicate that people are aware of the ecological threats that are around us, and that people understand that most of the threats are caused by human activities and can be reversed by human behavior (Environics, 2007a). However, most people continue to maintain the habits that cause harm to the environment, and most show low levels of PEB (Environics, 2007b). As we will see later, it is not only important to understand why people remain relatively inactive despite the large effort to make them aware of the importance of the situation, we must also examine how communication strategies could be made more effective to guide them in their attempts to adopt new PEBs.

The second broader intervention for promoting PEB has relied on incentives and disincentives (Dwyer et al., 1993; Geller, 1989). Creating incentives is usually perceived as a powerful approach because it can make PEB attractive to a person who lacks motivation to engage in PEB and does not otherwise feel concerned by environmental conditions (e.g., recycles tin cans only to get a monetary reward). Also, incentives can be used as barriers to actions that harm the environment (e.g., increasing the cost of buying gasoline can be an incentive to buy a smaller car).

But whether such an approach is truly effective remains to be sufficiently established. For one thing, under some conditions, incentives can have unintended consequences that are experienced as punishment (Gardner & Stern, 1996). For example, an increase in the cost of energy might force low-income people to make hard choices between heating their homes in winter and buying food or clothing. Second, incentives can lead to short-term effects, but lose their appeal over time, or are not adequate enough to instill much long-term change (Geller, Winett, & Everett, 1982; Katzev & Johnson, 1984; Winett, Leckliter, Chinn, Stahl, & Love, 1985; Witmer & Geller, 1976). Third, and more importantly, several researchers (e.g., Aronson & Gonzales, 1990; DeYoung, 1986; Wang & Katzev, 1990; Witmer & Geller, 1976) have observed that when incentives were discontinued, the PEB that was targeted returned to baseline levels, i.e. the level that existed before implementation of the intervention. This is precisely what is predicted by self-determination theory (Deci & Ryan, 1985, 1987)—that rewards and incentives typically promote target behaviors only as long as they are given to reinforce these behaviors. Moreover, in most circumstances, incentives aimed at changing the behavior of individuals have been unsuccessful when the individuals felt that the costs of the behavior change outweighed the benefits of the incentive, or when the larger social system posed significant barriers to action. As a consequence, when protecting the environment requires great effort or expense, behaviors become unlikely unless interventions to reduce the barriers are present as well.

But even making a behavior easier, like providing access to a curbside recycling program, has limitations. For example, close to 40% of citizens indicate that they recycle at home where the recycling bin is immediately accessible; however, this number drops to less than 10% when citizens are outside their homes, or do not have access to a recycling program (Oskamp, 1995). Finally, because the facilitation of recycling by providing access to a curbside recycling program targets only that behavior, it does not lead individuals to do other PEBs. The use of incentives does not generalize to all PEB, nor does it promote internalization of PEB into a sustainable lifestyle. In sum, these results suggest that providing incentives, combined with facilitating a specific behavior like recycling, may lead to a positive attitude toward recycling and to more recycling behaviors as long as these behaviors are not too costly and/or there are no barriers present. Providing incentives for a behavior or making a behavior easier does not seem to carry over to conditions where the behavior is not reinforced anymore, where the behavior is more difficult, or to other PEBs.

Thus, it appears that the overall response of psychological science to the problem of sustainable development has been eclectic and not very coherent. Although strategies designed to encourage people to act have been growing at a rapid pace, we might question the extent to which the field is moving forward. Research shows that some of the strategies used to motivate people can lead to PEB (Bamberg & Möser, 2007); however, long-term maintenance of these behaviors remains a serious problem. People seem to react positively to the strategies initially, but their behavior declines over time, and, more importantly, behavior returns to baseline if the source of "motivation" is withdrawn (Lehman & Geller, 2004). In sum, the response of psychological science combines different conclusions about the factors that could lead to PEB (see Clayton, 2009; Gardner & Stern, 1996, 2008; Geller, 1995; Kazdin, 2009; Swim et al., 2009), but these various conclusions are scattered across domains within psychology, and across theories within each domain. Having a plethora of researchers doing isolated research will only provide scattered pieces of the puzzle. In order for psychological science to truly make a difference with respect to environmental destruction, research needs to be strongly guided by a comprehensive theory that will address how we could conceptualize sustainability, how interventions should be designed, and how information should be provided to the population so that these strategies truly motivate people to act in a way that will lead to the integration of PEB into their lifestyles (i.e., to become "eco-citizens"). A theory-based approach could represent a vital ingredient in explaining why some strategies or interventions are more effective than others, and the type of psychological processes that are at work.

SDT and the Motivation for Pro-environmental Behaviors

One theoretical perspective of human motivation that has received a great deal of attention from researchers over the last decade—and also has implications for the issues of maintenance and integration of change—is self-determination theory (SDT), proposed by Deci and Ryan (1985, 2000, 2008). This theory holds the potential to significantly contribute to our understanding of the issues related to environmentally responsible behaviors for several reasons. To begin with, it distinguishes between different types of motivation that can have a distinct impact on the maintenance and integration of behaviors. Second, it presents clear hypotheses regarding the social, contextual, and interpersonal conditions that should hinder or facilitate individuals' motivation to adopt a new PEB. Furthermore, it outlines various consequences (cognitive, affective, and behavioral) that are associated with the different types of motivation. In addition, it addresses the issue of internalization, the process by which changes that were initially reinforced by external sources (e.g., incentives or a significant other) become integrated within the individual to form a permanent part of his or her character. Lastly, it provides the reasoning for the process by which people could internalize more than one PEB and truly become an eco-citizen.

As illustrated in this volume, SDT is a broad theory of human motivation that has been applied to a wide range of phenomena and a variety of life domains. The theory explains how different conditions promote different qualities of motivation, along a continuum from lesser to greater self-determination. SDT has also been a useful theory to explain why some strategies are problematic or ineffective in motivating behavior, and why some people may be motivated at first to do PEB, but do not maintain these behaviors over time. An overview of the theory is provided in the first chapter of this volume. For this reason, other than to briefly define the key concept we will be discussing, self-determined motivation will not be reviewed here. Instead, we will turn our attention first to the different ways SDT has been applied in the environmental context; then, we will examine new possible avenues for pivotal research.

Quality of Motivation and the Occurrence of PEB

Although the evidence that relates SDT to PEB is only beginning to appear, recent studies have supported the existence of the different types of motivation proposed by SDT in the environmental context (Osbaldiston & Sheldon, 2003; Pelletier, 2002; Pelletier, Tuson, Green-Demers, Noels, & Beaton, 1998; Villacorta, Koestner, & Lekes, 2003). In addition to these findings, other studies have examined how the different types of motivation for PEB relate to several indicators of PEB.

One set of studies in particular have shown that different types of motivation were related not only to pro-environmental concerns but also to several PEBs (such as recycling, conserving energy, purchasing specific products, and others; Pelletier et al., 1998; Villacorta et al., 2003) and environmental activism (Séguin, Pelletier, & Hunsley, 1998) in a manner that is consistent with research in other life domains. That is, the more that individuals report being self-determined for PEB, the more likely they are to report a higher frequency of PEB. Pelletier and Sharp (2007) have also reported that higher levels of self-determined motivation for PEB were associated with higher maintenance of behavior over time (e.g., sustained recycling over 2 months), along with behavioral patterns consistent with adopting not only one behavior, but several behaviors (e.g., recycling, conserving energy, conserving water, and buying biodegradable products) that are indicative of having integrated the PEB into one's lifestyle and becoming an eco-citizen.

Motivation for More and Less Difficult PEBs

Some authors have studied how self-determination relates to behaviors that have been made more easily accessible, behaviors for which barriers have been removed, or behaviors with different levels of difficulty. As mentioned before, environmentalists have previously proposed relying on strategies that reduce barriers by making an activity more accessible (e.g., a curbside recycling program), and therefore easier to achieve.

A study by Green-Demers, Pelletier, and Ménard (1997) examined the impact of the perceived level of difficulty of environmental behaviors on the magnitude of the relationship between environmental self-determination and the occurrence of three types of PEB with an increasing level of difficulty (recycling, purchasing environmentally friendly products, and educating oneself about what can be done for the environment). Results demonstrated that frequency of behaviors was higher when self-determination was higher, and lower when behavioral difficulty was higher. Moreover, the decrease in the frequency of self-reported PEB caused by the behavior's difficulty was less pronounced when people were self-determined. Third, the positive relationship between self-determination frequencies of PEB was greater for more difficult PEBs. In other words, everyone was more likely to do easier PEBs, but only self-determined people were likely to do more difficult PEBs

In another study, Pelletier and Sharp (2007) were able to isolate differences in the level of difficulty for the same behavior by examining the impact of the degree of self-determination and three levels of difficulty for recycling behavior on the amount of recycling. Residents of three municipalities were randomly selected to participate in a survey on PEB. In one of the municipalities, residents had access to a curbside recycling program (easy recycling); in the second municipality, residents had access to a recycling program, but had to bring their recyclables to one of the available local municipal depots (moderate recycling); in the third municipality, residents did not have access to a local municipal recycling program, but could dispose of their recyclables by driving 20 min to the next municipality that had a local recycling program (difficult recycling). Results revealed that, for the easy recycling condition, the quantity of recycling was not significantly different for self-determined and non self-determined individuals; however, for the moderate condition, the amount of recycling for self-determined and non self-determined individuals became significantly different, although both groups recycled less than participants in the easy condition. This trend held true for the difficult recycling condition as well. Additional analyses revealed that the ease of access to recycling had no relationship with the frequency of other PEBs, while peoples' degree of self-determination related positively to frequency of PEBs other than recycling. Apparently, the benefits of making recycling easier or accessible did not transfer to other PEB domains, while the benefits of self-determination did generalize to various PEB domains.

The investigators also examined the effects of self-determination and difficulty on the residents' perceived satisfaction with local environmental conditions, satisfaction with government environmental policy, and the importance of the environment. Self-determined residents were less satisfied with current environmental conditions and with government environmental policy, and considered the ecological situation more important than non self-determined individuals. These perceptions did not differ significantly as a function of the level of difficulty of recycling behaviors.

Finally, Aitken, Pelletier, and Baxter (2010) measured participants' frequency of PEBs and perceived difficulty of those PEBs in two contexts—at home and at one's school residence. Results indicated that for PEBs perceived as difficult, higher self-determined motivation was associated with more frequent PEB. When the behavior was perceived to be easy, degree of self-determined motivation had no influence on behavior frequency. This pattern was consistent across context. Furthermore, a mediation analysis showed that feeling competent regarding PEB had a positive indirect relation with frequency of difficult PEBs (via self-determined motivation), while the indirect effect of feeling competent on easy behaviors was not significant. In sum, this study suggests that a sense of competence and self-determined motivation regarding PEB are particularly effective at encouraging difficult PEBs, potentially leading to a larger environmental impact.

Altogether, these studies suggest that PEBs could be encouraged either by making them easier, or by fostering self-determination in people. Although it is possible to decrease the difficulty of a PEB, thereby increasing its occurrence, this raises questions about the extent to which the PEB will be maintained if the behavior ceases to be easy, and the extent to which it will generalize to other PEBs. Studies regarding SDT and PEB, however, suggest that PEB performed for self-determined reasons have a better chance of becoming more frequent and being maintained once they have been developed because as PEB become more integrated in the person's self-system and lifestyle, and the negative impact of the behavior's perceived difficulty diminishes.

The Search for Information About Health Risks

Another line of inquiry where motivation could play an important role is examining how people could be pro-active by searching for information and educating themselves about environmental issues so that they could make informed decisions about the PEB they may adopt. One class of specific determinants of PEB that has received some attention and appears to be an important predictor of PEB is the perception of health risks. Government and industry tend to use a different measurement of risk than does the general public, and this difference can lead to significantly different perceptions, with government and industry more prone to discount risk and the general public more likely to perceive risk. These differences can lead the government and industry to view the public as alarmist, while leading the public view the government and industry as untrustworthy and driven only by financial factors.

Individuals' perceptions of health risks can be affected by the specific information they obtain from different sources like the media, governments agencies, activist organizations, public groups, or scientists. In addition, the characteristics of the sources of information (e.g., the type of information given, its trustworthiness or credibility) could either amplify or attenuate the perceptions of environmental health risks and consequently lead to more or less PEB (Kasperson et al., 1988; Renn, Burns, Kasperson, Kasperson, & Slovic, 1992). The more confidence people have in a particular source of information on environmental health risks, the more they should perceive health risks in the environment, and the more they should try to correct a situation by becoming actively involved.

Séguin et al. (1998) proposed to test a model of environmental activism in which the combined contribution of self-determined motivation for the environment and perceptions of various environmental health risks would be examined. Participants completed measures of perceptions of problems in the local environment, perceptions of health risks related to environmental conditions, the information they were obtaining from different sources (e.g., university scientists, medical doctors, environmental groups, government officials), their perceptions of the level of responsibility of specific organization to prevent health risks (e.g., the government, private industry), and their personal level of environmental activism (e.g., participation in events organized by ecological groups, financial support to these groups, circulation of petitions, writing letters to industries that manufacture harmful products). Results showed that the more individuals were self-determined, the more they paid attention to information about health risks, to problems in their local environment, and to the responsibility of different organizations to prevent health risks. In turn, individuals with a higher sensitivity to information about environmental health risks, and individuals who were aware of possible problems in their environment, reported higher levels of perceived health risks. Finally, the more individuals perceived health risks in their environment, the more they engaged in environmental activism.

An important aspect of these findings pertains to the role of self-determined motivation as a factor leading individuals to be more proactive and to seek out information on environmental health risks, the condition of their local environment, and the organizations responsible for preventing health risks in the environment. Interestingly, the more individuals perceived that various organizations had responsibilities to prevent health risks in the environment, the higher was their perception of risks to their health. In other words, self-determined motivation may represent more than a reliable predictor of PEB, and may also be a predictor of the processes leading individuals to be more proactive and to take steps to prevent damage to their health or the environment.

In a second study, Séguin, Pelletier, and Hunsley (1999) more closely examined the above-mentioned relationships by asking participants to complete a survey about their perceptions of environmental health risks, the extent to which they were seeking information on health risks from different sources, their level of confidence in these sources, their motivation, and their frequency of PEB. The sources of information on health risks included federal government agencies, the government itself, public interest groups, environmental groups, the media, scientists, and industry. The authors observed that self-determination was associated with the amount of information individuals sought from various sources of information on health risks, which led to more confidence in these sources of information; in turn, the level of confidence in the different sources of information was a significant predictor of individuals' perceptions of environmental health risks and these perceptions were predictors of PEB. It is noteworthy that self-determination toward the environment was a much stronger predictor of PEB than perceptions of health risks (twice as great), even after controlling for the effect of motivation on the search for information on health risks.

In sum, the results of several studies reveal that people are not only engaging in pro-environmental behaviors for different reasons, but it appears that these reasons are related to important consequences. Consistent with SDT, the more individuals indicate that they are self-determined toward the environment, the more they engage in PEB, difficult PEB in particular, and mild activism, and the more they seek out information about health risks. These studies also suggest that higher levels of self-determined motivation for PEB are associated with higher maintenance of behavior over time, as well as behavioral patterns consistent with the adoption of multiple PEBs and thus indicative of being/becoming an eco-citizen.

Given the consequences linked to a more self-determined profile of motivation, it becomes worthwhile to investigate possible factors that could either enhance or possibly impair the development of this motivational orientation. In the next section, we turn our attention to studies that have examined the determinants of environmental motivation.

Determinants of Motivation for PEB

According to SDT, individuals are inherently motivated to integrate within themselves the regulation of activities that are useful for effective functioning in the social world, but that are not inherently interesting. Because our environment has important implications for our economy, our health, and the quality of our lives, people's desire to be effective in dealing with the challenges posed by the ecological situation should prompt them to take in the regulation of PEBs that are not interesting in their own right, but that they perceive to be important or valued. Like the internalization of activities in other life domains, the internalization of PEBs should be an active process through which people gradually transform socially valued behaviors into personally endorsed activities. SDT proposes that the satisfaction of innate psychological needs for competence, autonomy, and relatedness, as well as social contexts that support the satisfaction of these needs, promotes the internalization of autonomous or functional forms of regulation, and well-being (Deci & Ryan, 2000; Ryan & Deci, 2000). Although internalization of PEB is facilitated by people in a relatively close social environment (e.g., a spouse, friends, children, educators) that could represent a daily source of influence on motivation, we think that the impact that broader sources of influence, including the government, the media, and public role models, is especially critical. Therefore, actions from these broader sources of influence that are informative and support autonomy, such as providing a good rationale for PEB, pointing the way to being more effective in meetings environmental challenges, and letting people freely choose among different options, could foster the development of self-determined motivation. In contrast, actions that pressure people toward specific outcomes or that represent attempts to control behaviors, like financial incentives, punishments, or imposed rules, may produce temporary compliance, but will not lead to lasting commitment or investment, nor will it lead one PEB to generalize to other PEBs. Finally, situations where no rationale for acting is provided, where no guidance is provided about a solution to the perceived problem, and where people perceive solutions to be out of their reach all create a sense of helplessness that leads individuals to disengage from PEB (Pelletier, Dion, Tuson, & Green-Demers, 1999). With respect to the environment, a critical social-contextual factor is the government's approach toward the implementation of environmental programs and strategies that target PEB.

The Influence of Government Policies

As illustrated at the beginning of this chapter, citizens are increasingly aware of the precarious state of our environment. For instance, in a recent survey, while many Canadians (28.7%) recognize that they, as individuals, are primarily responsible for the protection of the environment, even more (43.1%) believe that the government is primarily responsible for implementing policies for the population in general (Environics, 2005).

Although citizens assign an important role to their government in the pursuit of environmental sustainability, little attention has been paid to the impact of the government's approach toward environmental policy on the environmental behaviors of individual citizens. Understanding this is important, as government environmental programs and policies are universally applied and, therefore, exert a systemic influence on every citizen. Besides providing the infrastructure for the facilitation of several large-scale PEBs such as curbside recycling programs or energy conservation, government is responsible for the development and the implementation of several programs and policies aimed at motivating individuals to engage in PEB (e.g., advertisements, transit pass tax credits, rebates for programmable thermostats, discounts on insurance of hybrid vehicles, etc.) at a community through to a national level. Yet, to date, few studies have examined the effects of the government's approach toward the introduction and implementation of such programs and policies on the motivation for PEB of individual citizens. Therefore, there is a need to examine if and how government environmental regulation affects the motivation for, and performance of, PEB at the level of the individual. There is also a need to examine what individuals perceive to be the most efficient ways to motivate people to act. That is, if the protection of the environment and climate change are perceived as real threats, and there is sense of urgency to do something about it, how do individuals believe the government should proceed to motivate people to act? The answer to this question is important because it may explain what type of government one chooses to support or vote for in a time of crisis.

By definition, environmental laws and policies are a form of control and, as SDT claims (Deci & Ryan, 1987), they should lead to controlled form of motivation and low levels of PEB integration in one's lifestyle if they are not implemented with an understanding of human needs and psychological functioning. In one study, Lavergne, Sharp, Pelletier, and Holtby (2010) tested a motivational model of PEB that used perception of government style in the implementation of environmental programs and policies as a predictor of motivation for PEB. As expected, autonomous motivation predicted a higher frequency of PEB, controlled motivation did not predict frequency of PEB, and amotivation predicted lower frequency of PEB. Congruent with previous studies, these findings lend support to the important role of self-determined motivation for the promotion of PEB at an individual level. In addition to these findings, the role of government support for the facilitation of self-determined PEB was also confirmed. That is, perception of the government as autonomy-supportive contributed to higher levels of self-determination, which was evidenced by a direct positive effect on autonomous motivation and a direct negative effect on amotivation. Perception of the government as controlling did not support participants' self-determination; instead, it had a strong direct positive effect on both controlled motivation and amotivation. In sum, the way that the government is perceived by the individual has a significant impact on that person's PEB, either in a positive direction if government is seen as autonomy-supportive, or in a negative direction if government is perceived as controlling. Since autonomous motivation is much more closely associated with PEB, the most valuable form of government would be one that is autonomy supportive, and thus fosters the type of motivation necessary to encourage the members of a society to become eco-citizens.

Lavergne et al. (in press) results provide a snapshot of the influence of perceived government style on environmental motivation and self-determined PEB. Because it is the perception of government as more or less autonomy-supportive or controlling that influences a person's motivation (Deci & Ryan, 1987), then one would expect that these perceptions might differ from one country to another, or that they may shift when governments change their leadership or when governments change their ideologies.

Hence, research on the influence of government policies could significantly contribute to the environmental literature in several ways. For instance, longitudinal research could uncover the role of government in the internalization (or diminution) of environmental motivation over the course of months or years. The implementation of new environmental policies or changes in existing ones may reveal fluctuations in the public's perception of government, which could also be associated with corresponding variations in environmental motivation. In addition, it would be fruitful to compare the effects of governments with different environmental orientations in the same country and across different countries.

The Influence of Information on Environmental Issues

Substantial effort is devoted to shaping the public's views on environmental conditions through information campaigns in the media. One strategy consist of providing extensive information about different ecological threats (e.g., global climate change, toxic pollution of air and water supplies, etc.), urging individuals to prevent further deterioration of the environment, and stressing the necessity of having individuals directly participate in PEBs in order to address current environmental degradation. These messages tend to focus on those behaviors that people do not commit on a regular basis but that are known to effect positive changes in the environment.

Describing the nature and the severity of a problem could make people more conscious of the situation. It can also make them aware that there is a discrepancy between the importance they attribute to the environmental situation and their level of activity to correct that situation. As a consequence, this may create discomfort or cognitive dissonance.

In this section, we first examine how providing knowledge about the seriousness of the situation can create discomfort or cognitive dissonance, but it can also lead to paradoxical effects in people with different motivational orientations. Second, we examine how information campaigns on the environment could take advantage of recent principles of persuasive communication strategies, principles of behavior change, and principles derived from SDT to make people aware of the importance of environmental conditions and lead them to change their behavior.

Motivation and the Reduction of Cognitive Dissonance

The psychological discomfort (i.e., negative affect) induced by the presence of a conflict (i.e., dissonance) between a cognition and a behavior has been shown to motivate individuals to adopt a strategy to reduce the dissonance. Several studies demonstrate that cognitive dissonance is an aversive state, and point toward an alleviation of psychological discomfort as the motivation underlying dissonance-induced attitude change (Higgins, Rhodewalt, & Zanna, 1978; Losch & Cacioppo, 1990; Zanna, Higgins, & Taves, 1976). However, Harmon-Jones (2000) conducted a large literature review on dissonance studies and found that the means of dissonance reduction people use most often is to change their attitude to be consistent with their behavior, rather than the other way around. In other words, when a person becomes aware of a discrepancy between their belief that environmental degradation has occurred and their lack of action to reduce that degradation, they may well choose to downplay the seriousness of the environmental situation rather than changing their behavior. This may occur because changing one's attitude or perception is perceived as being easier than changing one's behavior. This reinforces the necessity of having a clear strategy when a message is communicated to the public. It also raises questions about the effects of simply alarming the public about the seriousness of the environmental situation without giving them clear and accessible means to solve the situation or providing the psychological support needed to move toward the solution.

Recently, Lavergne, Pelletier, and Aitken (2010) tried to shed some light on this issue by examining whether people's level of self-determined motivation plays a role in the amount of dissonance people experience and in how they decide to reduce (or not reduce) this dissonance. In an initial study they assessed how people react when they detect dissonance about their perception of the importance of environmental sustainability and their PEB. Four types of reactions were identified: doing nothing, deflecting (i.e., thinking environmental problems are not their responsibility or hoping nobody notices their lack of action), self-bolstering (i.e., reminding themselves that they try the best they can but sometimes make mistakes), or using self-monitoring and bringing their behavior more in line with their beliefs (i.e., reminding themselves to pay more attention in the future, or planning to do more PEB). In a second study the authors examined how these four types of reactions were related to self-determined motivation and dissonance. The results revealed that a low level of self-determined motivation predicted the tendency to react to dissonance by inaction or deflection, while a high level of self-determined motivation predicted the tendency to use self-bolstering and especially self-monitoring and planning behavior change to address dissonance. In agreement with SDT, it appears that when self-determined people experience dissonance regarding an issue important to them, they reduce the dissonance by acting consistently with their values. In contrast, inducing dissonance in people with a low level of self-determined motivation seems to backfire, pushing them in the opposite direction of the goal intended by the message. In summary, the present program of research offers insight into some promising possibilities for new research. More studies are needed to examine the effects that messages which create discomfort have on people, and the long-term effects of messages that do little more than constantly remind people of the importance of dealing with environmental conditions.

The Use of Strategic Information

In response to the relatively low impact of information campaigns that have targeted PEB, Pelletier and Sharp (2008) proposed a global strategy for improving messages devoted to shaping the public's views on specific environmental issues, based on recent principles of persuasive communication strategies, principles of behavior change, and principles derived from SDT. First, the authors proposed that messages should be tailored in terms of three phases of behavior change (Burkholder & Evers, 2002; Rosen, 2000; Rothman & Salovey, 2007)—that is detection of a problem, decision to act on it, and implementation of the action. This should enhance self-determined motivation for the behaviors that people adopt, since these phases of behavior change represent a move from the absence of motivation, to motivation where one decides to act, to a motivation where one sees the value in the behavior. Once people are ready to act, progressively communicating information that supports individuals' basic needs by being framed in terms of intrinsic rather than extrinsic goals, and information on how individuals could implement their goals and intentions, could further enhance the internalization and maintenance of PEB.

More specifically, the detection phase is characterized by a state where people are primarily sensitive to messages that help them gather and interpret information needed to decide whether there is a problem. Once people have detected the presence of a problem and determined that this problem is important, they are in the decision phase where they are primarily sensitive to messages that help them decide whether to take action, and how to take action (Rothman & Salovey, 2007; Rothman, Baldwyn, & Hertel, 2004). Once people have decided to act, they become primarily sensitive to information about how to implement a behavior, and possibly how to maintain the behavior or integrate it in their lifestyle. Thus, one type of message could be effective for some people to help them move toward behavior change, while it could be ineffective for other people. For example, information about how to implement a behavior would not be helpful to somebody who is not aware that a problem exists. Likewise, further information on the existence of a problem is not likely to motivate people further once they are aware that a problem exists.

Once people are aware that a problem exists, messages should communicate information on the important actions that could be done to reduce the risks associated with a situation (i.e., to facilitate progress through the decision phase). The information presented at this phase specifically serves the purpose of identifying the specific behaviors that point the way to effectively meeting the challenges introduced in the first phase. In agreement with SDT, to facilitate the internalization of behaviors, the information should also provide a good rationale. That is, it should not only indicate possible actions, it should also explain why and how these actions improve the situation.

Finally, once people have decided to take action, they may become more interested in information about when, where, and how a specific behavior could be implemented. This information helps individuals translate their intentions into behavior (i.e., progress through the implementation phase). Whereas a goal that results from the decision phase specifies what one wants to achieve, implementation intentions involve specifying more precisely when, where, and how an action will lead to goal achievement. In sum, implementation intentions represent an important step to facilitate self-determined motivation because they help individuals set the conditions that will determine when they get started and how they stay on track (Koestner, Lekes, Powers, & Chicoine, 2002).

For these three phases of behavior change, principles derived from SDT research on intrinsic versus extrinsic goal orientations should be applied. For instance, consistent with the research on intrinsic vs. extrinsic goal framing (Vansteenkiste, Lens, & Deci, 2006; Vansteenkiste, Simons, Lens, Sheldon, & Deci, 2004), framing messages systematically in terms of intrinsic goals (i.e., health, well-being, altruism), as opposed to extrinsic goals (i.e., money, possessions, prestige, fame), should not only enhance peoples' self-determined motivation, it should also facilitate the maintenance of the behaviors that people adopt. The type of motive considered when a goal is framed is important because message framing influences what people attend to, what knowledge and attitudes become cognitively accessible, and what behaviors are considered. As a consequence, when a goal is framed as a function of extrinsic rather than intrinsic motives, it should lead to less self-determined motivation for an activity, less engagement in the activity, and less persistence. In fact, a recent study by Osbaldiston and Sheldon (2003) examined the relationship between autonomy support and goal performance with respect to PEB. The authors asked participants to perform certain environmental goals, such as taking shorter showers or saving electricity, in an autonomy-supportive manner (namely allowing choice, providing rationale, and acknowledging the other's perspective). Over the course of a week, participants gave daily reports via email on how they were performing with respect to their goal. Results demonstrated that, the more an individual perceived the experimenter as autonomy supportive, the higher their initial level of internalized motivation; this initial level of autonomous motivation, in turn, significantly predicted goal performance, final levels of internalized motivation, and future intentions to perform goals during the following week. Thus, framing messages to be autonomy supportive can have a significant impact on whether an individual will achieve and persist at their environmental goals.

Finally, it is likely that goal framing for a particular phase will influence the way that information is processed for the subsequent phase of behavior change (Rothman & Salovey, 2007). For example, the emphasis on the financial costs of ecological threats in the detection phase should raise the likelihood of goals and solutions that have financial implications in the decision phase, and then, the maintenance of financial incentives to initiate behavior in the implementation phase. In contrast, putting emphasis on the health risks of ecological threats in the detection phase should raise the likelihood of goals and solutions that have health implications in the decision phase, and then health related feedback to maintain behavior in the last phase. In other words, we need to be careful about how we frame messages in an early stage, because that angle tends to stay with that person for the stages that follow.

It is important to emphasize that very little research pertaining to PEB has examined the propositions that are described above. The test of these proposed principles should shed some lights on the role that motivation plays in the perception and the processing of persuasive messages, when individuals form judgments about risk, when they evaluate potential solutions, or when they decide to implement a new behavior. Finally, they should also help us determine if the different reasons for changing behavior are equally effective.

Conclusion: Toward Sustainable Development

All the proponents of sustainable development agree that society and its constituents (individual citizens) need to change, despite the fact that there are major debates over the best way(s) to achieve this change. Keeping the debate at the level of trade-offs between environmental issues and socio-economic issues, while generally ignoring the interplay between governments, the media and the individuals who will inevitably be the agents of change, may lead to counterproductive effects. To achieve environmental sustainability we must address the processes that will lead individuals to learn new PEB, adopt these behaviors, and more importantly, integrate these behaviors in their lifestyle. Self-determination theory offers a promising framework for understanding the social factors that could lead to, or interfere with, such behaviors. Furthermore, the study of PEB represents a domain with its own challenging characteristics that could further our knowledge on the causes, consequences, and mechanisms of motivation.

In this chapter we focused our attention on the difference that the quality of motivation makes when individuals deal with more or less difficult PEBs, as well as the pro-active role that self-determined motivation plays when individuals search for and process information on health risks. We also examined how government policies could affect motivation, we introduced a new avenue of research on the positive and negative strategies people use to reduce their cognitive dissonance regarding

PEB, and we examined how tailoring and framing messages could guide individuals and help them become more self-determined. Although the studies described in this chapter are consistent with SDT, more studies that use experimental methodologies are required to demonstrate causality. We also need more research that assesses behavioral indicators of PEB, and, more importantly, indicators that PEB have been integrated in one's lifestyle. Like the research on SDT in other life domains, the research on PEB should also examine how people from different countries and different cultures integrate PEB in their own lifestyle. Finally, we must find a way to address what we may call the "elephant in the room" in PEB—the impact that the growing population will have on the achievement of sustainability.

Motivating people to change behaviors that are harmful to the environment represents a challenging task. Below is a brief summary of the key lessons learned from self-determination theory and related research regarding the optimal ways to frame messages, implement local changes, implement government policies, educate children and adults, train educators, and promote autonomous, comprehensive, and enduring pro-environmental motivation and behavior:

- Be mindful of stages of change (detection, decision, and implementation), tailor the intervention to the stage where the recipient of the intervention is located, and aim to facilitate movement through the stage and transition to the next stage of change:
- When providing information about an environmental problem, simultaneously provide concrete steps for arriving at a solution;
- Act in a way that satisfies peoples' needs for autonomy, competence, and relatedness by providing them with good justification for their action, explaining how a specific behavior could be helpful, helping them figure out how they could implement new actions, and being careful about the reasons we provide to justify these changes;
- Give justifications in terms of intrinsic values and goals (i.e., health, well-being, altruism) rather than extrinsic ones (i.e., money, possessions, prestige, fame);
- Provide step-by-step procedures (i.e., implementation goals and implementation intentions), and means of tracking progress and providing feedback;
- Recognize that incentives are extrinsic motivators and thus double-edged swords, and implement them in a context that promotes eventual internalization of pro-environmental values.

References

Aitken, N., Pelletier, L. G., & Baxter, D. (2010, May). *Doing the hard stuff: Influence of self-determined motivation toward the environment on pro-environmental behaviours*. Paper presented at the Fourth international SDT conference, Ghent, Belgium.

Aronson, E., & Gonzales, M. H. (1990). Alternative social influence processes applied to energy conservation. In J. Edwards, R. S. Tindale, L. Heath, & E. J. Posavac (Eds.), *Social influence processes and prevention* (pp. 301–325). New York: Plenum Press.

Bamberg, S., & Möser, G. (2007). Twenty years after Hines, Hungerford, and Tomera: A new meta-analysis of psycho-social determinants of pro-environmental behavior. *Journal of Environmental Psychology, 27*, 14–25.

Burkholder, G. J., & Evers, K. E. (2002). Application of the transtheoretical model to several problem behaviors. In P. M. Burbank &D. Riebe (Eds.), *Promoting exercise and behavior change in older adults: Interventions with the transtheoretical model* (pp. 85–145). New York: Springer

Clayton, S. (2009). Promoting sustainable behavior. In S. Clayton & M. Myers (Eds.), *Conservation psychology: Understanding and promoting human care for nature* (pp. 143–161). Boston: Blackwell.

Darby, S. (2006). *The effectiveness of feedback on energy consumption: A review for DEFRA of the literature on metering, billing, and direct displays.* Oxford, England: Environmental Change Institute, University of Oxford. Retrieved March 2, 2010, from www.cci.ox.ac.uk/research/energy/downloads/smart-metering-report.pdf

De Young, R. (1986). Encouraging environmentally appropriate behavior: The role of intrinsic motivation. *Journal of Environmental Systems, 15*, 281–292.

Deci, E. L., & Ryan, R. M. (1985). *Intrinsic motivation and self-determination in human behavior.* New York: Plenum Press.

Deci, E. L., & Ryan, R. M. (1987). The support of autonomy and the control of behavior. *Journal of Personality and Social Psychology, 53*, 1024–1037.

Deci, E. L., & Ryan, R. M. (2000). The "what" and "why" of goal pursuits: Human needs and self-determination of behavior. *Psychological Inquiry, 11*, 227–268.

Deci, E. L., & Ryan, R. M. (2008). Facilitating optimal motivation and well-being across life's domains. *Canadian Psychology, 49*, 14–23.

Dwyer, W. O., Leeming, F. C., Cobern, M. K., Porter, B. E., & Jackson, J. M. (1993). Critical review of behavioral interventions to preserve the environment – Research since 1980. *Environment and Behavior, 25*, 275–321.

Eagly, A. H., & Kulesa, P. (1997). Attitudes, attitude structure, and resistance to change: Implications for persuasion on environmental issues. In M. H. Bazerman, D. M. Messick, A. E. Tenbrunsel, & K. A. Wade-Benzoni (Eds.), *Environment, ethics, and behavior* (pp. 154–168). San Francisco, CA: The New Lexington Press.

Environics Research Group. (2005). *2005 Environics focus Canada survey* (No. EFC051). Retrieved September 14, 2008, from http://www.queensu.ca/cora/5data.html

Environics. (2007a). *Canadian environmental barometer* (Poll). Ottawa: Environics.

Environics. (2007b). *Ontario consumer market research on attitudes and behavior toward electricity conservation.* Ottawa: Ontario Power Authority, Environics.

Gardner, G. T., & Stern, P. C. (1996). *Environmental problems and human behavior.* Needham Heights, MA: Allyn & Bacon.

Gardner, G. T., & Stern, P. C. (2002). *Environmental problems and human behavior* (2nd ed.). Boston: Pearson Custom Publishing.

Gardner, G. T., & Stern, P. C. (2008). The short list: Most effective actions US households can take to limit climate change. *Environment, 50*(5), 13–24.

Geller, E. S. (1989). Applied behavior analysis and social marketing: An integration for environmental preservation. *Journal of Social Issues, 45*, 17–36.

Geller, E. S. (1995). Integrating behaviorism and humanism for environmental protection. *Journal of Social Issues, 51*, 179–195.

Geller, E. S., Winett, R. A., & Everett, P. B. (1982). *Preserving the environment: New strategies for behavior change.* Elmsford, NY: Pergamon.

Gifford, R. (2007). *Environmental psychology: Principles and practice.* Coleville, WA: Optimal Books.

Goldstein, N. J., Cialdini, R. B., & Griskevicius, V. (2008). A room with a viewpoint: Using social norms to motivate environmental conservation in hotels. *Journal of Consumer Research, 35*, 472–482.

Green-Demers, I., Pelletier, L. G., & Ménard, S. (1997). The impact of behavioral difficulty on the saliency of the association between self-determined motivation and environmental behaviors. *Canadian Journal of Behavioral Sciences, 29,* 157–166.

Harmon-Jones, E. (2000). An Update on Cognitive Dissonance Theory, with a Focus on the Self. In A. Tesser, R. B. Felson, & J. M. Suls (Eds.) *Psychological Perspectives on Self and Identity* (pp. 119–144), Washington, DC: American Psychological Association.

Hines, J. M., Hungerford, H. R., & Tomera, A. N. (1987). Analysis and synthesis of research on responsible environmental behavior: A meta-analysis. *Journal of Environmental Education, 18,* 1–8.

Higgins, E. T., Rhodewalt, F., Zanna, M. P. (1978). Dissonance motivation: Its nature, persistence, and reinstatement. *Journal of Experimental Social Psychology, 15,* 16–34.

Hopwood, B., Mellor, M., & O'Brien, G. (2005). Sustainable development: Mapping different approaches. *Sustainable Development, 13,* 38–52.

Intergovernmental Panel on Climate Change [IPCC]. (2007). Summary for policymakers. In: S. Solomon, D. Qin, M. Manning, Z. Chen, M. Marquis, K. B. Averyt, M. Tignor, & H. L. Miller (Eds.), *Climate change 2007: The physical science basis.* Contribution of working Group I to the fourth assessment report of the Intergovernmental Panel on Climate Change. Cambridge/New York: Cambridge University Press. Retrieved February 12, 2010, from http://www.ipcc-wg2.org/

Kasperson, R. E., Renn, O., Slovic, P., Brown, H. S., Emel, J., Goble, R., et al. (1988). The social amplification of risk: A conceptual framework. *Risk Analysis, 8,* 177–187.

Katzev, R. D., & Johnson, T. (1984). Comparing the effects of monetary incentives and foot-in-the-door strategies in promoting residential electricity conservation. *Journal of Applied Social Psychology, 14,* 12–27.

Kazdin, A. E. (2009). Psychological science's contributions to a sustainable environment: Extending our reach to a grand challenge of society. *American Psychologist, 64,* 339–356.

Koestner, R., Lekes, N., Powers, T. A., & Chicoine, E. (2002). Attaining personal goals: Self-concordance plus implementation intentions equals success. *Journal of Personality and Social Psychology, 83,* 231–244.

Kollmuss, A., & Agyeman, J. (2002). Mind the gap: Why do people act environmentally and what are the barriers to pro-environmental behaviors? *Environmental Education Research, 8,* 239–252.

Lavergne, K. J., Pelletier, L. G., & Aitken, N. (2010, May). *The role of self-determined motivation in the dissonance process: An exploratory study.* Paper presented at the fourth international SDT conference, Ghent, Belgium.

Lavergne, K. J., Sharp, E. C., Pelletier, L. G., & Holtby, A. (2010). The role of perceived government style in the facilitation of self-determined and non self-determined pro-environmental behaviour. *Journal of Environmental Psychology, 30,* 169–177.

Lehman, P. K., & Geller, E. S. (2004). Behavioral analysis and environmental protection: Accomplishments and potential for more. *Behavioral and Social Issues, 13,* 13–24.

Losch, M. E., Cacioppo, J. T. (1990). Cognitive dissonance may enhance sympathetic tonus, but attitudes are changed to reduce negative affect rather than dissonance. *Journal of Experimental Social Psychology, 26,* 289–304.

McKenzie-Mohr, D., & Smith, W. (1999). *Fostering sustainable behavior: An introduction to community-based social marketing.* Gabriola Island, BC: New Society Publishers.

McKenzie-Morh, D. (2008). Fostering sustainable behavior: Beyond brochures. *International Journal of Sustainability Communication, 3,* 108–118.

McKenzie-Morh, D., & Oskamp, S. (1995). Psychology and sustain capacity: An introduction. *Journal of Social Issues, 51,* 1–14.

Osbaldiston, R. (2004). *Meta-analysis of the responsible environmental literature* (Ph.D. dissertation; UMI Number 3144447) University of Missouri-Columbia.

Osbaldiston, R., & Sheldon, K. M. (2003). Promoting internalized motivation for environmentally responsible behavior: A prospective study of environmental goals. *Journal of Environmental Psychology, 23,* 349–357.

Oskamp, S. (1995). Resource conservation and recycling: Behavior and policy. *Journal of Social Issues, 51*, 157–177.

Oskamp, S. (2000). Psychological contributions to achieving an ecologically sustainable future for humanity. *Journal of Social Issues, 56*, 373–390.

Pelletier, L. G. (2002). A motivational analysis of self-determination for pro-environmental behaviors. In E. L. Deci & R. M. Ryan (Eds.), *The handbook of self-determination research* (pp. 205–232). Rochester, NY: University of Rochester Press.

Pelletier, L. G., Dion, S., Tuson, K. M., & Green-Demers, I. (1999). Why do people fail to adopt environmental behaviors? Towards a taxonomy of environmental amotivation. *Journal of Applied Social Psychology, 29*, 2481–2504.

Pelletier, L. G., & Sharp, E. C. (2007, June). *From the promotion of pro-environmental behaviors to the Development of an Eco-Citizen: The self-determination theory perspective*. Paper presented at the annual conference of the Canadian Psychological Association, Ottawa, ON.

Pelletier, L. G., & Sharp, E. C. (2008). Persuasive communication and pro-environmental behaviors: How message tailoring and message framing can improve the integration of behaviours through self-determined motivation. *Canadian Psychology, 49*, 210–217.

Pelletier, L. G., Tuson, K. M., Green-Demers, I., Noels, K., & Beaton, A. M. (1998). Why are you doing things for the environment? – The motivation toward the environmental scale (MTES). *Journal of Applied Social Psychology, 28*, 437–468.

Renn, O., Burns, W. J., Kasperson, J. X., Kasperson, R. E., & Slovic, P. (1992). The social amplification of risk: Theoretical foundations and empirical applications. *Journal of Social Issues, 48*, 137–160.

Rosen, C. S. (2000). Is the sequencing of change processes by stage consistent by health problems? A meta-analysis. *Health Psychology, 19*, 593–604.

Rothman, A. J., Baldwyn, A., & Hertel, A. (2004). Self-regulation and behavior change: Disentangling behavioral initiation and behavioral maintenance. In K. Vohs & R. F. Baumeister (Eds.), *The handbook of self-regulation* (pp. 130–148). New York: Guilford Press.

Rothman, A. J., & Salovey, P. (2007). The reciprocal relation between principles and practice. In A. Kruglanski & E. T. Higgins (Eds.), *Social psychology: Handbook of basic principle* (2nd ed., pp. 826–849). New York: Guilford Press.

Ryan, R. M., & Deci, E. L. (2000). Self-determination theory and the facilitation of intrinsic motivation, social development, and well-being. *American Psychologist, 55*, 68–78.

Stern, P. C. (2000). Toward a coherent theory of environmentally significant behavior. *Journal of Social Issues, 56*, 407–424.

Swim, J., Clayton, S., Doherty, T., Gifford, R., Howard, G., Reser, J., et al. (2009). *Psychology and global climate change: Addressing a multi-faceted phenomenon and set of challenges*. A report by the American Psychological Association's Task Force on the Interface Between Psychology and Global Climate Change. Washington, DC: APA.

Séguin, C., Pelletier, L. G., & Hunsley, J. (1998). Toward a model of environmental activism. *Environment and Behavior, 30*, 628–652.

Séguin, C., Pelletier, L. G., & Hunsley, J. (1999). Predicting environmental behaviors: The influence of self-determination and information about environmental health risks. *Journal of Applied Social Psychology, 29*, 1582–1600.

United Nations Population Fund. (2009). *World population to exceed 9 billion by 2050*. http://www.un.org/esa/population/publications/wpp2008/pressrelease.pdf

Vansteenkiste, M., Lens, W., & Deci, E. L. (2006). Intrinsic versus extrinsic goal contents in self-determination theory: Another look at the quality of motivation. *Educational Psychologist, 41*, 19–31.

Vansteenkiste, M., Simons, J., Lens, W., Sheldon, K. M., & Deci, E. L. (2004). Motivating learning, performance, and persistence: The synergistic effects of intrinsic goal contents and autonomy-supportive contexts. *Journal of Personality and Social Psychology, 87*, 246–260.

Villacorta, M., Koestner, R., & Lekes, N. (2003). Further validation of the motivation toward the environment scale. *Environment and Behavior, 35*, 486–505.

Wang, T. H., & Katzev, R. (1990). Group commitment and resource conservation: Two field experiments on promoting recycling. *Journal of Applied Social Psychology, 20*, 265–275.

Winett, R. A., Leckliter, I. N., Chinn, D. E., Stahl, B., & Love, S. Q. (1985). Effects of television modeling on residential energy conservation. *Journal of Applied Behavior Analyses, 18*, 33–44.

Witmer, J. F., & Geller, E. S. (1976). Facilitating paper recycling: Effects of prompts, raffles, and contests. *Journal of Applied Behavior Analysis, 9*, 315–322.

Wood, W., Tam, L., & Guerrero-Witt, M. (2005). Changing circumstances, disrupting habits. *Journal of Personality and Social Psychology, 88*, 918–933.

World Commission on Economic Development. (1987). *Our common future*. New York: Oxford University Press.

Zanna, M. P., Higgins, E. T., Taves, P. A. (1976). Is dissonance phenomenologically aversive? *Journal of Experimental Social Psychology, 12*, 530–538.

Zelesny, L. C. (1999). Educational interventions that improve environmental behaviors: A meta-analysis. *Journal of Environmental Education, 31*, 5–14.

Index

A

Activity, 5, 10, 25, 49–50, 68–69, 73–75, 77, 126–127, 133–136, 142–144, 146–148, 155–156, 169, 194, 210, 215, 219, 224–225, 243, 257, 263, 269, 271

Advertising
 negative effects of advertising and violent media products, 220

Agency
 psychological and autonomous agency, 67

Agency, 9–14, 16–20, 67, 69–72, 74–77, 86, 243

Ancient Greece, 2, 4

Aristotle, 3, 6, 46–47, 55

Aspirations
 negative effects of unrealized aspirations on well-being, 213

Attachment theory, 98–99, 228

Authority
 legitimate, 244
 parental, 246

Autonomous self regulation, 23, 45, 52–53, 57, 119, 134, 136, 138–140, 142, 146–148

Autonomy
 biological, 67, 69–70, 73, 84–85
 human psychological, 22–23, 67, 71
 interpersonal, 13, 23, 33
 intrapsychic, 12–13
 motivational autonomy, 1, 3, 13, 67–69, 82–85, 125–127, 141, 146, 167, 228
 need for, 7, 12–13, 24, 36, 84, 96, 100–101, 104–106, 111–128, 133, 165, 169–171, 174–175, 204, 219, 243
 perceived, 37–38, 84, 101, 104, 111, 116, 121, 147
 personal autonomy/personal freedom, 2, 4, 7, 9–14, 24–26, 36, 67–68, 79–80, 133–157, 191, 207–229, 241–253, 257–273
 political autonomy, 67
 -promoting Schools, 24, 112, 120–128
 psychological, 10, 12–14, 21–23, 67, 69–71, 77
 support
  benefits of, 101, 116
  definition, 40, 84, 101–103, 119–120, 154
  political support for, 117
  value of, 7, 66–67
 -supportive social relationships, 84

B

Bar exams, 39

Basic psychological needs, 20, 23, 26, 36, 42–43, 45, 48–49, 56–57, 59–60, 78, 96, 98–99, 101, 105, 111, 120, 134, 143, 165, 177, 208, 215, 217, 219, 221, 224, 242

Baumol, 221

Boggle, 39

Brain, 1, 16, 23, 65–86, 217

C

Capability
 approach, 216

Capitalism, 25, 191–204

Christianity, 4

Circumplex models, 195–198

Civic engagement, 213, 242

Cognitive dissonance, 269, 272

Confucian teaching/ethics, 2, 6

Controlled motivation, 82–83, 97, 107, 114, 143–144, 150–151, 268

Controlled self regulation, 141, 148–149

Controlling, 36, 40–41, 46, 50–52, 54, 57–59, 78, 86, 101–103, 112–116,

Controlling (cont.)
    118–122, 125–128, 139, 142, 146,
    153, 174, 176, 191, 198, 214,
    217–219, 222, 251, 266, 268
Cross-cultural, 9, 23–25, 41–43, 81, 84–85,
    104, 107, 112, 127–128, 135, 138,
    142, 147, 155, 163–164, 166, 168,
    172, 174, 176–178, 194–195, 249,
    251–252
Cross-cultural psychology, 83
Cultural relativism, 18, 20, 66
Cultural systems, 10, 25, 200, 204
Cultural universalism, 66
Culture
    of horizontality, 23, 78–79, 81, 84–85
    of verticality, 23, 78–79, 81

D
Democracy/liberal democracy/democratic
    societies, 242, 250
Democratic/non-democratic government, 250
Determinants of motivation, 266–267
Determinism, 14, 16, 18, 65–67, 70–71
Deterministic trend, 15–16
Developmental psychology, 242
Difficulty of pro-environmental behaviors, 259

E
Easterlin paradox, 210, 212
Economic growth, 26, 194, 198, 203–204,
    208–210, 212–215, 218–221,
    223–225, 227, 229, 257
Economics, 26, 58, 207–209, 212–218,
    223, 228
    and materialism, 223
Economy, 25–27, 141, 164, 207–229, 258, 266
    effects of economic production and
        consumption on community
        ties, 220
Education, 135, 154, 217, 220–221, 225–228,
    248–250, 259
    strategies, 259
Egalitarian
    countries, 24, 128
    nations, 117
    social institutions, 117
    societies, 77
    structure, 117
    values, 117
Emergent properties, 67, 71–72, 74
Employee engagement, 25, 163–178
Eudaimonia, 2–3, 6, 20–21
    eudaimonic happiness, 3, 19, 21–22, 66–67
Eudaimonic approach, 226

Evolution, 33–34, 60, 65, 69–70, 72–74, 124,
    163, 224
External regulation, 7, 50–52, 144, 146
Extrinsic goals, 35, 56–58, 60, 144, 195, 198,
    270–271

F
Flourishing, 6, 18, 20–23
Foster Inner Directed Valuing Processes (FIV),
    121–124
Framing of information, 259, 272–273
Freedom and free will, 67
    freedom of choice and actions, 10, 69
Frontal lobes, 73–75

G
Giovanni Rico della Mirandola, 4
Goals, 1–3, 6–7, 9–11, 13, 17, 21–22, 24–25,
    35, 42, 45–46, 52, 55–60, 69,
    74, 76, 78, 82, 85, 100, 111–112,
    118–127, 133, 143–146, 155,
    173–174, 194–195, 198–199, 212,
    215, 217–219, 225, 258, 270–273
Good life/moral life, 2, 6–9, 14, 19–21, 27,
    45–47, 53, 56
Government policies, 27, 267–268, 272–273

H
Happiness
    happiness economics, 207, 209, 212–214,
        216, 223, 228
    and national income across countries,
        207–209
    trend of happiness, 210
Health and culture, 20, 22, 24–25, 42, 51,
    65, 68, 72, 75, 82–83, 85, 95–107,
    133–135, 138–139, 141–142,
    146–147, 149, 155–157, 168, 171,
    173, 176
Health-related behaviors, 25, 134
Health risks, 85, 137, 259, 264–266, 272
Hedonic adaptation, 209, 213, 223–224
Hedonic approach, 47
Hierarchical
    countries, 24, 128
    nations, 117
    social institutions, 112, 118–119
    societies, 24, 121
    structure, 112, 118, 120
    values, 111, 117
Homo economicus, 215–218
Homunculus, 15–16, 71
Horizontal collectivism, 78–79, 85
Horizontal individualism, 79–80

Human capabilities, 19–20, 23, 81, 86, 216
Humanism, 20, 22

I
Identified regulation, 51–52, 140, 145, 148
Income
    income inequality, 221–222
    relative income, 212, 214, 223–224
    and well-being, 26, 207–210, 224
Indicators of pro-environmental behaviors, 26, 258–259, 261–262, 266, 273
Inequality, 219, 221–222, 247
    income inequality, 221–222
Information on environmental issues, 268–272
Information strategies, 259
Inner compass, 111, 119–120, 124–125
Insecurity
    effects of insecurity and stress on people's autonomy, 208, 221
    job insecurity, 221–222
Integrated regulation, 51, 144, 153
Interests, 6, 9–11, 22, 24, 40, 42, 47, 50, 53–54, 59–60, 68, 82, 85, 100, 102, 105–106, 111, 119–120, 122–126, 140–141, 144, 146, 149–150, 153, 163, 165, 170–171, 177, 191–194, 198–200, 209, 212, 217–218, 222, 229, 241–243, 245–246, 248–250, 257, 265–266, 271
Internalization, 7–8, 24, 26, 36, 43, 51–52, 54, 57, 60, 101, 119, 124, 134–135, 137–138, 155, 170, 174, 247, 260–261, 266, 268, 270–271, 273
Intrinsic motivation, 37, 40, 49–50, 52, 57, 60, 68, 82, 101, 105, 116, 126, 135–136, 141–143, 145–149, 166, 174, 176, 198, 201
Introjected regulation, 51, 144–146, 149

J
Job design, 25, 163–164, 166–168, 171–172, 175, 177–178

K
Kant, 1, 5–6, 21, 67, 77

L
Law schools, 37–38
Learning climate questionnaire, 38
Lingua franca, 43

M
Maslow, Abraham, 14, 20–22
Materialism
    strengthening of, 219
May, Rollo, 14, 20, 22
Mindfulness, 84, 105, 224
Motivation
    autonomous, 23, 53, 58, 68, 82–85, 96–98, 100, 104, 106–107, 145–146, 150–151, 169, 171, 175, 268, 271
    controlled, 82–83, 97, 107, 114, 143–144, 150–151, 268
    environmental, 258, 266, 268, 273
    exercise, 143, 148
    extrinsic, 49–52, 57, 136, 149, 198
    human, 35, 134, 261–262
    individual's, 10, 215, 225, 261
    internalized, 140, 271
    intrinsic, 37, 40, 49–50, 52, 57, 60, 68, 82, 101, 105, 116, 126, 135–136, 141–143, 145–149, 166, 174, 176, 198, 201
    optimal, 33, 204
    quality, 148, 262–266, 272
    self-determined, 38, 41, 69, 82, 145, 262, 264–266, 268–272
    work, 165–167, 169–170, 172

N
Needs
    basic psychological needs, 20, 23, 26, 36, 42–43, 45, 48–49, 56–57, 59–60, 78, 96, 98–99, 101, 105, 111, 120, 134, 143, 165, 177, 208, 215, 217, 219, 221, 224, 242
    substitute needs, 217–218, 220–221, 223–224
Neurophenomenology, 70
Non-Western societies, 134, 247, 249
Nussbaum, 19, 216, 241–242
Nutrition, 133–136, 216

O
Obesity, 1, 145, 147, 149, 223
Organismic valuing process, 35

P
Parenting, 24, 40, 78, 81, 95–107, 149, 209, 217, 220–221, 226–228
Participation/democratic voice, 123, 216, 248–250
Participative management, 164, 173–175
Passivity, 5, 223
Perceived autonomy, 37–38, 84, 101, 104, 111, 116, 121, 147
Perceived competence, 53, 116, 134–138, 142, 145, 150

Perceived locus of causality, 82, 143
Performance monitoring, 176
Personal autonomy, 2, 4, 7, 9–14, 24–26, 36, 67–68, 79–80, 133–157, 191, 207–229, 241–253, 257–273
Personal choice, 241–247, 251, 253
Physical activity, 133–136, 142–148, 155–156
Physical well-being, 24–25, 116–117, 133, 135–136, 142
Policy, 225–229
    policies in support of people's personal autonomy, 225
Positive psychology, 19, 22–23, 33–43
Pro-environmental behaviors, 26, 258–259, 261–272
Pro-social behavior, 173, 201
Psychological freedom, 19–21, 54, 60
Psychological needs, 13, 20, 23, 26, 36, 41–43, 45, 48–49, 54, 56–57, 59–60, 69, 78, 96, 98–99, 101, 105, 111, 120–125, 133–134, 143, 165, 177, 200, 208, 215, 217, 219, 221, 224, 229, 241–243, 248, 266
Psychological self
    familial, 12
    individualized, 12
    personal, 12
    spiritual, 12

R

Reason, 3, 5, 7–11, 14, 24, 33, 40, 46, 51–52, 65, 68–69, 81–82, 84, 96–98, 101, 104, 113, 119, 124, 140–141, 143, 147, 155, 165, 193, 196, 199, 202, 215–216, 221, 227, 243–245, 249–250, 261–262, 264, 266, 272–273
Relatedness, 20, 23, 27, 35–39, 41, 48–50, 52–54, 56–60, 96, 98–101, 104–106, 111, 124, 134, 145–146, 167, 215, 224, 243–244, 248, 266, 273
Relationships
    causal, 16, 137–138
    dialectical, 22–23, 65–86
    interpersonal, 24–25, 56
    peer, 225
    romantic, 97–98, 106
    social, 13, 26, 73, 78, 84, 213–214, 222, 224–225, 241, 248
Relative income, 212, 214, 223–224
    changing the importance of relative income, 224

Renaissance, 2, 4
Rights/freedoms, 26, 163, 198, 241–248
Rogers, Carl, 14, 20–21, 34, 97, 123, 213

S

Schools, 24, 34, 37–39, 41, 50–52, 54, 57–58, 78, 84, 102, 111–128, 137, 142, 221, 226, 228, 245, 249–250, 252, 257, 264
Scientific perspectivism, 17
Scitovsky, 218
Self-determination theory (SDT), 2, 8, 15, 20, 22–26, 33–43, 45–52, 54–60, 65, 67–69, 81–86, 95–107, 111, 117, 120, 133–138, 141–142, 145–146, 150–156, 164–166, 168–169, 173, 176–177, 191, 195, 198–199, 204, 208, 215, 217–218, 224, 226, 229, 241–244, 247–248, 251, 253, 258–262, 264, 266–267, 269–273
Self-enhancing values, 194–196, 198, 200–201, 203–204
Self Regulation, 17, 23, 36, 39, 45, 49, 52–53, 57, 68, 72, 113, 116, 119, 134–136, 138–142, 144–149, 156, 175
Self-reinforcement in decision making, 218
Sen, 79, 207, 216–217, 226, 241–242
Skinner, 14–16
Social capital, 78, 213, 222
Social constructionism
    'macro' social constructionism, 17–18
    'micro' social constructionism, 17–19
    'strong' social constructionism, 17
    'weak' social constructionism, 17
Social domain theory, 243
Social norms, 24, 42, 114, 128, 253, 259
Social relationships
    deterioration of, 213–214
    negative externalities on, 214
Socio-cultural environment, 22–23, 65, 73, 75–76, 84
Socrates, 1–3
South Asian societies, 2
Spinoza, 1, 4–5, 21, 67, 77
Standard social science model, 18
The Stoics, 67, 77
Stress, 38, 47, 75, 121, 145, 163, 166, 171, 173, 176, 208, 216, 219–223
Students, 24, 36–39, 41, 54–55, 57–58, 84–85, 102, 112–116, 118–128, 140, 142, 191, 194, 219, 223, 228, 245, 249, 252
Substantia individua rationalis, 4
Substitute needs, 217–218, 220–221, 223–224

Index

Support of Reflective Value/Goal Exploration (SVE), 121–124
Sustainable environment, 258–261
Symbolic mental representations, 70
Symbolic reflective actions, 73, 75
Systems theory/approach, 67, 71, 75

T

Teachers, 36, 43, 54, 57–58, 84, 86, 104, 113–116, 118–128, 191, 194, 228, 244, 249
Theory of planned behavior, 114–115, 128
Tobacco, 53, 58, 133–138, 142, 155–156
Trust, 20–21, 55, 57, 78, 85, 122, 125, 172, 213–214, 222, 229, 264

U

Unemployment, 211, 221, 224, 228

V

Values
    cultural, 35, 54, 83, 119, 128, 177–178, 195
    extrinsic, 120, 134, 195–196, 198, 200, 203–204
    hierarchical, 111, 117
    individual, 195–196
    materialistic, 200–201, 219
    moral, 3, 7–8, 79–80, 124
    personal, 45, 52, 66, 123, 194, 199
    TSRQ, 152–153
Vertical collectivism, 7, 80
Vertical individualism, 80, 85
Virtue, 3, 5–6, 8, 30, 42, 61, 83

W

Weight Control, 147–148
Well-being
    and income, 208–210, 224
    objective measures of, 211–212
    valuable information in the survey question on, 209–210
Western societies, 14, 134, 147, 247, 249
Work hours, 171, 200–201

CPSIA information can be obtained at www.ICGtesting.com
233786LV00008B/24/P